Healthy Heart Sourcebook for Women

Heart Diseases & Disorders
Sourcebook, 2nd Edition

Household Safety Sourcebook

Immune System Disorders Sourcebook

Infant & Toddler Health Sourcebook

Infectious Diseases Sourcebook

Injury & Trauma Sourcebook

Kidney & Urinary Tract Diseases &
Disorders Sourcebook

Learning Disabilities Sourcebook,
2nd Edition

Leukemia Sourcebook

Liver Disorders Sourcebook

Lung Disorders Sourcebook

Medical Tests Sourcebook, 2nd Edition

Men's Health Concerns Sourcebook,
2nd Edition

Mental Health Disorders Sourcebook,
2nd Edition

Mental Retardation Sourcebook

Movement Disorders Sourcebook

Obesity Sourcebook

Osteoporosis Sourcebook

Pain Sourcebook, 2nd Edition

Pediatric Cancer Sourcebook

Physical & Mental Issues in Aging
Sourcebook

Podiatry Sourcebook

Pregnancy & Birth Sourcebook,
2nd Edition

Prostate Cancer

Public Health Sourcebook

Reconstructive & Cosmetic Surgery
Sourcebook

Rehabilitation Sourcebook

Respiratory Diseases & Disorders
Sourcebook

Sexually Transmitted Diseases
Sourcebook, 2nd Edition

Skin Disorders Sourcebook

Sleep Disorders Sourcebook

Sports Injuries Sourcebook, 2nd Edition

Stress-Related Disorders Sourcebook

Stroke Sourcebook

Substance Abuse Sourcebook

Surgery Sourcebook

Transplantation Sourcebook

Traveler's Health Sourcebook

Vegetarian Sourcebook

Women's Health Concerns Sourcebook,
2nd Edition

Workplace Health & Safety Sourcebook

Worldwide Health Sourcebook

Teen Health Series

Cancer Information for Teens

Diet Information for Teens

Drug Information for Teens

Fitness Information for Teens

Mental Health Information
for Teens

Sexual Health Information
for Teens

Skin Health Information
for Teens

Sports Injuries Information
for Teens

DATE DUE

Muscular Dystrophy
SOURCEBOOK

Health Reference Series

First Edition

Muscular Dystrophy SOURCEBOOK

Basic Consumer Health Information about Congenital, Childhood-Onset, and Adult-Onset Forms of Muscular Dystrophy, Such as Duchenne, Becker, Emery-Dreifuss, Distal, Limb-Girdle, Facioscapulohumeral (FSHD), Myotonic, and Ophthalmoplegic Muscular Dystrophies, Including Facts about Diagnostic Tests, Medical and Physical Therapies, Management of Co-Occurring Conditions, and Parenting Guidelines

Along with Practical Tips for Home Care, a Glossary, and Directories of Additional Resources

Edited by
Joyce Brennfleck Shannon

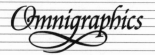

615 Griswold Street • Detroit, MI 48226

Bibliographic Note

Because this page cannot legibly accommodate all the copyright notices, the Bibliographic Note portion of the Preface constitutes an extension of the copyright notice.

Edited by Joyce Brennfleck Shannon

Health Reference Series

Karen Bellenir, *Managing Editor*
David A. Cooke, MD, *Medical Consultant*
Elizabeth Barbour, *Permissions Associate*
Dawn Matthews, *Verification Assistant*
Laura Pleva Nielsen, *Index Editor*
EdIndex, Services for Publishers, *Indexers*

* * *

Omnigraphics, Inc.

Matthew P. Barbour, *Senior Vice President*
Kay Gill, *Vice President—Directories*
Kevin Hayes, *Operations Manager*
Leif Gruenberg, *Development Manager*
David P. Bianco, *Marketing Director*

* * *

Peter E. Ruffner, *Publisher*

Frederick G. Ruffner, Jr., *Chairman*

Copyright © 2004 Omnigraphics, Inc.

ISBN 0-7808-0676-X

Library of Congress Cataloging-in-Publication Data

Muscular dystrophy sourcebook : basic consumer health information about congenital, childhood-onset, and adult-onset forms of muscular dystrophy, such as Duchenne, Becker, Emery-Dreifuss, distal, limb-girdle, facioscapulohumeral (FSHD), myotonic, and ophthalmoplegic muscular dystrophies, including facts about diagnostic tests, medical and physical therapies, management of co-occurring conditions, and parenting guidelines; along with practical tips for home care, a glossary, and directories of additional resources / Joyce Brennfleck Shannon, editor.-- 1st ed.
    p. cm.
Includes index.
ISBN 0-7808-0676-X (hard cover)
1. Muscular dystrophy--Popular works. I. Shannon, Joyce Brennfleck.
RC935.M7M876 2004
616.7'48--dc22

2004010217

Table of Contents

Visit www.healthreferenceseries.com to view *A Contents Guide to the Health Reference Series*, a listing of more than 10,000 topics and the volumes in which they are covered.

Preface ix

Part I: Overview of Muscular Dystrophy

Chapter 1—What Are Muscular Dystrophies? 3

Chapter 2—Myopathies: Diseases of the Muscles 11
    Section 2.1—Facts about Myopathies 12
    Section 2.2—Facts about Mitochondrial
                Myopathies 26

Chapter 3—Metabolic Diseases of the Muscles 43

Chapter 4—Myositis: Inflammatory Diseases of the
    Muscles 59

Part II: Congenital and Childhood-Onset Muscular Dystrophies

Chapter 5—Congenital Muscular Dystrophy 69

Chapter 6—Duchenne Muscular Dystrophy 77

Chapter 7—Becker Muscular Dystrophy 87

Chapter 8—Emery-Dreifuss Muscular Dystrophy 95

Part III: Adult-Onset Muscular Dystrophies

Chapter 9—Distal Muscular Dystrophy 103

Chapter 10—Facioscapulohumeral Muscular Dystrophy (FSHD) 107

Chapter 11—Limb-Girdle Muscular Dystrophy 121

Chapter 12—Myotonic Muscular Dystrophy............................ 133

Chapter 13—Ophthalmoplegic Muscular Dystrophy 151

Part IV: Diagnostic Tests

Chapter 14—Accurate and Affordable Diagnosis of Duchenne Muscular Dystrophy 159

Chapter 15—New Test for Myotonic Muscular Dystrophy...... 163

Chapter 16—Creatine Kinase Test 167

Chapter 17—Muscle Biopsy... 171

Chapter 18—Electromyography (EMG) 177

Chapter 19—Gene Testing.. 181

Part V: Treatment and Management of Muscular Dystrophies and Related Concerns

Chapter 20—Osteoporosis: A Serious, but Manageable Effect of Muscular Dystrophy 189

Chapter 21—The Heart Is a Muscle, Too: Cardiac Problems in Muscular Diseases 201

Chapter 22—Anesthesia Risks with Muscular Dystrophy 213

Chapter 23—Inflammation in Neuromuscular Disease........... 219

Chapter 24—Progress in Treatments for Muscular Dystrophy.. 223

Chapter 25—Physical Therapy: Flexibility, Fitness, and Fun 233

Chapter 26—Managing Breathing Difficulties 245

    Section 26.1—Making Breathing Easier 246

    Section 26.2—Noninvasive Ventilation 254

Chapter 27—Pain Control and Neuromuscular Disease 267

Chapter 28—Treating Scoliosis in Muscular Dystrophy 279

Chapter 29—Achilles Tendon Release 289

Chapter 30—Treatment for Duchenne Muscular Dystrophy 293

    Section 30.1—Therapy and Bracing 294

    Section 30.2—Nutritional Issues,
                  Supplements, Steroids,
                  and Antibiotics 299

    Section 30.3—Stretching, Exercises,
                  and Postural Correction
                  in Duchenne Muscular
                  Dystrophy 308

Part VI: Care and Management of Muscular Dystrophy at Home

Chapter 31—Handling Disability 329

Chapter 32—Home Adaptations for Living with
              Muscular Dystrophy 333

Chapter 33—101 Hints to Help Patients with Muscular
              Dystrophy 349

Chapter 34—Wheelchairs for Children and Adults with
              Muscular Dystrophy 363

Chapter 35—Home Health Care 379

Chapter 36—Feeding Tubes 387

Chapter 37—Managing Toileting and Hydration 393

Part VII: Parenting Children with Muscular Dystrophy

Chapter 38—You Are Not Alone: Dealing with a
              Muscular Dystrophy Diagnosis 405

Chapter 39—Discussing Muscular Dystrophy with
              Family and Friends 415

Chapter 40—Daily Life with Muscular Dystrophy 421

Chapter 41—Age and Mobility Stages 429

Chapter 42—Education Rights and Responsibilities of
              Parents of Children with Muscular Dystrophy 437

    Section 42.1—Individuals with Disabilities
                  Education Act (IDEA) 438

    Section 42.2—Your Rights in the Special
                  Education Process 465

Section 42.3—Integration of the
Student with Muscular
Dystrophy into a School
Physical Program 471

Chapter 43—Estate Planning Issues When Parents
Have a Disabled Child 477

Section 43.1—Overview of Estate
Planning 478

Section 43.2—The Letter of Intent 486

Section 43.3—The Special Needs Trust 493

Part VIII: Additional Information

Chapter 44—Glossary of Important Muscular Dystrophy
Terms 511

Chapter 45—Directory of Organizations with Muscular
Dystrophy Information 519

Chapter 46—Directory of On-Line Providers of
Information and Equipment for People
with Muscular Dystrophy 523

Index 531

Preface

About This Book

Muscular dystrophy causes degeneration of the muscles that control movement. Different kinds of muscular dystrophy have different genetic causes, affect people at different ages, and involve different muscles. The many forms of muscular dystrophy affect approximately 250,000 American children and adults. Currently there are no cures; however, treatments and therapies exist to help with the painful and disabling symptoms. Although the severity of disease and prognosis vary, each type of muscular dystrophy has a significant impact on the individual patient, their family members, and caregivers.

This *Sourcebook* provides health information about childhood-onset and adult-onset muscular dystrophies including congenital, Duchenne, Becker, Emery-Dreifuss, distal, limb-girdle, facioscapulohumeral, myotonic, and ophthalmoplegic muscular dystrophy. Readers will learn about the causes, diagnosis, treatment, and management of muscular dystrophy. Tips for parenting children with muscular dystrophy and for home care are also included, along with a glossary and directories of additional resources.

How to Use This Book

This book is divided into parts and chapters. Parts focus on broad areas of interest. Chapters are devoted to single topics within a part.

Part I: Overview of Muscular Dystrophy presents basic information about the muscular dystrophies and other diseases of muscles, including myopathies (which cause problems with the tone and contraction of skeletal muscles), metabolic diseases that cause chemical changes within muscle cells and impair normal functioning, and inflammatory myopathies (caused by immune system attacks on muscles).

Part II: Congenital and Childhood-Onset Muscular Dystrophies describes muscular dystrophies which are evident from birth or which typically manifest themselves in childhood or adolescence. These include congenital, Duchenne, Becker, and Emery-Dreifuss muscular dystrophies. Detailed information about these diseases helps families to understand their causes, progression, and effects.

Part III: Adult-Onset Muscular Dystrophies explains the causes, affected muscles, symptoms, prognosis, and management of distal, facioscapulohumeral, limb-girdle, myotonic, and ophthalmoplegic muscular dystrophies. Depending on the form of adult-onset muscular dystrophy, affected adults may notice symptoms as early as age 25 or as late as in their 60s.

Part IV: Diagnostic Tests describes muscle biopsy, electromyography, and blood tests for creatine kinase and gene mutations. These tests, along with descriptions of physical symptoms, allow doctors to diagnose, treat, and counsel individuals and families affected by muscular dystrophy.

Part V: Treatment and Management of Muscular Dystrophies and Related Concerns presents information about how muscular dystrophy affects the heart, bones, breathing, pain response, and digestive system. Management strategies include physical, respiratory, and drug therapies, and surgical treatments.

Part VI: Care and Management of Muscular Dystrophy at Home gives practical advice for handling disability and managing essential home health care issues, including feeding tubes, hydration, and personal hygiene, along with tips for hiring caregivers, adapting living environments, and selecting wheelchairs.

Part VII: Parenting Children with Muscular Dystrophy offers advice for parents about dealing with a muscular dystrophy diagnosis, coping with daily life, finding support, and understanding disease progression.

Information about education for children with disabilities and estate planning is also included.

Part VIII: Additional Help and Information includes a glossary of important terms and directories of organizations and on-line providers of information and equipment for people with muscular dystrophy.

Bibliographic Note

This volume contains documents and excerpts from publications issued by the following U.S. government agencies: Educational Resources Information Center (ERIC) Clearinghouse on Disabilities and Gifted Education, National Information Center for Children and Youth with Disabilities (NICHCY), National Institute of Arthritis and Musculoskeletal and Skin Diseases (NIAMS), National Institute of Neurological Disorders and Stroke (NINDS), and U.S. Department of Energy Human Genome Program and the Human Genome Management Information System at Oak Ridge National Laboratory.

In addition, this volume contains copyrighted documents from the following organizations and individuals: Center for Human Genetics at the Duke University Medical Center, Cleveland Clinic Foundation, FacioScapuloHumeral Society (FSH Society), Joe F. Jabre, M.D., McKesson Health Solutions L.L.C., Muscular Dystrophy Association–Australia, Muscular Dystrophy Association–USA, Muscular Dystrophy Association of Canada, Muscular Dystrophy Campaign, Muscular Dystrophy Family Foundation, Myotonic Dystrophy Support Group, Parent Project Muscular Dystrophy, and University of Iowa's Virtual Hospital.

Full citation information is provided on the first page of each chapter. Every effort has been made to secure all necessary rights to reprint the copyrighted material. If any omissions have been made, please contact Omnigraphics to make corrections for future editions.

Acknowledgements

Special thanks go to the many organizations, agencies, and individuals who have contributed materials for this *Sourcebook* and to managing editor Karen Bellenir, medical consultant Dr. David Cooke, permissions specialist Liz Barbour, artist Alison DeKleine, verification assistant Dawn Matthews, indexer Edward J. Prucha, and document engineer Bruce Bellenir. Estate planning review was done by attorney Douglas A. Cox.

About the Health Reference Series

The *Health Reference Series* is designed to provide basic medical information for patients, families, caregivers, and the general public. Each volume takes a particular topic and provides comprehensive coverage. This is especially important for people who may be dealing with a newly diagnosed disease or a chronic disorder in themselves or in a family member. People looking for preventive guidance, information about disease warning signs, medical statistics, and risk factors for health problems will also find answers to their questions in the *Health Reference Series*. The *Series*, however, is not intended to serve as a tool for diagnosing illness, in prescribing treatments, or as a substitute for the physician/patient relationship. All people concerned about medical symptoms or the possibility of disease are encouraged to seek professional care from an appropriate health care provider.

Locating Information within the Health Reference Series

The *Health Reference Series* contains a wealth of information about a wide variety of medical topics. Ensuring easy access to all the fact sheets, research reports, in-depth discussions, and other material contained within the individual books of the series remains one of our highest priorities. As the *Series* continues to grow in size and scope, however, locating the precise information needed by a reader may become more challenging.

A *Contents Guide to the Health Reference Series* was developed to direct readers to the specific volumes that address their concerns. It presents an extensive list of diseases, treatments, and other topics of general interest compiled from the Tables of Contents and major index headings. To access *A Contents Guide to the Health Reference Series*, visit www.healthreferenceseries.com.

Medical Consultant

Medical consultation services are provided to the *Health Reference Series* editors by David A. Cooke, M.D. Dr. Cooke is a graduate of Brandeis University, and he received his M.D. degree from the University of Michigan. He completed residency training at the University of Wisconsin Hospital and Clinics. He is board-certified in Internal Medicine. Dr. Cooke currently works as part of the University of Michigan Health System and practices in Brighton, MI. In his free time, he enjoys writing, science fiction, and spending time with his family.

Our Advisory Board

We would like to thank the following board members for providing guidance to the development of this series:

Dr. Lynda Baker,
Associate Professor of Library and Information Science,
Wayne State University, Detroit, MI

Nancy Bulgarelli,
William Beaumont Hospital Library, Royal Oak, MI

Karen Imarisio,
Bloomfield Township Public Library, Bloomfield Township, MI

Karen Morgan,
Mardigian Library, University of Michigan-Dearborn, Dearborn, MI

Rosemary Orlando,
St. Clair Shores Public Library, St. Clair Shores, MI

Health Reference Series *Update Policy*

The inaugural book in the *Health Reference Series* was the first edition of *Cancer Sourcebook* published in 1989. Since then, the *Series* has been enthusiastically received by librarians and in the medical community. In order to maintain the standard of providing high-quality health information for the layperson the editorial staff at Omnigraphics felt it was necessary to implement a policy of updating volumes when warranted.

Medical researchers have been making tremendous strides, and it is the purpose of the *Health Reference Series* to stay current with the most recent advances. Each decision to update a volume will be made on an individual basis. Some of the considerations will include how much new information is available and the feedback we receive from people who use the books. If there is a topic you would like to see added to the update list, or an area of medical concern you feel has not been adequately addressed, please write to:

Editor
Health Reference Series
Omnigraphics, Inc.
615 Griswold Street
Detroit, MI 48226
E-mail: editorial@omnigraphics.com

Part One

Overview of
Muscular Dystrophy

Chapter 1

What Are Muscular Dystrophies?

The muscular dystrophies are a group of diseases which weaken the skeletal muscles that we use to move voluntarily. These disorders vary in their age of onset, in severity, and in the pattern of which muscles are affected. All forms of muscular dystrophy, however, grow worse as muscles progressively degenerate. In some types of muscular dystrophy, the heart, the gastrointestinal system, endocrine glands, the skin, the eyes, and other organs may be affected. All of the muscular dystrophies are genetic disorders, although the types of inheritance vary, and Duchenne muscular dystrophy, the most common and best known of the childhood muscular dystrophies, often arises from new mutations.

Can We Treat Muscular Dystrophies?

Research has revealed most—but not yet all—of the gene defects that cause the different forms of muscular dystrophy. Unfortunately, the life expectancy and quality of life for people with muscular dystrophy have not improved substantially since those discoveries. There is still no specific treatment that can stop or reverse the progression of any form of muscular dystrophy. For Duchenne muscular dystrophy,

This chapter includes excerpts from "Testimony on Muscular Dystrophy," by Audrey S. Penn, M.D., Acting Director, National Institute of Neurological Disorders and Stroke (NINDS), February 27, 2001; and "Faulty Muscle Repair Implicated in Muscular Dystrophies," by Tania Zeigler, National Institute of Neurological Disorders and Stroke (NINDS), May 21, 2003.

corticosteroids may help, but have side effects that can be especially troubling with children. Symptomatic treatment, though not able to stop the disease process, may improve the quality of life for some people with muscular dystrophy through physical therapy, wheelchairs and braces used for support, corrective orthopedic surgery, and drugs.

The failure so far to produce a definitive therapy for any form of muscular dystrophy reflects the difficulty of the problems that we must confront to cure these diseases. Some of these problems are unique to a particular type of muscular dystrophy, some common to all muscular dystrophies, and others are shared by many genetic disorders. The National Institute of Neurological Disorders and Stroke (NINDS) and the National Institute of Arthritis and Musculoskeletal and Skin Diseases (NIAMS) lead efforts of several components of National Institutes of Health (NIH) against these diseases. The shared responsibility recognizes the value that various medical specialties and disciplines bring to research and treatment. The muscular dystrophies affect many aspects of physiology, benefit from a wide range of fundamental biological research, and require exploration of diverse strategies for treatment. What is most encouraging is the range of scientific approaches that research is bringing to bear on these diseases. Molecular biology has given us a foothold to understand what goes wrong. To examine the list of therapies being explored for the muscular dystrophies is tantamount to taking a tour through the most active frontiers of modern medicine, including gene therapy, cell replacement, and innovative approaches to drug development.

Three Common Types of Muscular Dystrophy

Myotonic Muscular Dystrophy

Myotonic muscular dystrophy (MMD) is probably the most common adult form of muscular dystrophy, partly because people with this disorder can live a long life, with variable but slowly progressive disability. Myotonia refers to impaired muscle relaxation which is associated with MMD along with muscle wasting and weakness. This form of muscular dystrophy affects many body systems in addition to skeletal muscles. These include the heart, endocrine organs, eyes, and gastrointestinal tract.

Myotonic muscular dystrophy follows an autosomal dominant pattern of inheritance. This means that the disorder can occur in either sex when a person inherits a single defective gene from either parent.

The gene defect that causes MMD is a triplet repeat expansion in the untranslated region of a gene that encodes a protein kinase (DM-PK). This means that the inherited gene defect arises from a long repetition of a three-letter "word" in the part of the genetic code that carries the instructions for making a protein. The protein is one of a class called kinases that help regulate the function of other proteins. In this case the "word" is not in the part of the gene that specifies the makeup of the protein itself, but in a region that may help control when the gene is turned on and off. We do not yet understand how this genetic defect leads to muscle degeneration, but the triplet repeat mechanism has now been found in at least 15 other disorders. Scientists have found some clues, both for myotonic dystrophy and triplet repeat disorders in general, and research is continuing. The fact that the repetition in the genetic code tends to get longer with each generation explains the phenomenon of anticipation in which the disease shows itself earlier and more severely in each generation.

Facioscapulohumeral Muscular Dystrophy

Facioscapulohumeral muscular dystrophy (FSHD) initially affects muscles of the face (facies), shoulders (scapulas), and upper arms (humeral) with progressive weakness. Symptoms usually develop in the teenage years. Life expectancy is normal, but some affected individuals become severely disabled. The pattern of inheritance is, like myotonic muscular dystrophy, autosomal dominant, but the underlying genetic defect is poorly understood. Most cases are associated with a deletion—that is, a missing piece of chromosome—near the end of chromosome number 4. These deletions do not appear to disrupt a particular gene, but may affect the activity of nearby genes. This complicates the search for the relevant gene and suggests a novel mechanism may be involved.

Research registry: In September of 2000, the NIAMS and the NINDS funded a research registry for FSHD and myotonic dystrophy. The long-term goal of the registry is to facilitate research in FSHD and myotonic dystrophy by serving as a liaison between families affected by these diseases who are eager to participate in specific research projects, and investigators interested in studying these disorders. The registry, based at the University of Rochester, will recruit and classify patients, and store medical and family history data for individuals with clinically diagnosed FSHD and myotonic dystrophy. Scientists will be provided with statistical analyses of the registry data, as well as access to registry members who have agreed to assist with particular research studies. The national registry will serve as a resource for scientists seeking a cure for these diseases, in addition to enhancing research to understand what changes occur in muscular dystrophy.

Duchenne and Becker Muscular Dystrophy

Duchenne muscular dystrophy (DMD) is the most common childhood form of muscular dystrophy, affecting approximately 1 in 3,000 male births. About one-third of cases reflect new mutations and the rest are familial. Because inheritance is X-linked recessive, DMD affects primarily boys, though girls and women who carry one defective gene may show some mild symptoms.

DMD is a particularly devastating and lethal form of muscular dystrophy. When the body's attempts to regenerate muscle cannot keep up with the destructive process, muscle wasting and progressive weakness result. DMD usually becomes evident when children begin to walk. Boys typically require a wheelchair by age 10 to 12, and usually die in late teens or early 20s. Becker muscular dystrophy (BMD) is a less severe but closely related disease. DMD results from an absence of the protein dystrophin, and BMD reflects a partly functional version of the same protein.

Understanding the disease: More than 15 years ago, researchers supported by the NIH and the Muscular Dystrophy Association identified the gene for dystrophin that, when defective, causes DMD and BMD. The identification of the dystrophin gene stimulated research that provided new insights and directions for research on the biology of muscle and the mechanisms of disease, as evident in thousands of high quality scientific publications and several promising leads for developing new therapies.

One challenge the dystrophin gene presents is its enormous size. The gene is the largest gene yet identified in humans. Most vectors (usually modified viruses) available for gene replacement cannot incorporate a gene of this magnitude. The size probably also contributes to the high rate of new mutations in the gene and to the large number of different mutations that can occur within the gene. Definitive therapy may require precise knowledge of the particular gene defect in each patient.

The dystrophin protein was unknown before the discovery of its link to DMD. Subsequent studies have revealed that dystrophin is part of a complex structure involving several other protein components. The "dystrophin-glycoprotein complex" helps anchor the contents of muscle cells through the cells' outer enclosing membrane to the material in which muscle cells are embedded. Defects in this assembly lead to structural problems that can disrupt the integrity of the outer membrane of muscle cells, resulting eventually in degeneration. One of the most remarkable spin-offs from the elucidation of the complex has been clarification of the interrelationships among DMD and other forms of muscular dystrophy. Several other forms of muscular dystrophy, whose relationships to DMD were obscure, result from mutations in other protein components of the same dystrophin-glycoprotein complex. These include several forms of limb-girdle muscular dystrophy, named for the characteristic pattern of muscle weakness. Research to more fully understand the normal and abnormal functions of the dystrophin complex, and of other proteins closely related to dystrophin, is ongoing, and evidence is accumulating that these proteins play important roles in the brain as well as in muscles.

Therapeutic approaches: Several new approaches have emerged for developing therapies to stop or reverse muscle degeneration in Duchenne muscular dystrophy. All of these strategies rely upon increased understanding of the underlying biology of the disease. However, one point made at the May 2000 workshop is the extent to which novel therapeutic strategies for DMD arise from research that is not focused on muscular dystrophy, muscle biology, or even therapeutics in general.

Logically, the simplest approach to treating DMD might seem to be to supply a good copy of the defective gene. An important advantage in studying DMD is the availability of the mdx mouse which is a useful model of the human disease. Results in mice with the same gene defect as DMD show that modified virus "vectors," such as the adeno-associated virus, can carry the therapeutic genes into muscle cells and partially reverse the disease. Recent experiments have also shown that a genetically engineered "mini-dystrophin," while much smaller than the natural form, seems able to carry out its essential functions. However, considerable advances are needed to make gene replacement workable for children with MD. The technology of gene replacement is just beginning to yield clinical success in some of the simplest diseases to treat. Treating DMD presents special problems not only because of the large size of the gene, but also due to the need to deliver the gene reliably and safely to muscle cells throughout the body. Improving the delivery of genes to muscle, optimizing the control elements that regulate the activity of therapeutic genes, and minimizing immunological and other potential safety problems are ongoing areas of research. The first preliminary gene replacement trials for any form of muscular dystrophy have been designed by MDA for a form of limb-girdle muscular dystrophy caused by a defect in a component of the dystrophin-glycoprotein complex.

Several other approaches to counteracting the gene defect, besides gene transfer by viral vectors, also show promise for DMD. The use of "naked DNA" is one approach under investigation for several diseases that may be applicable to DMD. Another approach uses chimeraplasts. These specifically designed synthetic molecules are hybrids of DNA and RNA that can guide the muscle cells' own repair machinery to correct some types of defect in the dystrophin gene. "Antisense" nucleotides are another type of synthetic molecule that has therapeutic potential. These molecules, which are designed to bind specifically to certain parts of genetic material, alter how the cells' internal machinery reads a gene to make protein, thus compensating for certain types of defects in dystrophin. Another strategy uses aminoglycoside antibiotics. Some children with DMD (perhaps 15%) carry a mutation in the dystrophin gene that creates an erroneous DNA code signal to stop making the protein. Dr. Sweeney did experiments in mice with the same types of errors in dystrophin and found that antibiotics can cause the protein synthesizing machinery to ignore stop signals and allow muscle cells to make enough dystrophin. Gentamicin, an antibiotic of this type, is now being tested in clinical trials for DMD in children.

Finally, drug therapy for DMD has also been a focus of research efforts. One approach has used high throughput screening (HTS) to try to find drugs that increase the muscle production of another protein, utrophin, that can help compensate for the loss of dystrophin. High throughput screening employs robotics and miniaturized assays (tests) to screen thousands of chemical compounds quickly to find leads for further drug development. Other pharmacological research areas of continued interest for DMD relate to the use of corticosteroids in the disease and to strategies informed by increased understanding of immunology and its relation to DMD.

Faulty Muscle Repair Implicated in Muscular Dystrophies

Researchers have revealed what may be a totally new cause for muscular dystrophy (MD). A recent study shows that a protein defective in two types of late-onset MD plays a critical role in the normal repair of muscles.

The researchers found that the defective protein dysferlin causes a glitch during normal muscle repair, suggesting that faulty muscle repair, rather than an inherent weakness in the muscles' structural integrity, leads to the progressive muscle degeneration seen in these two forms of MD. The study, conducted by Kevin Campbell, Ph.D., of the University of Iowa in Iowa City, and colleagues, appeared in the May 8, 2003, issue of *Nature*.[1] It identifies the first known component of the membrane-repair machinery in muscle cells.

"Muscles are continuously being damaged and repaired, and to find a particular protein that's involved in the process is very exciting," says study co-author Steven Vogel, Ph.D., acting chief of the section on cellular biophotonics at the National Institute of Alcohol Abuse and Alcoholism. This work was done while Dr. Vogel was a grantee of the National Institute of Neurological Disorders and Stroke (NINDS) at The Medical College of Georgia in Augusta.

The muscular dystrophies are a group of genetic diseases characterized by progressive weakness and degeneration of the muscles that control movement. Adults with either of the two types of MD in this study—Miyoshi myopathy and limb-girdle MD type 2b—have slowly progressing weakness and wasting of muscles of the hands, forearms, and lower legs. An earlier study showed that mutations affecting dysferlin activity are associated with both Miyoshi myopathy and limb-girdle MD type 2b, but little was known until now about how the absence of dysferlin caused disease.

Most genetic mutations that cause MD have been linked to errors in a large protein complex that controls the structural integrity of muscle cells. Dysferlin does not appear to be associated with this protein complex. Instead, dysferlin is normally found throughout the membranes of muscle cells and in vesicles. Some researchers believe vesicles—bubbles within muscle cells—might play a role in cell membrane repair.

Dr. Vogel's colleagues at the University of Iowa and the Howard Hughes Medical Institute engineered mice that lacked the dysferlin gene. As they aged, these mice developed MD similar to humans with either Miyoshi or limb-girdle MD. Interestingly, treadmill tests showed that their muscles were not much more susceptible to damage than the muscles of normal mice, demonstrating that the absence of dysferlin did not seem to interfere with the structural integrity of the muscles.

Under a microscope, the researchers saw that in the mice lacking dysferlin, unusually high numbers of vesicles accumulated at damaged membrane sites. The abnormal number of vesicles seemed to indicate that an error in membrane resealing might be responsible for the MD. To observe the protein's normal activity, the researchers tagged dysferlin with a dye marker. They saw patches enriched with dysferlin, which formed when dysferlin-containing vesicles that traveled to the damaged site fused. These dysferlin patches seemed to play a critical role in the sealing of damaged membranes.

Dr. Vogel says this new information about dysferlin's role in muscle repair opens a new pathway for understanding the causes of the muscular dystrophies, as well as other diseases that affect cardiac and skeletal muscles. "It's become clear that errors in membrane trafficking are linked to human disease," says Dr. Vogel. "A lot of progress has been made, and there's a lot more that needs to be learned in terms of the molecular mechanisms of membrane repair."

Reference

1. Bansal D, Miyake K, Vogel S, Groh S, Chen C, Williamson R, McNeil P, Campbell K. "Defective repair of membranes in dysferlin-deficient muscular dystrophy." *Nature*, Vol. 423, No. 6936, May 8, 2003, pp. 168-172.

Chapter 2

Myopathies:
Diseases of the Muscles

Chapter Contents

Section 2.1—Facts about Myopathies 12
Section 2.2—Facts about Mitochondrial Myopathies 26

Section 2.1

Facts about Myopathies

Excerpted from "Facts about Myopathies" with permission from the Muscular Dystrophy Association, www.mdausa.org © 2001 The Muscular Dystrophy Association. For additional information, call the Muscular Dystrophy Association National Headquarters toll-free at (800) 572-1717. To find an MDA office in your area, look in your local telephone book, or click on "Clinics and Services" on the MDA website.

What Are the Myopathies?

The word myopathy means disease of muscle. More specifically, myopathies are diseases that cause problems with the tone and contraction of skeletal muscles (muscles that control voluntary movements). These problems range from stiffness (called myotonia) to weakness, with different degrees of severity.

Some myopathies, especially when they're present from birth, have life-threatening complications. But, with time and physical therapy, some people born with myopathies can gain muscle strength. Others often can manage their symptoms through medication, lifestyle modifications, or use of orthopedic and respiratory equipment.

This section focuses on six inheritable myopathies (myopathies that can be passed from parent to child).

- myotonia congenita (Thomsen's disease and Becker type)
- paramyotonia congenita (Eulenburg's disease)
- periodic paralysis (hyperkalemic, hypokalemic, normokalemic)
- central core disease
- nemaline myopathy (rod body disease)
- myotubular myopathy (centronuclear myopathy)

This section also contains information on two non-inheritable myopathies caused by abnormal activity of the thyroid gland—hypothyroid myopathy and hyperthyroid myopathy.

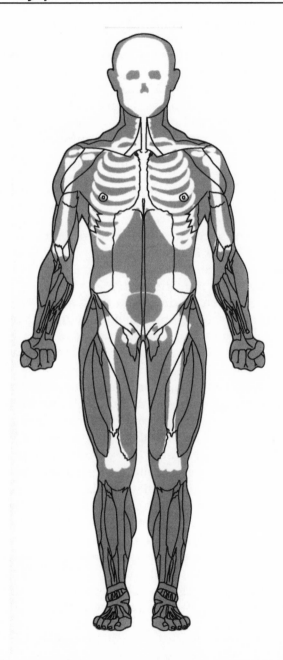

Figure 2.1. *Myopathies can cause weakness or stiffness in all of the body's voluntary muscles. Because muscles support the body's posture, severe muscle weakness can lead to skeletal deformities.*

What Causes the Inheritable Myopathies?

These inheritable myopathies are caused by mutations, or changes, in genes—the blueprints for making proteins that are necessary for our bodies to function correctly. Genes are responsible for building our bodies; we inherit them—along with any mutations or defects they have—from our parents, and pass them on to our children.

In the inheritable myopathies, genetic mutations cause defects in various proteins necessary for muscle tone and contraction.

What Are Muscle Tone and Contraction, and What Controls Them?

Contraction is the forceful shortening or tightening of muscle, which pulls on the joints to cause movement. In other words, when your brain "tells" a muscle to move, you cause it to contract, and it's then able to do what you're asking.

Muscle tone refers to a readiness for contraction that makes resting muscle resistant to stretching. Or, a toned muscle holds its shape and its elasticity and is able to respond by contracting when you want it to move. Bodies with poor muscle tone appear floppy. Good muscle tone is important for posture and coordination.

A skeletal muscle's tone and contraction depend on its ability to respond to stimulation from nerve cells, which are responding to signals sent from the brain, such as your decision to move your hand or leg. A muscle is actually a bundle of individual muscle cells, each one stimulated by a single nerve cell.

The process of muscle contraction begins when the nerve cells release chemical signals onto the muscle cells. These signals cause the opening of ion channels, pores in each muscle cell's outer surface that open and close to regulate ion movement. Ion channels allow certain ions—charged molecules of sodium, calcium, potassium, or chloride— to pass into and out of the muscle cell, creating electrical currents. Opening of sodium and calcium channels causes an electrical excitation that will lead to contraction, while opening of potassium and chloride channels keeps the excitation from occurring.

The purpose of the electrical excitation is to stimulate the opening of still more channels that release calcium from internal compartments in the muscle cell. Finally, the freed calcium ions trigger muscle contraction by stimulating the sliding action of filament proteins.

These rodlike proteins run lengthwise within the muscle cell and are anchored at opposite ends by scaffolds called Z-discs. When the filament proteins slide past each other—by an energy-dependent, ratchet-like mechanism—they cause shortening of the muscle cell and shortening (contraction) of the whole muscle.

If this process is disrupted at any stage between the nerve's signaling the muscle and the filament proteins' action, the muscle loses its normal capacity for tone and contraction. At one extreme, the muscle might be limp and weak, and at the other extreme, the muscle may be unable to relax.

Many of the inheritable myopathies are caused by mutations that interfere with ion channels, preventing necessary ions from flowing

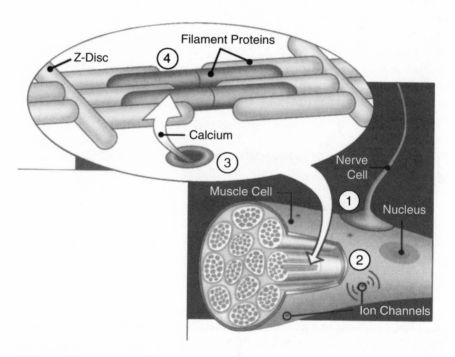

Figure 2.2. A muscle cell is stimulated to contract by chemical signals sent from an adjoining nerve cell (1). Those signals open ion channels at the muscle cell's surface, causing an inward/outward flow of ions that acts as an electrical current (2). Inside the muscle cell, the current spreads and causes opening of ion channels that line calcium storage compartments, releasing the calcium ions trapped within (3). The freed calcium ions trigger nearby filament proteins to slide past each other, pulling the Z-discs closer together and shortening the muscle cell (4).

15

through the muscle cells. These disorders (myotonia congenita, paramyotonia congenita, periodic paralysis, and central core disease) are sometimes called channelopathies.

Central core disease seems to damage, and thus weaken, muscles by causing an excess release of internal calcium. The other channelopathies interfere with normal muscle tone and contraction by causing over- or underexcitation. A fifth myopathy, nemaline myopathy, is caused by mutations that affect filament proteins. When the filament proteins fail to do their jobs, muscles can't contract properly, causing a loss of tone and strength.

At least one myopathy (a type of myotubular myopathy) is caused by mutations in a muscle protein required for normal muscle development. When this protein is absent or inactive, the muscles don't form properly. Some of the inheritable myopathies are congenital, meaning they cause problems from the time of birth. Others have a later onset, with symptoms appearing in childhood or adulthood.

By the way, myopathies aren't contagious, and they aren't caused by overexertion. However, exercise can aggravate some of the myopathies, because of mutations that change the way muscles respond to activity.

What Happens to Someone with an Inheritable Myopathy?

Some of the congenital inheritable myopathies cause severe, general muscle weakness that creates problems with basic activities like swallowing and breathing. These problems can be fatal if not dealt with, but they can be treated with assistive medical devices like feeding tubes and mechanical ventilators.

Other inheritable myopathies cause episodes of muscle weakness or stiffness that are milder and more localized and temporary in nature. These episodes often can be managed through medication, or by careful control of exercise and diet.

Unlike muscular dystrophies, myopathies usually don't cause muscles to die but just keep them from working properly. Also, myopathies are usually nonprogressive—that is, a myopathy usually doesn't grow worse over a person's lifetime. In fact, some children with myopathies gain strength as they grow older.

Finally, some myopathies can give people a listless facial expression, caused by weakness of muscles in the face. Myopathies have no effect on intelligence.

Special Issues in Inheritable Myopathies

Anesthesia: People with myopathies can experience adverse reactions to certain anesthetic drugs used during surgery. Although these drugs sometimes just aggravate the myopathy, they also can produce a potentially fatal reaction called malignant hyperthermia, which refers to a dangerously high increase in body temperature. People with central core disease are especially at risk for malignant hyperthermia because the two conditions are sometimes caused by the same ion channel defects.

Malignant hyperthermia is triggered by certain inhaled anesthetics (like halothane) and certain muscle relaxants (like succinylcholine). These drugs can intensify ion channel defects and boost muscle metabolism—the set of chemical reactions that provides energy to muscle. The increased metabolism raises body temperature, and causes excessive contraction and rhabdomyolysis—a process of acute muscle breakdown. The resulting leakage of ions and muscle proteins into the circulatory system can cause life-threatening damage to the heart, lungs, and kidneys.

People with central core disease are not always susceptible to malignant hyperthermia. Those who are susceptible won't experience malignant hyperthermia unless they're exposed to triggering anesthetics. Before having surgery, people who have a personal or family history of central core disease—or any other myopathy—should consult their doctors about the risks of anesthesia and about the availability of nontriggering anesthetics.

Respiratory care: Nemaline myopathy and congenital (X-linked) myotubular myopathy cause weakening of the respiratory muscles (those that control the lungs). Therefore, people with either of these diseases probably will need to use mechanical ventilation to support breathing, and should have their breathing monitored regularly by a specialist. Also, weak lungs are susceptible to infection, so signs of respiratory illness should be taken seriously.

Cardiac care: The myopathies almost never affect heart muscle directly, but sometimes they can cause indirect damage to the heart. In nemaline myopathy and congenital myotubular myopathy, an inadequate oxygen supply to the body during severe bouts of respiratory weakness can lead to heart problems. In hyperkalemic periodic paralysis, certain conditions can trigger potassium elevation in the blood, which can interfere with contraction of the heart. People with these diseases should be wary of potential heart problems and have their cardiac function checked by a specialist.

What Are the Symptoms and Treatments for Each Inheritable Myopathy?

Myotonia Congenita

Cause: This disease is caused by mutations in the gene for a chloride channel that's necessary for shutting off the electrical excitation that causes muscle contraction.

Inheritance: Autosomal recessive (Becker-type), autosomal dominant (Thomsen's).

Onset: Early to late childhood.

Symptoms: The main problems faced by people with this disease are delayed muscle relaxation and muscle stiffness, typically provoked by sudden movements after rest. The stiffness can interfere with simple activities like walking, grasping, and chewing, but is usually manageable by doing warm-up movements. The disease doesn't cause any muscle wasting; instead, it can sometimes cause muscle enlargement and increased muscle strength. Becker-type myotonia is the most common form of myotonia congenita, while Thomsen's disease is a very rare, relatively mild form.

Treatment: Someone who has myotonia congenita can lead a long, productive life, and can even excel at sports where strength is more important than agility. Your Muscular Dystrophy Association (MDA) clinic director can tell you about appropriate exercises, and if necessary, appropriate medications for dealing with muscle stiffness.

Paramyotonia Congenita

Also called: Eulenburg's disease. (Some researchers regard paramyotonia congenita as a form of periodic paralysis.)

Cause: Sodium channels normally open to cause muscle excitation, and then close to end the excitation. In paramyotonia congenita, mutations in the muscle sodium channel gene prolong the channel's opening, causing higher-than-normal muscle excitation.

Inheritance: Autosomal dominant.

Onset: Congenital.

Symptoms: Paramyotonia congenita causes episodes of muscle stiffness and weakness—mostly in the face, neck, and upper extremities—that can last from minutes to hours. The stiffness is sensitive to exercise and cold. During brief exercise, overexcitation of muscles can cause stiffness, and with prolonged exercise, the overexcitation can occasionally lead to a fatigue-like weakness or even complete paralysis. Cold exposure can have similar effects, but some people experience muscle stiffness, weakness, or sometimes, temporary paralysis even when they're warm.

Treatment: By avoiding strenuous exercise and cold, most people with this condition can largely escape disability. But medications can be beneficial, especially for those who experience symptoms independent of exercise and cold. Your MDA clinic director can give you more information about these medications.

Periodic Paralyses

In these diseases, faulty ion channels cause attacks of temporary muscle weakness that can result in temporary paralysis when severe. There are different types of periodic paralysis, distinguished by what happens to potassium levels in the blood (specifically the fluid portion of the blood, or serum). In the hyperkalemic type (hyperKPP), high serum potassium levels can cause attacks. In the hypokalemic type (hypoKPP), low serum potassium levels can trigger attacks. (Kalemic refers to potassium; hyper means too much and hypo too little.) Unlike the case for most myopathies, many people with hypoKPP and some people with hyperKPP experience progressive, permanent muscle damage that occurs independently of the attacks.

Hyperkalemic Periodic Paralysis

Cause: This disease is caused by distinct mutations in the muscle sodium channel gene. These mutations cause very slow closing of the sodium channel, leading to episodes of prolonged muscle excitation and weakness, and myotonia (muscle stiffness) in some people. It's not fully understood just how high levels of potassium interact with the defective sodium channels to trigger attacks.

19

Inheritance: Autosomal dominant.

Onset: Childhood.

Symptoms: Attacks of weakness usually last 15 minutes to an hour, but can last for a day or more. They can recur daily in severe cases. The attacks commonly occur after rest that was preceded by vigorous exercise, and can be aggravated by stress, pregnancy, or foods high in potassium. During attacks not caused by excess potassium intake, a person can become hyperkalemic or remain normokalemic (with no change in serum potassium levels). The frequency of attacks usually declines after middle age.

Treatment: To keep hyperKPP attacks to a minimum, stick to a diet rich in carbohydrates and low in potassium, and avoid strenuous exercise. When you do exercise, be sure to cool down with mild activity before resting. During an attack, certain prescription drugs can be used to alleviate symptoms. Your MDA clinic director can give you more specific information on how to manage hyperKPP through appropriate exercise, diet, and medication.

Hypokalemic Periodic Paralysis

Causes: This disease seems to be caused by a reduced availability of the sodium channels necessary for muscle excitation. That condition can be brought about by certain genetic defects in the sodium channels themselves, or strangely, by genetic defects in a channel that acts like a key to the muscle's calcium stores.

Inheritance: Autosomal dominant.

Onset: Early childhood to adulthood.

Symptoms: Attacks of weakness can occur daily and usually happen in the morning (during waking) or at night. Some people with the disease might experience only a few mild attacks in their lifetime. But the most severe attacks cause nearly full-blown paralysis.

Treatment: As in hyperKPP, attacks of hypoKPP can be prevented by avoiding strenuous activity and alleviated by medications. The dietary precautions, however, are nearly opposite. High-carbohydrate foods can trigger hypokalemia and contribute to an attack, while potassium intake can restore serum potassium levels and stem an oncoming attack. Ask your MDA clinic director for specific recommendations about diet, exercise, and medications.

Central Core Disease

Causes: This rare disease appears to have multiple origins. But it's commonly caused by defects in a channel that acts like a gate to internal calcium stores. The defect causes leakage of calcium from the stores, which appears to damage muscle cells.

Inheritance: Autosomal dominant, possibly autosomal recessive in rare cases.

Onset: Congenital.

Symptoms: The disease is named for damaged areas within muscle cells (the cores), where the filament proteins are disorganized, and mitochondria (the tiny energy-producing factories that power muscle contraction) are missing. The impact of the cores on disease severity isn't clear.

This disease causes poor muscle tone (hypotonia) and persistent muscle weakness in infants. In rare cases, toddlers with the disease fail to walk at all, but usually they just reach motor milestones late. Older children and adults typically experience mild disabilities that worsen slowly with time, if at all. Due to chronic muscle weakness, many people develop skeletal deformities, including joint dislocations and scoliosis, or curvature of the spine that can compress vital internal organs.

People with this disease should be cautious about surgery because they face an especially high risk of malignant hyperthermia, a potentially fatal reaction to certain anesthetic drugs.

Treatment: Someone with a severe form of central core disease might need a walker or other support devices for mobility, but many people require none. Unlike the case for other myopathies, people with this disease can benefit from exercise. Scoliosis and other skeletal problems can usually be corrected by use of orthopedic devices or by surgery. Your doctor or MDA clinic director can tell you more about the risks of surgery, and about anesthetic drugs that are safe.

Nemaline Myopathy

Also called: Rod body disease.

Causes: This disease is caused by a variety of genetic defects, each one affecting one of the filament proteins required for muscle tone and contraction.

Inheritance: Autosomal recessive, autosomal dominant.

Onset: Congenital to adulthood.

Symptoms: The disease gets its name from the fact that the muscle cells contain abnormal clumps of threadlike material—probably disorganized filament proteins—called nemaline bodies (nema is Greek for thread). It causes weakness and poor tone (hypotonia) in the muscles of the face, neck, and upper limbs, and often affects the respiratory muscles (those that control breathing).

The infantile-onset cases tend to be the most severe. Usually, infants with the disease lack the muscle strength and tone required for simple postures and movements. They also have serious difficulties with feeding and respiration. Although many infants with the disease die from respiratory failure or lung infections, some survive to adulthood. Affected children usually attain motor milestones slowly, and at puberty they might experience further weakening, necessitating use of a wheelchair.

For adults, even noncongenital forms of the disease can cause life-threatening respiratory problems. Adults also might experience swallowing and speech problems, and those with restricted mobility might develop scoliosis. However, even people who have had the disease since birth can lead active lives.

Treatment: An infant with nemaline myopathy usually requires a feeding tube to deliver nutrition and mechanical ventilation to support respiration. Children and adults also can benefit from respiratory support, since respiratory failure during sleep can be a persistent danger. Mobility and strength can be improved significantly by physical and orthopedic therapies. If you or your child has nemaline myopathy, your MDA clinic director can provide further information about treatments.

Myotubular Myopathy

Also called: Centronuclear myopathy.

Causes: The most common form (X-linked) is caused by defects or deficiencies of myotubularin, a protein thought to promote normal muscle development.

Inheritance: X-linked, autosomal recessive, autosomal dominant.

Onset: Congenital (X-linked); infancy to early adulthood (autosomal recessive); childhood to adulthood (autosomal dominant).

Symptoms: X-linked myotubular myopathy usually affects only boys, and causes severe muscle weakness and hypotonia noticeable at birth and sometimes before. The weakness and hypotonia interfere with posture and movement, and cause life-threatening difficulties with feeding and respiration. Sometimes, failure or infection of the lungs causes death in early infancy, but about two-thirds of boys survive to at least 1 year of age. Usually, these boys require a feeding tube and a mechanical ventilator. Most attain motor milestones slowly, and some might not walk at all. However, most boys gradually gain muscle strength, and a few grow up with little disability. Independent of skeletal muscle problems, some boys with X-linked myotubular myopathy experience problems in other organ systems. These include anemia, gallstones, accelerated growth, and serious liver abnormalities.

The autosomal forms affect boys and girls equally. They cause muscle problems similar in quality to those of the X-linked form, but the autosomal dominant form is considered mild and the recessive form intermediate. In these forms muscle problems grow worse with age. Problems with other organs haven't been reported.

Treatment: Until recently, nearly all infants with X-linked myotubular myopathy were expected to die within their first few months of life. But it's now clear that intensive, continuous support of feeding and ventilation can significantly improve their life expectancy and allow a high quality of life.

Respiratory support and monitoring also might be necessary for children and adults diagnosed with autosomal forms of myotubular myopathy. Also, most people with this disease benefit from physical and orthopedic therapies. Your MDA clinic director can give you more information about treatment.

How Are These Six Inheritable Myopathies Diagnosed?

Usually, diagnosis begins with evaluation of the patient's personal and family history, and proceeds with physical and neurological examinations that test reflexes and strength. The exams can detect problems with muscle tone and contraction, and the histories can bring to light patterns of inheritance and conditions that might have aggravated the muscle problems in the past. Given this information, a doctor can sometimes distinguish an inheritable myopathy from other diseases that affect muscle function, such as muscular dystrophies and neurological disorders. But to accurately identify the myopathy and plan an appropriate course of treatment, the doctor can use several specialized tests.

A muscle biopsy, the removal of a small piece of muscle tissue, is used to look for physical signs of muscle disease. Under the microscope, muscles affected by central core disease, nemaline myopathy, or myotubular myopathy have fairly distinctive appearances.

Also, muscle biopsy can be used to see how isolated muscles respond to different potentially harmful conditions. For example, to determine a patient's susceptibility to malignant hyperthermia, a biopsied muscle can be tested for its reaction to potentially dangerous anesthetic drugs.

A muscle's activity can be measured by electromyography (EMG), which involves observing the electrical signals that a muscle produces during contraction. A needlelike electrode inserted into the muscle reads the electrical signals and sends them to a monitor called an oscilloscope. The technique usually causes some discomfort, but is useful for diagnosing channelopathies, which can show telltale abnormal signals on the oscilloscope.

Because the channelopathies sometimes just cause temporary muscle problems induced by changes in exercise, diet, or temperature, the affected muscles might appear normal during a visit to the doctor's office. Therefore, the doctor might use a provocative test to elicit and evaluate a mild occurrence of the muscle problem. An exercise test, which can involve anything from repeatedly making a fist to riding a stationary bicycle, usually can reveal symptoms of a channelopathy. Also, a doctor might test for periodic paralysis by having the patient consume safe doses of carbohydrate or potassium, or for paramyotonia congenita by immersing the patient's arm in cold water. Doctors frequently administer a thyroid-stimulating hormone (THS) test to determine whether the myopathy is endocrine-related or to rule out the endocrine myopathies.

Finally, with just a blood sample, genetic tests can check for specific genetic defects that give rise to some of the inheritable myopathies.

These tests are safe, relatively painless, and very accurate. However, because some of the genetic defects that cause inheritable myopathies remain to be discovered, a negative test result doesn't necessarily mean a person doesn't have a myopathy.

Endocrine Myopathies

Endocrine myopathies can occur when a gland produces too much or too little of a hormone. Hormones travel through the bloodstream and affect metabolism (a set of vital chemical reactions) in a variety of tissues, including muscle. Overproduction of the hormone thyroxine by the thyroid gland causes hyperthyroid myopathy, while underproduction causes hypothyroid myopathy.

A common cause of both myopathies is autoimmunity, a condition in which the immune system turns against part of the body—in this case, the thyroid. Sometimes, the endocrine myopathies occur with myasthenia gravis, another autoimmune disease that causes muscle weakness. Both myopathies can be almost completely alleviated by restoring normal thyroid activity, called the euthyroid state.

Hyperthyroid Myopathy

Also called: Thyrotoxic myopathy.

Symptoms: This disease commonly involves weakness and wasting of muscles around the shoulders and sometimes the hips. There also can be weakness in muscles of the face and throat, and in the respiratory muscles. Severe cases can cause rhabdomyolysis (acute muscle breakdown). Some people with hyperthyroid myopathy develop Grave's disease, damage to muscles that control movement of the eye and eyelids, which can lead to vision loss. Others develop thyrotoxic periodic paralysis, which involves temporary, but severe attacks of muscle weakness.

Treatment: Restoring normal thyroxine levels can be achieved with anti-thyroid drugs, but sometimes requires partial or complete surgical removal of the thyroid (thyroidectomy).

Hypothyroid Myopathy

Symptoms: The most common symptoms include weakness around the hips and sometimes the shoulders, and a slowing of reflexes. Some people also experience muscle stiffness and painful muscle cramps. Severe cases can cause rhabdomyolysis.

Sometimes, the disease causes muscle enlargement along with muscle weakness. In adults, this condition is called Hoffman's syndrome, and in children, it's called Kocher-Debre-Semelaigne syndrome.

Treatment: Thyroxine levels can be brought up to normal with oral thyroxine pills.

Section 2.2

Facts about Mitochondrial Myopathies

Reprinted from "Facts about Mitochondrial Myopathies" with permission from the Muscular Dystrophy Association, www.mdausa.org. © 2001 The Muscular Dystrophy Association. For additional information, call the Muscular Dystrophy Association National Headquarters toll-free at (800) 572-1717. To find an MDA office in your area, look in your local telephone book, or click on "Clinics and Services" on the MDA website.

What Are Mitochondrial Diseases?

Mitochondrial myopathy (MM) is a disease with many different faces. Dozens of varieties of mitochondrial diseases have been identified, with a complex array of symptoms. Some symptoms can be so mild as to be hardly noticeable, while others are life-threatening.

From this section you will learn a few encouraging things about MM. For example, although this is a very rare disorder, many of its symptoms are common in the general population, such as heart problems, seizures, and diabetes. Therefore, good medical treatments already exist to help manage many symptoms.

Always remember that researchers are continually moving toward better treatments and, ultimately, cures for mitochondrial diseases. In addition, people with disabilities have greater opportunities than ever before to make the most of their abilities, as well as legal rights to equal employment opportunity and access to public places. Children with physical and cognitive disabilities are guaranteed by law a public education with whatever supports they need.

Just as some diseases are named for the part of the body they affect (like heart disease), mitochondrial diseases are so-named because they affect a specific part of the cells of which our bodies are made. Specifically, mitochondrial diseases affect the mitochondria—tiny energy factories found inside almost all our cells.

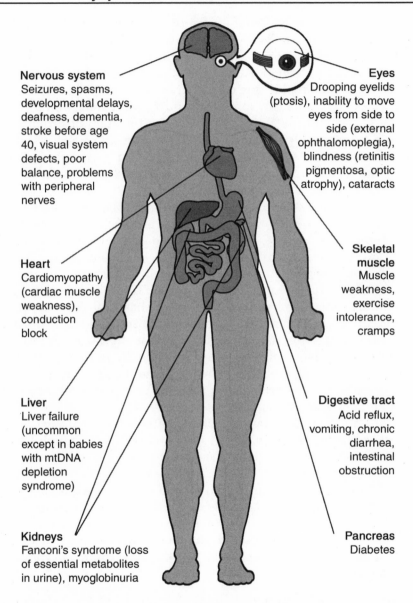

Nervous system
Seizures, spasms, developmental delays, deafness, dementia, stroke before age 40, visual system defects, poor balance, problems with peripheral nerves

Eyes
Drooping eyelids (ptosis), inability to move eyes from side to side (external ophthalomoplegia), blindness (retinitis pigmentosa, optic atrophy), cataracts

Heart
Cardiomyopathy (cardiac muscle weakness), conduction block

Skeletal muscle
Muscle weakness, exercise intolerance, cramps

Liver
Liver failure (uncommon except in babies with mtDNA depletion syndrome)

Digestive tract
Acid reflux, vomiting, chronic diarrhea, intestinal obstruction

Kidneys
Fanconi's syndrome (loss of essential metabolites in urine), myoglobinuria

Pancreas
Diabetes

Figure 2.3. *Mitochondrial Diseases. The main problems associated with mitochondrial disease—low energy, free radical production, and lactic acidosis—can result in a variety of symptoms in many different organs of the body. This diagram depicts common symptoms of mitochondrial disease, of which most affected people have a specific subset. Many of these symptoms are very treatable.*

Mitochondria are responsible for producing most of the energy that's needed for our cells to function. In fact, they provide such an important source of energy that a typical human cell contains hundreds of them. A mitochondrial disease can shut down some or all the mitochondria, cutting off this essential energy supply.

Nearly all our cells rely on mitochondria for a steady energy supply, so a mitochondrial disease can be a multisystem disorder affecting more than one type of cell, tissue, or organ. The exact symptoms aren't the same for everyone, because a person with mitochondrial disease can have a unique mixture of healthy and defective mitochondria, with a unique distribution in the body.

Because muscle cells and nerve cells have especially high energy needs, muscular and neurological problems—such as muscle weakness, exercise intolerance, hearing loss, trouble with balance and coordination, seizures, and learning deficits—are common features of mitochondrial disease. Other frequent complications include cataracts, heart defects, diabetes, and stunted growth. Usually, a person with a mitochondrial disease has two or more of these conditions, some of which occur together so regularly that they're grouped into syndromes.

A mitochondrial disease that causes prominent muscular problems is called a mitochondrial myopathy (*myo* means muscle, and *pathos* means disease); while a mitochondrial disease that causes both prominent muscular and neurological problems is called a mitochondrial encephalomyopathy (*encephalo* refers to the brain).

Despite their many potential effects, mitochondrial diseases sometimes cause little disability. Sometimes, a person has enough healthy mitochondria to compensate for the defective ones. Also, because some symptoms of mitochondrial disease (such as diabetes or heart arrhythmia) are common in the general population, there are effective treatments for those symptoms (such as insulin or anti-arrhythmic drugs).

This section describes general causes, consequences, and management of mitochondrial diseases, with an emphasis on myopathies and encephalomyopathies and a close look at the most common syndromes. These include:

- Kearns-Sayre syndrome (KSS)

- Leigh's syndrome

- mitochondrial DNA depletion syndrome (MDS)

- mitochondrial encephalomyopathy, lactic acidosis and strokelike episodes (MELAS)

- myoclonus epilepsy with ragged red fibers (MERRF)

- mitochondrial neurogastrointestinal encephalomyopathy (MNGIE)
- neuropathy, ataxia, and retinitis pigmentosa (NARP)
- Pearson syndrome
- progressive external ophthalmoplegia (PEO)

What Causes Mitochondrial Diseases?

First, mitochondrial diseases aren't contagious, and they aren't caused by anything a person does. They're caused by mutations, or changes, in genes—the cells' blueprints for making proteins.

Genes are responsible for building our bodies, and are passed from parents to children, along with any mutations or defects they have. That means that mitochondrial diseases are inheritable, although they often affect members of the same family in different ways.

The genes involved in mitochondrial disease normally make proteins that work inside the mitochondria. Within each mitochondrion (singular of mitochondria), these proteins make up part of an assembly line that uses fuel molecules derived from food to manufacture the energy molecule ATP. This highly efficient manufacturing process requires oxygen; outside the mitochondrion, there are less efficient ways of producing ATP without oxygen.

Proteins at the beginning of the mitochondrial assembly line act like cargo handlers, importing the fuel molecules—sugars and fats—into the mitochondrion. Next, other proteins break down the sugars and fats, extracting energy in the form of charged particles called electrons.

Proteins toward the end of the line—organized into five groups called complexes I, II, III, IV and V—harness the energy from those electrons to make adenosine 5'-triphosphate (ATP). Complexes I through IV shuttle the electrons down the line and are therefore called the electron transport chain, and complex V actually churns out ATP, so it's also called ATP synthase.

A deficiency in one or more of these complexes is the typical cause of a mitochondrial disease. (In fact, mitochondrial diseases are sometimes named for a specific deficiency, such as complex I deficiency.)

When a cell is filled with defective mitochondria, it not only becomes deprived of ATP—it can accumulate a backlog of unused fuel molecules and oxygen, with potentially disastrous effects. Excess fuel molecules are used to make ATP by inefficient means, which can generate potentially harmful byproducts such as lactic acid. (This also occurs when a cell has an inadequate oxygen supply, which can happen to muscle cells during strenuous exercise.) The buildup of lactic acid in the blood—called lactic acidosis—is associated with muscle fatigue, and might actually damage muscle and nerve tissue. Meanwhile, unused oxygen in the cell can be converted into destructive compounds called reactive oxygen species. (These are the targets of so-called antioxidant drugs and vitamins.)

ATP derived from mitochondria provides the main source of power for muscle cell contraction and nerve cell firing. So, muscle cells and nerve cells are especially sensitive to mitochondrial defects. The combined effects of energy deprivation and toxin accumulation in these

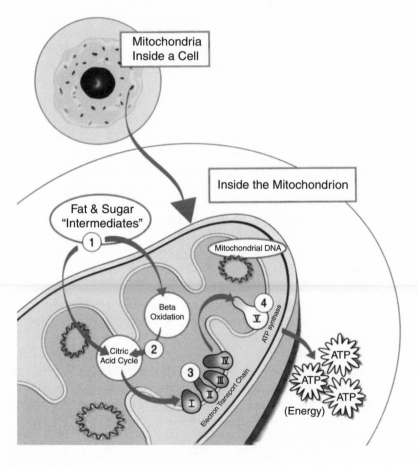

Figure 2.4. Inside the Mitochondrion

cells probably give rise to the main symptoms of mitochondrial myopathies and encephalomyopathies.

What Happens to Someone with a Mitochondrial Disease?

Myopathy

The main symptoms of mitochondrial myopathy are muscle weakness and wasting, and exercise intolerance. It's important to remember that the severity of any of these symptoms varies greatly from one person to the next, even in the same family.

Weakness and wasting usually are most prominent in muscles that control movements of the eyes and eyelids. Two common consequences are the gradual paralysis of eye movements, called progressive external ophthalmoplegia (PEO), and drooping of the upper eyelids, called ptosis. Often, people automatically compensate for PEO by moving their heads to look in different directions, and might not even notice any visual problems. Ptosis is potentially more frustrating because it can impair vision and also cause a listless expression, but it can be corrected by surgery, or by using glasses that have a "ptosis crutch" to lift the upper eyelids.

Mitochondrial myopathies can also cause weakness and wasting in other muscles of the face and neck, which can lead to slurred speech and difficulty with swallowing. In these instances, speech therapy or changing the diet to easier-to-swallow foods can be useful. Sometimes, people with mitochondrial myopathies experience loss of muscle strength in the arms or legs, and might need braces or a wheelchair to get around.

Exercise intolerance, also called exertional fatigue, refers to unusual feelings of exhaustion brought on by physical exertion. The degree of exercise intolerance varies greatly among individuals. Some people might only have trouble with athletic activities like jogging, while others might experience problems with everyday activities like walking to the mailbox, or lifting a milk carton.

Sometimes, exercise intolerance is associated with painful muscle cramps and/or injury-induced pain. The cramps are actually sharp contractions that may seem to temporarily lock the muscles, while the injury-induced pain is caused by a process of acute muscle breakdown called rhabdomyolysis. Cramps or rhabdomyolysis usually occur when someone with exercise intolerance "overdoes it," and can happen during the overexertion or several hours afterward.

31

Encephalomyopathy

A mitochondrial encephalomyopathy typically includes some of the mentioned symptoms of myopathy plus one or more neurological symptoms. Again, these symptoms show a great deal of individual variability in both type and severity.

Hearing impairment, migraine-like headaches, and seizures are among the most common symptoms of mitochondrial encephalomyopathy. In at least one syndrome, headaches and seizures are accompanied by stroke (interruption of the brain's blood supply).

Fortunately, there are good treatments for some of these conditions. Hearing impairment can be managed using hearing aids and alternate forms of communication. Often, headaches can be alleviated with medications and seizures can be prevented with drugs used for epilepsy (anti-epileptics). Several drugs are currently under investigation for treating stroke.

In addition to affecting the musculature of the eye, a mitochondrial encephalomyopathy can affect the eye itself and parts of the brain involved in vision. (For instance, cataracts—thickening of the lenses that focus light in the eye—are a common symptom of mitochondrial encephalomyopathy.) Compared to muscle problems, these effects are more likely to cause serious visual impairment.

Often, mitochondrial encephalomyopathy causes ataxia, or trouble with balance and coordination. People with ataxia are usually prone to dizzy spells and falls, but can partly avoid those problems through physical and occupational therapy, and the use of supportive aids such as railings, a walker or—in severe cases—a wheelchair.

Special Issues in Mitochondrial Myopathies and Encephalomyopathies

Respiratory Care

Sometimes, these diseases can cause significant weakness in the muscles that support breathing. Also, mitochondrial encephalomyopathies sometimes cause brain abnormalities that alter the brain's control over breathing.

A person with mild respiratory problems might require occasional supplemental oxygen, while someone with more severe problems might require permanent support from a ventilator. If you have a mitochondrial disorder, you should watch for signs of respiratory insufficiency (such as shortness of breath or morning headaches), and have your breathing checked regularly by a specialist.

Cardiac Care

Sometimes, mitochondrial diseases directly affect the heart. In these cases, the usual cause is an interruption in the rhythmic beating of the heart, called a conduction block. Though dangerous, this condition is treatable with a pacemaker, which stimulates normal beating of the heart. If you have a mitochondrial disorder, you may need to have regular examinations by a cardiologist.

Other Potential Health Issues

Some people with mitochondrial disease experience serious kidney problems, gastrointestinal problems, and/or diabetes. Some of these problems are direct effects of mitochondrial defects in the kidneys, digestive system, or pancreas (in diabetes), and others are indirect effects of mitochondrial defects in other tissues.

For example, rhabdomyolysis can lead to kidney problems by causing a protein called myoglobin to leak from ruptured muscle cells and build up in the bloodstream. This condition, called myoglobinuria, strains the kidneys' ability to filter waste from the blood into urine, and can cause kidney damage.

Special Issues in Children

Vision: Though progressive external ophthalmoplegia (PEO) and ptosis typically cause mild visual impairment in adults, they're potentially more harmful in children with mitochondrial myopathies. The brain's visual system can be affected in children with mitochondrial myopathy. Because the development of the brain is sensitive to childhood experiences, PEO or ptosis during childhood can sometimes cause permanent damage to the brain's visual system. For this reason, it's important for children with signs of PEO or ptosis to have their vision checked by a specialist.

Developmental delays: Due to muscle weakness, brain abnormalities, or a combination of both, children with mitochondrial diseases may have difficulty developing certain skills. For example, they might take an unusually long time to reach motor milestones (such as sitting, crawling, and walking). As they get older, they may be unable to get around as easily as other children their age, and they might have speech problems and/or learning disabilities. If your child is severely affected by these problems, he or she may benefit from physical therapy, speech therapy, and possibly an individualized education program (IEP) at school.

How Are Mitochondrial Diseases Treated?

While mitochondrial myopathies and encephalomyopathies are relatively rare, some of their potential manifestations are common in the general population. Consequently, those complications (including heart problems, stroke, seizures, migraines, deafness, and diabetes) have highly effective treatments (including medications, dietary modifications, and lifestyle changes).

It's fortunate that these treatable symptoms are often the most life-threatening complications of mitochondrial disease. With that in mind, people affected by mitochondrial diseases can do a great deal to take care of themselves by monitoring their health and scheduling regular medical exams.

Instead of focusing on specific complications of mitochondrial disease, some newer, less-proven treatments aim at fixing or bypassing the defective mitochondria. These treatments are dietary supplements based on three natural substances involved in ATP production in our cells.

One such substance, creatine, normally acts as a reserve for ATP by forming a compound called creatine phosphate. When a cell's demand for ATP exceeds the amount its mitochondria can produce, creatine can release phosphate (the "P" in ATP) to rapidly enhance the ATP supply. In fact, creatine phosphate (also called phosphocreatine) typically provides the initial burst of ATP required for strenuous muscle activity.

Another substance, carnitine, generally improves the efficiency of ATP production by helping import certain fuel molecules into mitochondria, and cleaning up some of the toxic byproducts of ATP production. Carnitine is available as an over-the-counter supplement called L-carnitine.

Finally, coenzyme Q10, or coQ10, is a component of the electron transport chain, which uses oxygen to manufacture ATP. Some mitochondrial diseases are caused by coQ10 deficiency, and there's good evidence that coQ10 supplementation is beneficial in these cases. Some doctors think that coQ10 supplementation might also alleviate other mitochondrial diseases.

Creatine, L-carnitine, and coQ10 supplements are often combined into a "cocktail" for treating mitochondrial disease. Although there's little scientific evidence that this treatment works, many people with mitochondrial disease have reported modest benefits. At the very least, there appear to be almost no harmful side effects to the three supplements when they're taken in moderation, but you should consult your doctor or MDA clinic director before taking any of them.

What Syndromes Occur with Mitochondrial Disease?

Note: Typically, these syndromes are inherited in either a maternal pattern (*) or a so-called Mendelian pattern (**), and/or they're sporadic (***), which means occurring with no family history.

Kearns-Sayre Syndrome (KSS) *

Onset: Before age 20.

Features: This disorder is defined by PEO (usually as the initial symptom) and pigmentary retinopathy, a "salt-and-pepper" pigmentation in the retina that can affect vision, but often leaves it intact. Other common symptoms include conduction block (in the heart) and ataxia. Less typical symptoms are mental retardation or deterioration, delayed sexual maturation, and short stature.

Leigh's Syndrome: Subacute Necrotizing Encephalomyopathy * and **

MILS: Maternally inherited Leigh's syndrome.

Onset: Infancy.

Features: Leigh's syndrome causes brain abnormalities that can result in ataxia, seizures, impaired vision and hearing, developmental delays, and altered control over breathing. It also causes muscle weakness, with prominent effects on swallowing, speech, and eye movements.

Mitochondrial DNA Depletion Syndrome (MDS) **

Onset: Infancy.

Features: This disorder typically causes muscle weakness and/or liver failure, and more rarely, brain abnormalities. "Floppiness," feeding difficulties, and developmental delays are common symptoms; PEO and seizures are less common.

Mitochondrial Encephalomyopathy, Lactic Acidosis, and Strokelike Episodes (MELAS) *

Onset: Childhood to early adulthood.

Features: MELAS causes recurrent strokes in the brain, which manifest as migraine type headaches, vomiting, and (less often) seizures, and can lead to permanent brain damage. Other common symptoms include PEO, general muscle weakness, exercise intolerance, hearing loss, diabetes, and short stature.

Myoclonus Epilepsy with Ragged Red Fibers (MERRF) *

Onset: Late childhood to adolescence.

Features: The most prominent symptoms are myoclonus (muscle spasms), seizures, ataxia, and muscle weakness. The disease can also cause hearing impairment and short stature.

Mitochondrial Neurogastrointestinal Encephalomyopathy (MNGIE) **

Onset: Usually before age 20.

Features: This disorder causes PEO, ptosis, limb weakness, and gastrointestinal (digestive) problems, including chronic diarrhea and abdominal pain. Another common symptom is peripheral neuropathy (a malfunction of the nerves that can lead to sensory impairment and muscle weakness).

Neuropathy, Ataxia, and Retinitis Pigmentosa (NARP) *

Onset: Infancy to adulthood.

Features: NARP causes neuropathy, ataxia, and retinitis pigmentosa (degeneration of the retina in the eye, with resulting loss of vision). It can also cause developmental delay, seizures, and dementia.

Pearson Syndrome ***

Onset: Infancy.

Features: This syndrome causes severe anemia and malfunction of the pancreas. Children who survive the disease usually go on to develop KSS.

Progressive External Ophthalmoplegia (PEO) * and ** and ***

Onset: Usually in adolescence or early adulthood.

Features: As noted, PEO is often a symptom of mitochondrial disease, but sometimes it stands out as a distinct syndrome. Often, it's associated with exercise intolerance.

How Are Mitochondrial Diseases Diagnosed?

None of the hallmark symptoms of mitochondrial disease—muscle weakness, exercise intolerance, hearing impairment, ataxia, seizures, learning disabilities, cataracts, heart defects, diabetes, and stunted growth—are unique to mitochondrial disease. However, a combination of three or more of these symptoms in one person strongly points to mitochondrial disease, especially when the symptoms involve more than one organ system.

To evaluate the extent of these symptoms, a physician usually begins by taking the patient's personal history, and then proceeds with physical and neurological exams.

The physical exam typically includes tests of strength and endurance, such as an exercise test, which can involve activities like repeatedly making a fist, or climbing up and down a small flight of stairs. The neurological exam can include tests of reflexes, vision, speech, and basic cognitive (thinking) skills.

Depending on information found during the personal history and exams, the physician might proceed with more specialized tests that can detect abnormalities in muscles, brain, and other organs.

The most important of these tests is the muscle biopsy, which involves removing a small sample of muscle tissue to examine. When treated with a dye that stains mitochondria red, muscles affected by mitochondrial disease often show ragged red fibers—muscle cells (fibers) that have accumulated mitochondria. Other stains can detect the absence of essential mitochondrial enzymes in the muscle. It's also possible to extract mitochondrial proteins from the muscle and measure their activity.

In addition to the muscle biopsy, noninvasive techniques can be used to examine muscle without taking a tissue sample. For instance, a technique called muscle phosphorus magnetic resonance spectroscopy (MRS) can measure levels of phosphocreatine and ATP (which are often depleted in muscles affected by mitochondrial disease). Also, CT scans or magnetic resonance imaging (MRI) are tools for visualizing the overall structure of muscles.

CT scans and MRI can also be used to visually inspect the brain for signs of damage, and surface electrodes placed on the scalp can be used to produce a record of the brain's activity called an electroencephalogram (EEG).

Table 2.1. Diagnostic Tests in Mitochondrial Diseases

Type	Test	What It Shows
Family History	Clinical exam or oral history of family members	Can sometimes indicate inheritance pattern by noting "soft signs" in unaffected relatives. These include deafness, short stature, migraine headaches, and PEO.
Muscle Biopsy	1. Histochemistry	1. Detects abnormal proliferation of mitochondria and deficiencies in cytochrome C oxidase (COX, which is complex IV in the electron transport chain).
	2. Immuno-histochemistry	2. Detects presence or absence of specific proteins. Can rule out other diseases or confirm loss of electron transport chain proteins.
	3. Biochemistry	3. Measures activities of specific enzymes. A special test called polarography measures oxygen consumption in mitochondria.
	4. Electron microscopy	4. May confirm abnormal appearance of mitochondria. Not used much today.
Blood Enzyme Test	1. Lactate and pyruvate levels	1. If elevated, may indicate deficiency in electron transport chain; abnormal ratios of the two may help identify the part of the chain that is blocked.
	2. Serum creatine kinase	2. May be slightly elevated in mitochondrial disease but usually only high in cases of mitochondrial DNA depletion.
Genetic Test	1. Known mutations	1. Uses blood sample or muscle sample to screen for known mutations, looking for common mutations first.
	2. Rare or unknown mutations	2. Can also look for rare or unknown mutations but may require samples from family members; this is more expensive and time-consuming.

A blood test might be ordered so the lab can look for a buildup of lactate or unused fuel molecules in the blood or cerebrospinal fluid (fluid that bathes the brain and spinal cord).

Similar techniques might be used to examine the functions of other organs and tissues in the body. For example, an electrocardiogram (EKG) can monitor the heart's activity, and a blood test can detect signs of kidney malfunction.

Finally, a genetic test can determine whether someone has a genetic mutation that causes mitochondrial disease. Ideally, the test is done using genetic material extracted from blood and from a muscle biopsy. It's important to realize that, although a positive test result can confirm diagnosis, a negative test result isn't necessarily meaningful.

Does It Run in the Family?

Often, a mitochondrial disease can be difficult to trace through a family tree. But since they're caused by defective genes, mitochondrial diseases do run in families.

To understand how mitochondrial diseases are passed on through families, it's important to know that there are two types of genes essential to mitochondria. The first type is housed within the nucleus—the part of our cells that contains most of our genetic material, or DNA. The second type resides exclusively within DNA contained inside the mitochondria themselves. Mutations in either nuclear DNA (nDNA) or mitochondrial DNA (mtDNA) can cause mitochondrial disease.

Most nDNA (along with any mutations it has) is inherited in a Mendelian pattern, loosely meaning that one copy of each gene comes from each parent. Also, most mitochondrial diseases caused by nDNA mutations (including Leigh's syndrome, MNGIE, and even MDS) are autosomal recessive, meaning that it takes mutations in both copies of a gene to cause disease.

Unlike nDNA, mtDNA passes only from mother to child. That's because during conception, when the sperm fuses with the egg, the sperm's mitochondria—and its mtDNA—are destroyed. Thus, mitochondrial diseases caused by mtDNA mutations are unique because they're inherited in a maternal pattern.

Another unique feature of mtDNA diseases arises from the fact that a typical human cell—including the egg cell—contains only one nucleus, but hundreds of mitochondria. The upshot is that a single cell can contain both mutant mitochondria and normal mitochondria, and the balance between the two will determine the cell's health. This helps explain why the symptoms of mitochondrial disease can vary so much from person to person, even within the same family.

Imagine that a woman's egg cells (and other cells in her body) contain both normal and mutant mitochondria, and that some have just a few mutant mitochondria, while others have many. A child conceived from a "mostly healthy" egg cell probably won't develop disease, and a child conceived from a "mostly mutant" egg cell probably will. Also,

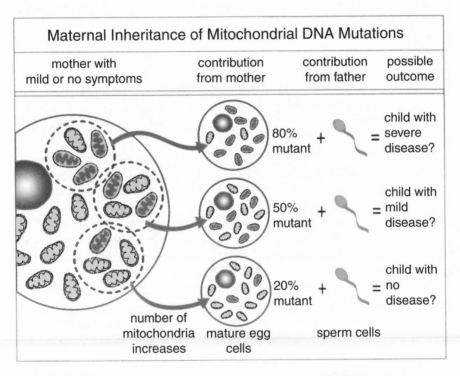

Figure 2.5. *Maternal Inheritance of Mitochondrial DNA Mutations*

the woman may or may not have symptoms of mitochondrial disease herself.

The risk of passing on a mitochondrial disease to your children depends on many factors, including whether the disease is caused by mutations in nDNA or mtDNA. A good way to find out more about these risks is to talk to a doctor or genetic counselor at your local MDA clinic.

MDA's Search for Treatments and Cures

With MDA's support, scientists continue to make significant progress in their quest to fully understand and treat mitochondrial diseases.

Because mitochondrial diseases can cause very diverse symptoms, they can be challenging to diagnose, and have historically been misdiagnosed as other diseases. MDA-funded scientists have helped improve diagnosis by carefully identifying the hallmark features of mitochondrial disease.

In an ongoing effort, MDA-funded scientists also have identified many of the genetic defects that cause mitochondrial diseases. They've used knowledge of those genetic defects to create animal models of mitochondrial disease, which can be used to investigate potential treatments. They've also designed genetic tests that allow accurate diagnosis of mitochondrial defects and provide valuable information for family planning. Perhaps most important, knowing the genetic defects that cause mitochondrial disease opens up the possibility of one day repairing those defects via gene therapy.

While some of MDA's scientists pursue gene therapy for mitochondrial diseases, others are conducting clinical trials to evaluate the benefits of dietary supplements (such as creatine, carnitine, and coQ10) and certain drugs (such as dichloroacetate, which can reduce lactic acidosis).

For people who have diseases caused by mtDNA mutations, MDA-funded scientists are working on several novel treatment strategies. For example, mtDNA isn't readily accessible to conventional gene therapy (because it's trapped inside mitochondria), so scientists are developing new gene therapy techniques to overcome that obstacle. Also, some scientists are investigating drug treatments and certain types of exercise to increase cellular levels of normal mtDNA relative to mutant mtDNA.

Additional Information

Muscular Dystrophy Association

3300 E. Sunrise Drive
Tucson, AZ 85718-3208
Toll-Free: 800-572-1717
Phone: 520-529-2000
Fax: 520-529-5300
Website: http://www.mdausa.org
E-mail: mda@mdausa.org

The Muscular Dystrophy Association offers a vast array of services to help you and your family deal with a mitochondrial myopathy. The Association's services include:

- a nationwide network of 230 hospital-affiliated clinics staffed by top neuromuscular disease specialists,

- week-long MDA summer camps for kids with neuromuscular diseases,

- support groups for those affected, spouses, parents or other caregivers,

- assistance with purchase and repair of wheelchairs and leg braces,

- evaluations for physical, occupational and respiratory therapy,

- flu shots to help protect the respiratory system, and

- equipment loan closets.

Chapter 3

Metabolic Diseases of the Muscles

What Are Metabolic Diseases of Muscle?

Metabolic diseases of muscle were first recognized in the second half of the 20th century. Each of these disorders is caused by a different genetic defect that impairs the body's metabolism, the collection of chemical changes that occur within cells during normal functioning.

Specifically, the metabolic diseases of muscle interfere with chemical reactions involved in drawing energy from food. Normally, fuel molecules derived from food must be broken down further inside each cell before they can be used by the cells' mitochondria to make the energy molecule adenosine 5'-triphosphate (ATP).

The mitochondria inside each cell could be called the cell's engines. The metabolic muscle diseases are caused by problems in the way certain fuel molecules are processed before they enter the mitochondria, or by the inability to get fuel molecules into mitochondria.

Muscles require a lot of energy in the form of ATP to work properly. When energy levels become too low, muscle weakness and exercise intolerance with muscle pain or cramps may occur. In a few

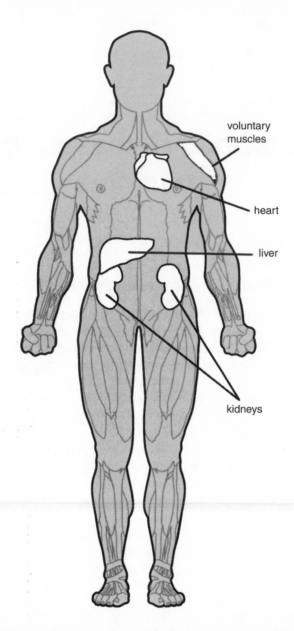

Figure 3.1. Metabolic diseases of muscle can affect all the body's voluntary muscles, such as those in the arms, legs, and trunk. Some can also involve increased risk of heart or liver diseases, and the effects can damage the kidneys.

metabolic muscle disorders, symptoms are not caused so much by a lack of energy, but rather by unused fuel molecules that build up inside muscle cells. This buildup may damage the cells, leading to chronic weakness.

Metabolic muscle diseases that have their onset in infancy tend to be the most severe, and some forms are fatal. Those that begin in childhood or adulthood tend to be less severe, and changes in diet and lifestyle can help most people with the milder forms adjust.

There are 10 metabolic diseases of muscle (myopathies) in Muscular Dystrophy Association's (MDA) program. Each one gets its name from the substance that is lacking:

- acid maltase deficiency (Pompe's disease)
- carnitine deficiency
- carnitine palmityl transferase deficiency
- debrancher enzyme deficiency (Cori's or Forbes' disease)
- lactate dehydrogenase deficiency
- myoadenylate deaminase deficiency
- phosphofructokinase deficiency (Tarui's disease)
- phosphoglycerate kinase deficiency
- phosphoglycerate mutase deficiency
- phosphorylase deficiency (McArdle's disease)

What Causes Metabolic Diseases?

Nine of the diseases in this chapter are caused by defects in the enzymes that control chemical reactions used to break down food. Enzyme defects are caused by flaws in the genes that govern production of the enzymes.

The 10th disease, carnitine deficiency, is caused by lack of a small, naturally occurring molecule that's not an enzyme but is involved in metabolism.

Enzymes are special types of proteins that act like little machines on a microscopic assembly line, each performing a different function to break down food molecules into fuel. When one of the enzymes in the line is defective, the process goes more slowly or shuts down entirely.

Our bodies can use carbohydrates (starches and sugars), fats, and protein for fuel. Defects in the cells' carbohydrate and fat-processing pathways usually lead to weakness in the voluntary muscles, but may also affect the heart, kidneys, or liver. Although defects in protein-processing pathways can occur as well, these usually lead to different kinds of disorders that affect other organs.

A gene is a recipe or set of instructions for making a protein, such as an enzyme. A defect in the gene may cause the protein to be made incorrectly or not at all, leading to a deficiency in the amount of that enzyme. Genes are passed from parents to children. Therefore, gene defects can be inherited.

The metabolic muscle diseases are not contagious, and they are not caused by certain kinds of exercise or lack of exercise. However, exercise or fasting (not eating regularly) may bring on episodes of muscle weakness in a person who has the disease because of a genetic flaw.

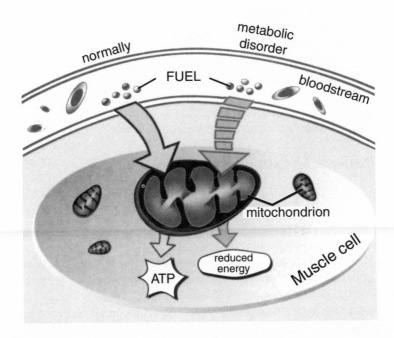

Figure 3.2. In normal metabolism, food provides fuel that is processed inside the cells, producing energy (ATP) for muscle contraction and other cellular functions. In metabolic myopathies, missing enzymes prevent mitochondria from properly processing fuel, and no energy is produced for muscle function.

What Happens to Someone with a Metabolic Disease?

Exercise Intolerance

The main symptom of most of the metabolic myopathies is difficulty performing some types of exercise, a situation known as exercise intolerance, in which the person becomes tired very easily.

The degree of exercise intolerance in the metabolic myopathies varies greatly between disorders and even from one individual to the next within a disorder. For instance, some people may run into trouble only when jogging, while others may have trouble after mild exertion such as walking across a parking lot or even blow-drying their hair. Each person must learn his activity limitations.

In general, people with defects in their carbohydrate-processing pathways tend to become very tired at the beginning of exercise, but may experience a renewed feeling of energy after 10 or 15 minutes. On the other hand, those with carnitine palmityl transferase deficiency (CPT) may experience fatigue only after prolonged exercise.

A person with exercise intolerance may also experience painful muscle cramps and/or injury-induced pain during or after exercising. The exercise-induced cramps (actually sharp contractions that may seem to temporarily lock the muscles) are especially noted in many of the disorders of carbohydrate metabolism and, rarely, in myoadenylate deaminase deficiency. The injury-induced pain is caused by acute muscle breakdown, a process called rhabdomyolysis, which may occur in any metabolic muscle disorder and is particularly noted in CPT.

Episodes of rhabdomyolysis usually occur when a person with a metabolic myopathy overdoes it (sometimes unknowingly). These episodes, often described as "severe muscle pain," may occur during exercise or several hours afterward. In those with carbohydrate-processing disorders, rhabdomyolysis may be triggered by aerobic exercise (such as running or jumping) or isometric exercise (like pushing or pulling heavy objects, squatting, or standing on tiptoes). In people with CPT, rhabdomyolysis is usually brought on by prolonged, moderate exercise, especially if an affected person exercises without eating. In CPT, rhabdomyolysis may also be triggered by illness, cold, fasting, stress, or menstruation.

Because rhabdomyolysis is painful and can cause extensive kidney damage, many people with metabolic muscle diseases try to avoid triggering these episodes by modifying their physical activities or diet. An MDA clinic director can help you work out a lifestyle plan to optimize your health and abilities.

Muscle Weakness

In acid maltase deficiency, carnitine deficiency, and debrancher enzyme deficiency, progressive muscle weakness, rather than exercise intolerance, is the primary symptom. Over time, people with acid maltase deficiency or debrancher enzyme deficiency may eventually need a wheelchair to get around and, as respiratory muscles weaken, may require ventilatory assistance to provide extra oxygen at night. All three of these disorders may be associated with heart problems.

It is important to realize that, although the metabolic muscle diseases characterized by exercise intolerance aren't generally prone to muscle weakness, some chronic or permanent weakness can develop in response to repeated episodes of rhabdomyolysis and to the normal loss of strength that occurs with aging. The degree of muscle weakness that develops in these disorders is extremely variable and may depend on such factors as genetic background and the number of episodes of rhabdomyolysis experienced. The diseases involving exercise intolerance do not usually progress to the degree that a wheelchair or any other mechanical assistance is needed.

Special Issues in Metabolic Disorders

Myoglobinuria: Myoglobinuria refers to rust-colored urine caused by the presence of myoglobin (a muscle protein). When overexertion triggers acute muscle breakdown (rhabdomyolysis), muscle proteins like creatine kinase and myoglobin are released into the blood and ultimately appear in the urine. Myoglobinuria can cause severe kidney damage if untreated. Incidences of myoglobinuria should be dealt with as emergencies and may require intravenous fluids to avoid renal failure.

Emergencies: The metabolic muscle diseases are so rare that emergency room staffs are frequently unfamiliar with them. As a result, they may not treat episodes properly (with fluids and pain medications) or may give the patient food or anesthesia that could trigger further problems. People with these disorders may want to consider carrying a treatment protocol that lists their doctor's phone number, the patient's current medications and dietary requirements, and guidelines for handling emergency situations. A Medic Alert bracelet can also be worn.

Anesthesia: People with metabolic muscle disorders may be at higher risk for a potentially fatal reaction to certain common general anesthetics (typically combinations of halothane and succinylcholine). This reaction, called malignant hyperthermia, can be avoided in planned surgeries by using lower-risk anesthetics. However, it is a good idea to wear a Medic Alert bracelet stating this susceptibility in case of an emergency.

Cardiac Care: People with debrancher enzyme deficiency, carnitine deficiency, and acid maltase deficiency may develop significant heart problems. In the case of primary carnitine deficiency, the only symptom may be heart failure; however, this disorder responds well to carnitine supplementation. If you are at risk for cardiac problems, a cardiologist who is familiar with your disorder should monitor your heart function.

Respiratory Care: Acid maltase deficiency and debrancher enzyme deficiency tend to weaken the respiratory muscles, those that operate the lungs, meaning that a person with one of these disorders may require supplemental oxygen at some point. If you are at risk for respiratory problems, your breathing should be monitored regularly by a specialist. Also, be conscious of symptoms such as unusual shortness of breath on exertion or morning headaches that may indicate that your breathing is compromised.

How Are the Metabolic Diseases of Muscle Treated?

For many people with metabolic muscle diseases, the only treatment needed is to understand what activities and situations tend to trigger attacks of rhabdomyolysis. A small percentage of adults with metabolic disorders may experience painful muscle cramps that have no obvious triggers—painkillers and meditation techniques may be effective under these circumstances.

In addition, some people with metabolic disorders have benefited from dietary changes. There is evidence that those with carbohydrate-processing problems may be helped by a high-protein diet, while those with difficulty processing fats may do well on a diet high in carbohydrates and low in fat. Carnitine supplements are usually given for carnitine deficiency and can be very effective in reversing heart failure in this disorder.

Please consult your doctor before undertaking any special diets. An MDA clinic director can help you design a specific plan suited for your metabolic disorder and your individual needs.

Also, there is emerging evidence that people with some carbohydrate-processing disorders, such as McArdle's disease, may benefit from light exercise. Researchers believe that people who are physically fit are

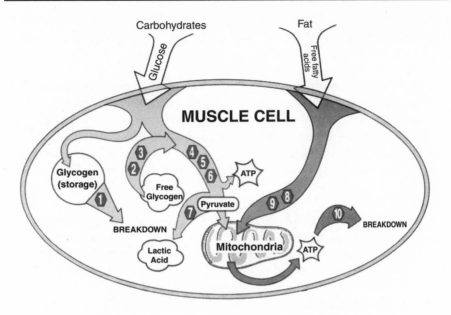

Figure 3.3. *Fueling the Muscles: Roadblocks Lead to Disorders. Where the Problems Lie in Each Disease.*

1.   *Acid maltase deficiency*
2.   *Muscle phosphorylase deficiency*
3.   *Debrancher enzyme deficiency*
4.   *Phosphofructokinase deficiency*
5.   *Phosphoglycerate kinase deficiency*
6.   *Phosphoglycerate mutase deficiency*
7.   *Lactate dehydrogenase deficiency*
8.   *Carnitine palmityl transferase deficiency*
9.   *Carnitine deficiency*
10.   *Myoadenylate deaminase deficiency*

Skeletal muscles normally depend on energy from carbohydrates and fats. These fuels can be stored in the muscle (glycogen) or imported directly from the bloodstream (glucose and fatty acids). When a genetic defect interferes with the processing of specific fuels, energy shortages can occur and toxic byproducts may build up. Some people may be able to bypass their defects by adjusting diet or exercise to draw energy more efficiently from unaffected pathways.

better able to use alternative fuel sources to make energy. Because overexertion can trigger muscle breakdown, you should only undertake an exercise program under the supervision of a doctor who is familiar with your disorder.

It is unclear whether regular exercise is beneficial in the fat-metabolizing disorders, such as carnitine palmityl transferase deficiency. Because of their rarity, the characteristics of several of these diseases are not known well.

Carbohydrate-Processing Disorders

These disorders affect the breakdown of glycogen or glucose (complex and simple carbohydrates) and are also called glycogenosis disorders.

Acid Maltase Deficiency

Also called: Glycogenosis type 2, Pompe's disease (infantile form), or lysosomal storage disease.

Onset: Infancy to adulthood.

Inheritance: Autosomal recessive.

Symptoms: Causes slowly progressive weakness, especially of the respiratory muscles and those of the hips, upper legs, shoulders, and upper arms. Enlargement of the tongue occurs in the infantile form, but rarely in the older forms. Cardiac involvement may occur in the childhood form, but is less common in adults. The childhood and adult-onset forms are less severe than the infantile form, but may require use of mechanical ventilation for breathing support as the disease progresses.

The infantile form of Pompe's disease often leads to death by age 2. An infant with this condition usually requires mechanical ventilation and a feeding tube to help with nourishment. If your infant's condition has been diagnosed as Pompe's disease, an MDA clinic director will keep you abreast of ongoing clinical trials for the disease and work with you to make the best decisions for care.

Debrancher Enzyme Deficiency

Also called: Cori's or Forbes' disease or glycogenosis type 3.

Onset: Childhood to adulthood.

Inheritance: Autosomal recessive.

Symptoms: Principally affects the liver, causing swelling of the liver, slowing of growth, low blood sugar levels, and sometimes, seizures. In children, these symptoms often improve around puberty. Muscle weakness may develop later in life, and is most pronounced in the muscles of the forearms, hands, lower legs, and feet. Weakness is often accompanied by loss of muscle bulk. The heart can be affected as well, and heart function should be monitored closely.

Phosphorylase Deficiency

Also called: Myophosphorylase deficiency, McArdle's disease, or glycogenosis type 5.

Onset: Childhood to adulthood.

Inheritance: Autosomal recessive.

Symptoms: Causes exercise intolerance, cramps, muscle pain, and weakness shortly after the beginning of exercise. A person with this disorder may tolerate light-to-moderate exercise such as walking on level ground, but strenuous exercise will usually bring on symptoms quickly. Resting may lead to a second wind, in which activity is then better tolerated. Isometric exercises that require strength, such as lifting heavy objects, squatting, or standing on tiptoe, also may cause muscle damage.

The symptoms of McArdle's disease vary in severity among people and even within the same person from day to day. Symptoms usually do not persist between attacks, although fixed weakness later in life is possible.

Phosphofructokinase Deficiency

Also called: Glycogenosis type 7 or Tarui's disease.

Onset: Childhood to adulthood.

Inheritance: Autosomal recessive.

Symptoms: Causes exercise intolerance, with pain, cramps, and occasionally, myoglobinuria. Symptoms are very similar to those of phosphorylase deficiency, but people with this disorder are less likely to experience the second wind phenomenon.

A carbohydrate meal typically worsens exercise capacity in this condition by lowering blood levels of fats, which are the major muscle energy fuels for those with the disorder. A partial deficiency of phosphofructokinase in the red blood cells results in the breakdown of those cells and an increase in blood levels of bilirubin, though the person usually experiences no symptoms.

Phosphoglycerate Kinase Deficiency

Also called: Glycogenosis type 9.

Onset: Infancy to early adulthood.

Inheritance: X-linked recessive.

Symptoms: May cause anemia, enlargement of the spleen, mental retardation, and epilepsy. More rarely, weakness, exercise intolerance, muscle cramps, and episodes of myoglobinuria also occur.

Phosphoglycerate Mutase Deficiency

Also called: Glycogenosis type 10.

Onset: Childhood to early adulthood.

Inheritance: Autosomal recessive.

Symptoms: Causes exercise intolerance, cramps, muscle pain, and sometimes, myoglobinuria. Permanent weakness is rare.

Lactate Dehydrogenase Deficiency

Also called: Glycogenosis type 11.

Onset: Early adulthood.

Inheritance: Autosomal recessive.

Symptoms: Causes exercise intolerance and episodes of myoglobinuria. A skin rash is common, probably because skin cells need lactate dehydrogenase.

Fat-Processing Disorders

Carnitine Deficiency

Onset: Childhood.

Inheritance: Autosomal recessive.

Symptoms: This slowly progressive disorder causes cardiac disease and muscle weakness in the hips, shoulders, upper arms, and legs. The neck and jaw muscles may also be weak. Carnitine deficiency may occur secondary to other metabolic diseases (secondary carnitine deficiency) or in response to a genetic mutation (gene defect) in the protein responsible for bringing carnitine into the cell (primary carnitine deficiency). Primary carnitine deficiency can often be treated successfully with carnitine supplements.

Carnitine Palmityl Transferase Deficiency

Onset: Childhood to early adulthood.

Inheritance: Autosomal recessive.

Symptoms: Symptoms are usually brought on by prolonged and intense exercise, especially in combination with fasting, but may not appear for several hours after activity stops. Short periods of exercise usually do not provoke symptoms. Symptoms can also be brought on by illness, cold, stress, or menstruation. This disorder causes muscle pain, stiffness, and tenderness, while weakness is less common. Breakdown of muscle tissue during an attack can cause myoglobinuria.

Disorder Affecting ATP Recycling

Myoadenylate Deaminase Deficiency

Onset: Adulthood.

Inheritance: Autosomal recessive.

Symptoms: Interferes with the recycling of the major energy molecule of the cell (called ATP). It may cause exercise intolerance, cramps, and muscle pain, although, in many cases people with deficiencies in this enzyme may experience no symptoms.

How Are the Metabolic Diseases of Muscle Diagnosed?

It is important to get an accurate diagnosis of a specific metabolic myopathy so the affected person can modify diet and exercise and monitor potentially serious disease effects. Because these diseases are rare, many people with metabolic disorders of muscle have spent some time trying to find out what caused their muscle weakness, myoglobinuria, or other symptoms. The diagnostic process usually begins with a careful medical history, a physical exam, and a neurological exam to test reflexes, strength, and the distribution of weakness. Several specialized tests are used to confirm a suspected diagnosis of metabolic disease.

- Blood tests can be used to detect the presence of certain chemicals in the blood that may indicate some metabolic diseases.

- An exercise test is used to monitor a person's response to intense or moderate exercise. Blood samples are taken during exercise for testing.

- Electromyography (EMG) uses small needle electrodes to measure the electrical currents in a muscle as it contracts. While an EMG cannot definitively diagnose metabolic disease, it can be used to rule out a number of other types of neuromuscular disease that cause similar patterns of weakness.

- A muscle biopsy requires the removal of a small piece of muscle tissue for microscopic analysis. The procedure is done either surgically, with an incision to expose the target muscle, or with a needle. A skin biopsy is also sometimes performed.

- Other tests that may be needed include an electrocardiogram to test heart function, and brain imaging studies such as CT or MRI scans.

- Genetic tests, using a blood sample, can analyze the person's genes for particular defects that cause metabolic disease, but these tests often are not necessary for diagnosis or for determining treatment.

Does It Run in the Family?

On being told they have a genetic disorder such as a metabolic muscle disease, bewildered patients often ask, "But it doesn't run in the family, so how could it be genetic?"

Metabolic myopathies can run in a family, even if only one person in the biological family has it. This is because of the ways in which genetic diseases are inherited.

Most of the metabolic diseases of muscle are inherited in an autosomal recessive pattern, meaning that a person needs two defective genes in order to have the disease. One copy is inherited from each parent, neither of whom would normally have symptoms.

Thus, the disease appears to have occurred out of the blue, but in reality, both parents may be carriers, silently harboring the genetic mutation (a flaw in the gene). Many parents have no idea they are carriers of a disease until they have a child who has the disease.

Other metabolic disorders have X-linked or autosomal dominant patterns of inheritance, each of which carries different risks for transmission to children. In some cases, a single disorder is associated with more than one pattern of inheritance.

Finally, metabolic disorders actually can occur out of the blue when a new mutation appears with a baby's conception. These are called spontaneous mutations, and after they occur they can be passed on to the next generation.

The risk of passing on a metabolic myopathy to your children depends on many circumstances, including exactly which type of metabolic disease has been diagnosed. A good way to find out more about these risks is to talk to an MDA clinic physician or ask to see the genetic counselor at the MDA clinic.

Additional Information

Muscular Dystrophy Association
3300 E. Sunrise Drive
Tucson, AZ 85718-3208
Toll-Free: 800-572-1717
Phone: 520-529-2000
Fax: 520-529-5300
Website: http://www.mdausa.org
E-mail: mda@mdausa.org

The Muscular Dystrophy Association offers a vast array of services to help you and your family deal with a mitochondrial myopathy. The Association's services include:

- a nationwide network of 230 hospital-affiliated clinics staffed by top neuromuscular disease specialists,

- week-long MDA summer camps for kids with neuromuscular diseases,
- support groups for those affected, spouses, parents or other caregivers,
- assistance with purchase and repair of wheelchairs and leg braces,
- evaluations for physical, occupational and respiratory therapy,
- flu shots to help protect the respiratory system, and
- equipment loan closets.

Chapter 4

Myositis: Inflammatory Diseases of the Muscles

Polymyositis and dermatomyositis are related diseases, both involving inflammation—swelling or irritation—of the voluntary muscles, those that normally govern movement, such as the muscles of the arms and legs.

Myositis means inflammation of muscle. Polymyositis means inflammation of many muscles, and dermatomyositis means inflammation of muscle and skin. The results of either condition are weakened muscles and often muscle pain. These conditions are seldom fatal, but in the most severe cases a person may need a wheelchair or require assistance with activities of daily living.

As early as 1863, a disease involving muscle inflammation and a reddish rash on the face and upper body was described and given the name polymyositis. In 1887, an apparent case of polymyositis without any rash was described by the German physician P. Hepp. Another German, H. Unverricht, then proposed using the name dermatomyositis for cases of muscle inflammation with skin changes and polymyositis for those without them. This terminology remains in use today. Both conditions are among the 40 neuromuscular diseases in the Muscular Dystrophy Association's (MDA) program.

Excerpted from "Facts about Polymyositis and Dermatomyositis" with permission from the Muscular Dystrophy Association, www.mdausa.org. © 1999 The Muscular Dystrophy Association. For additional information, call the Muscular Dystrophy Association National Headquarters toll-free at (800) 572-1717. To find an MDA office in your area, look in your local telephone book, or click on "Clinics and Services" on the MDA website.

The muscle inflammation in these two forms of myositis results from a disturbance in the body's immune system, the mechanisms that normally protect the body against infection and foreign substances. Research on the workings of the immune system and what causes it to malfunction is the key to knowledge about the treatment of the two disorders, and MDA-funded scientists are coming closer to understanding the many factors involved.

What Are Polymyositis and Dermatomyositis?

Polymyositis (PM) and dermatomyositis (DM) are two forms of inflammatory myopathies, diseases of muscle caused by an immune response. They cause muscle weakness as their major symptom. Dermatomyositis also causes a skin rash. Both are thought to be autoimmune diseases, in which the body's immune system attacks the muscles. Because the causes, symptoms, and treatments are similar, PM and DM are often discussed as a pair. They are contrasted with other types of inflammatory myopathies, including inclusion body myositis and myositis caused by infection or drug reactions.

Who Gets PM/DM?

It is estimated that PM and DM combined affect about 20,000 people in the United States, with approximately 1,400 new adult cases per year. PM and DM are two to three times as common among blacks as whites, and twice as common among women as men. They may appear at any age, but begin most commonly between the ages of 40 and 60. A juvenile form of dermatomyositis also occurs, with approximately 2,000 new cases per year in the United States. It appears most commonly in middle childhood to early adolescence.

What Causes PM/DM?

PM and DM are thought to be autoimmune diseases. An autoimmune disease occurs when the immune system, normally responsible for fighting infection, attacks the body's own tissues. Other examples of autoimmune diseases are rheumatoid arthritis, systemic lupus erythematosus, and myasthenia gravis. The weakness of PM and DM occur when the immune system attacks muscle cells and associated tissue. The trigger for this autoimmune attack is unknown.

Neither PM nor DM is a contagious disease, and they cannot be spread from person to person. Nor are they directly inherited, although some genetic factors may increase susceptibility. While there are families with more than one case of PM or DM, these are extremely rare.

What Are the Symptoms of Polymyositis?

Muscle weakness is the main symptom of PM. Weakness usually develops very gradually, over months or years, and many people find it difficult to state exactly when they first noticed their symptoms. Some people, however, develop weakness very rapidly, over a period of several weeks. The weakness is most prominent in the proximal muscles, those closest to the trunk, such as the muscles of the hips, thighs, neck, shoulders, and upper arms. The more distant, or distal, muscles are not usually affected, although they may become weak after many years of disease.

Muscle weakness can lead to difficulty climbing stairs, walking distances, arising from a chair or bed, or reaching for objects overhead. This weakness may cause a general reduction in physical activity.

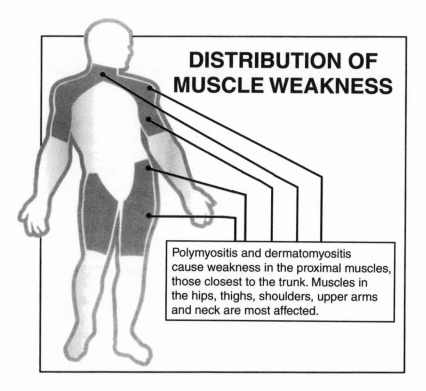

DISTRIBUTION OF MUSCLE WEAKNESS

Polymyositis and dermatomyositis cause weakness in the proximal muscles, those closest to the trunk. Muscles in the hips, thighs, shoulders, upper arms and neck are most affected.

Figure 4.1. Muscle Weakness in Polymyositis and Dermatomyositis

Swallowing difficulty (dysphagia) is also common in PM and may lead to weight loss or aspiration (entrance of food into the lungs) which can cause pneumonia.

Along with weakness, common symptoms of PM include fatigue and pain in the joints or muscles. Fatigue may lead to an increase in resting or napping. Pain may vary in intensity and location over time.

What Are the Symptoms of Dermatomyositis?

Dermatomyositis causes weakness, pain, and fatigue similar to that of polymyositis. In addition, DM is marked by a skin rash, which can precede weakness by weeks or months. In fact, some people who develop the skin rash do not develop muscle weakness for years, and may not be diagnosed with DM as a result. The rash is red or violet, hardened or scaly. It may appear on almost any body surface, but is most common on the face, eyelids, neck, chest, knuckles, knees, and elbows. The eyes may become puffy. Exposure to sun can worsen existing areas or lead to development of new ones. Hard nodules of calcium deposits under the skin (calcinosis) are common in juvenile dermatomyositis, but not in the adult form.

What Other Medical Conditions Are More Common in a Person with PM or DM?

People with PM or DM are more likely to have other autoimmune diseases. Arthritis is common, as is Raynaud's phenomenon, a condition causing temporary blanching of extremities exposed to cold. Others include systemic lupus erythematosus and Sjögren's syndrome.

Interstitial lung disease occurs in 10 percent to 30 percent of all people with PM or DM, almost all of whom carry antibodies against Jo-1. This condition causes fibrous scarring of lung tissue, leading to a dry, unproductive cough and shortness of breath with exertion.

Is Cancer More Common for People with PM and DM?

This question has been difficult for researchers to answer precisely. Some studies have indicated higher rates, especially for those with DM, while others show no significant increases. No increase in rates has been found in juvenile DM.

Mild cardiac disease can occur in PM/DM, but does not usually lead to complications. The most common problems are heart rhythm defects and myocarditis (muscle inflammation).

The Immune System in PM and DM

The immune system is a group of organs and cells located throughout the body. Its members include the thymus, spleen, bone marrow, and circulating white blood cells. When the immune system detects foreign substances, such as viruses or bacteria, the immune system attacks the invaders. Some white blood cells attack directly; others release proteins called antibodies which attack the outsider.

In normal human development, self-reactive immune cells are destroyed keeping the immune system from attacking the body's own tissues. Researchers think that in some people a few of these autoimmune cells may survive setting the stage for an autoimmune disease such as PM or DM.

Another theory of autoimmunity is that normally protective cells may mistakenly attack healthy cells that look similar to those of outside invaders. There is also some evidence that genetic factors can make a person more likely to develop one or more autoimmune diseases. These factors may combine to contribute to the development of autoimmune diseases such as PM and DM.

In polymyositis, the muscle damage is caused principally when white blood cells called T cells directly attack the muscle fiber. In dermatomyositis, antibodies attack the capillaries within the muscle. The resulting loss of blood supply then damages the muscle cells.

Almost all people with PM or DM have detectable levels of self-reactive antibodies in their bloodstreams. About three in 10 carry autoantibodies to an important cellular protein called amino-acyl tRNA synthetase, and in particular to one form of it called Jo-1. The presence of antibodies against Jo-1 is correlated with a high rate of interstitial lung disease and other inflammatory conditions. In some cases, a rise in antibody levels has been observed before a period of worsening symptoms. Malignancy is less commonly found in patients with these antibodies.

How Is Myositis Diagnosed?

If your doctor thinks you may have polymyositis or dermatomyositis, you should contact your local MDA office to arrange an examination at an MDA clinic.

Diagnosis of PM and DM begins with a careful medical history and a physical exam. A neurological exam is used to test reflexes, strength, and the distribution of weakness. Several specialized tests are used to confirm a suspected diagnosis of PM or DM. Electromyography (EMG) uses small needle electrodes to measure the electrical currents in a muscle as it contracts. While an EMG cannot definitively diagnose PM or DM, it can be used to rule out a number of other types of neuromuscular disease that cause similar patterns of weakness.

A creatine kinase (CK) test is a blood test for a muscle protein whose concentration in the blood rises with muscle damage. A blood sample is also used for antibody testing to determine whether self-reactive (autoimmune) antibodies are present.

A muscle biopsy requires the removal of a small piece of muscle tissue for microscopic analysis. The procedure is done either surgically with an incision to expose the target muscle or with a needle. A needle biopsy is faster and does not leave a scar, but removes less tissue making its diagnostic value somewhat lower.

Magnetic resonance imaging (MRI) may be used to identify areas of inflammation or replacement of muscle with fatty or fibrous tissue.

None of these tests can by itself definitively establish a diagnosis of PM or DM, although consistent results among all of them are highly informative. Diagnosis of dermatomyositis for those with a typical rash is usually not difficult. Establishing a firm diagnosis of polymyositis in cases without consistent findings can be a frustrating experience for both the doctor and the patient. Misdiagnosis is relatively common for polymyositis, and is one important reason for taking advantage of the diagnostic services of an MDA clinic.

How Is Myositis Treated?

The first line of treatment for both PM and DM is almost always oral prednisone, a corticosteroid hormone that suppresses the immune system. A high initial dose is continued long enough to improve strength and to reduce the CK levels in the blood, usually one to two months. The dose is then tapered over several months to a lower level which may be maintained for a year or more to prevent recurrence. Prednisone can cause significant side effects, including weight gain, puffy features, osteoporosis (brittle bones), diabetes, and mood changes.

Up to one-half of those with PM or DM do not have an adequate response to prednisone and require other immunosuppressive drugs. The most common agents are azathioprine and methotrexate. Cyclophosphamide, chlorambucil, and cyclosporine are also sometimes prescribed. The prednisone dose can often be reduced when another immunosuppressant is used. In some cases, intravenous methylprednisolone or methotrexate may be used to treat the disease more aggressively.

Intravenous immunoglobulin (IVIg) is used for those who have severe weakness or are unresponsive to other therapy. IVIg is a mixture of human blood proteins injected in large quantity into the bloodstream over two to five days. Improvements last only four to six weeks, although the treatment can be repeated. Despite its effectiveness and minimal side effects, the high expense of IVIg prevents it from becoming a standard initial treatment for PM or DM.

Plasmapheresis is a blood-filtering procedure pioneered by MDA in the 1970s. It is occasionally used to treat PM or DM when other treatments do not work, but it has had greater success in another autoimmune disease, myasthenia gravis.

Several other treatments are still considered experimental and are likely to be offered only as a last resort. These include whole-body irradiation and removal of the thymus gland (thymectomy).

How Are the Skin Disorders of Dermatomyositis Treated?

The DM rash usually improves with immunosuppressive treatment. For persistent rash, hydroxychloroquine may be effective. Topical corticosteroids may also be prescribed. Since the rash may worsen with sun exposure, avoidance of direct sunlight and use of sunscreen are recommended.

The calcinosis seen most often in juvenile dermatomyositis is difficult to treat. Colchicine is the most commonly prescribed drug. Nodules that are accessible can be removed surgically, although the pain or disability caused by their presence must be weighed against the risk of infection from surgery.

How Can Pain Be Treated?

The most common treatments for pain are the non-steroidal anti-inflammatory drugs, or NSAIDs. These include aspirin, ibuprofen, acetaminophen, and naproxen. When these are inadequate, a codeine-based pain reliever may be prescribed. Many non-drug methods can also relieve pain, including hot baths, application of hot or cold packs, stretching, or exercise.

How Can a Person with PM or DM Maintain and Improve Mobility?

Regular stretching exercises, prescribed by a physical therapist, help to maintain the range of motion in weakened limbs. This prevents the development of contractures, or permanent muscle shortening.

For people whose weakness limits their mobility, aids such as a cane, walker, or wheelchair can increase their ability to remain mobile in the home, community, or workplace. Braces for the legs, neck, or wrist are also commonly used. An occupational therapist can recommend the type of device best suited to the needs of the person with PM or DM.

How Are Swallowing Difficulties Treated?

A speech therapist can evaluate swallowing difficulties and may be able to recommend strategies to improve swallowing. Dietary changes or special food preparation techniques may be useful. In some cases, surgical removal of some muscle tissue in the throat (cricopharyngeal myotomy) can improve swallowing. If swallowing remains difficult and becomes unsafe (because of the risk of aspirating food into the lungs), a gastrostomy tube can be used to introduce food directly into the stomach.

What Treatments Are Used for Other Associated Conditions?

Interstitial lung disease is treated with the same range of immunosuppressive drugs as myositis. The treatment of cancer depends on the type and location of tumor detected.

What Is the Usual Course of PM and DM?

Studies have shown that prompt and aggressive treatment of PM and DM can help prevent worsening of the disease and improve the prospects for recovery of strength. Early treatment of juvenile dermatomyositis may help prevent calcinosis.

Most people with PM and DM respond well to treatment, especially if it is begun early. Nonetheless, there may be some residual weakness and relapses do occur. Lifespan may be reduced in the presence of cancer, significant heart disease, dysphagia, or interstitial lung disease.

Pregnancy may be a special concern for a woman with PM or DM. Women with active disease may worsen during pregnancy and are at increased risk for premature delivery or stillbirth. Women with their disease in remission during pregnancy often do not have flare-ups and are more likely to have a successful pregnancy.

Part Two

Congenital and Childhood-Onset Muscular Dystrophies

Chapter 5

Congenital Muscular Dystrophy

The congenital muscular dystrophies (CMD) are a group of the lesser known neuromuscular disorders. Diagnosis and recognition of this group of conditions has improved over the past few years following work done by a number of researchers around the world on the identification of the protein involved in CMD in a group of patients.

This protein is called merosin (otherwise known as laminin-m) and it is missing in the muscles of roughly half the patients diagnosed as having classical congenital MD. Work is presently under way to try and further identify the genetic fault responsible for CMDs, with a view to providing effective prenatal diagnosis and ultimately offering a treatment for the disorder. In the meantime, much can be done to assist a child who has CMD.

What Is Congenital Muscular Dystrophy?

Congenital means from birth and, indeed, one of the signs of congenital MD is that symptoms show as soon as the baby is born or in the first six months of life. Sometimes, however, a child is not diagnosed with congenital MD until much later.

These symptoms are likely to be hypotonia (floppiness), poor head control, muscle weakness, delayed motor milestones (e.g., when a baby first stands holding on to something, or learns to crawl or walk), and contractures (or tightness) in the ankles, hips, knees, and elbows. The baby's hips may be dislocated (out of joint) at birth. The contractures can sometimes be severe and affect several joints (known as arthrogryposis). They happen because the baby has not had the muscle strength to move freely enough in the womb.

There seem to be three main types of congenital muscular dystrophy:

1. Children who only have muscle weakness (dystrophy) involving all the muscles.

2. Children who have muscle weakness and learning difficulties, with or without epilepsy.

3. Children who have muscle weakness, learning difficulties, and abnormalities of the eye. Learning difficulties may be subtle, moderate, or severe.

Is Congenital Muscular Dystrophy Inherited?

Yes. The pattern of inheritance is known as autosomal recessive. This means that both parents are carriers of the condition (although clinically unaffected) and they have a risk of 25%, or 1 in 4 in each pregnancy, of passing the condition on to their children. Occasionally a case may be sporadic with little risk of recurrence in other children. There is no accurate way of predicting who is and who is not a carrier.

Table 5.1. Autosomal Recessive Inheritance

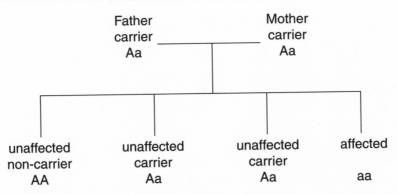

How Is Congenital Muscular Dystrophy Diagnosed?

A baby with congenital MD is usually first diagnosed as a floppy baby. Doctors can see the symptoms described, but as these could be due to a number of different conditions, they have to conduct a series of tests to try and make an accurate diagnosis.

First, a blood test is taken and the level of a muscle enzyme assessed (the creatine kinase or CK level). In over 75% of cases of congenital MD this level is 5–20 times higher than normal. However, at this stage, the diagnosis still needs to be backed up with a muscle biopsy. When the muscle is studied through a microscope there are three tell-tale signs which indicate that the child has congenital MD.

1. The muscle fibers, instead of being evenly sized, show great variation in size.

2. Some of the muscle fibers have been replaced by fat and fibrous tissue. Although some fat and fibrous tissue is found in normal muscle, in the case of congenital muscular dystrophy, the amount is greatly increased.

3. Some fibers are degenerating (breaking down).

In the merosin deficient cases, a skin biopsy rather than a muscle biopsy may be used to diagnose this type of CMD. This followed the discovery that the protein merosin was present in both skin and muscle and was absent from both tissues in these patients. A skin biopsy means only having to remove a very small skin sample from the patient and may be done under a local anesthetic. In addition, skin cells can easily be grown in tissue culture, and it is thought that in the future the cells which have been grown in the tissue culture might be used to discover exactly where the gene fault lies within the gene of an individual patient.

An electromyography (EMG) test may also be taken before a muscle biopsy is done. In EMG, a needle is inserted into muscle and the electrical activity recorded. An unusual level of activity could be either due to a myopathic (muscle related) or neuropathic (nerve related) condition.

An electromyogram gives a broad indication of a muscle problem, but a muscle biopsy must also be taken to pinpoint the precise diagnosis. An abnormal EMG cannot show any difference between a congenital myopathy and congenital muscular dystrophy; only a muscle biopsy can do this.

Is There a Treatment or a Cure?

At the moment there is no cure for congenital MD, but there are ways of helping to alleviate the effects of the condition.

Is Congenital Muscular Dystrophy Progressive and Is It Life-Threatening?

Sometimes the condition is fairly stable and the child even appears to gain strength as he or she gets older, although this is really a result of growing and developing rather than the muscle fibers regenerating and strengthening. If the condition is not progressive, there is no reason why a person should not live a normal lifespan. Sometimes the muscle weakness progresses quite rapidly and can lead to respiratory failure because the muscles which assist breathing are affected. This may happen in children of any age.

Can a Child with Congenital Muscular Dystrophy Learn to Walk?

The severity of this condition varies greatly from person to person. Some children will walk although this can be delayed until five years of age or older. Leg splints (braces) are often used to assist a child to walk. Children who have successfully walked may lose the ability later on because as they grow older and heavier the muscles are unable to cope with the greater strain. Other children never achieve walking. As the severity of congenital MD varies so much from child to child, it is important not to assume that certain developments will or will not take place, but to work with the child to achieve the goals which are in his or her power.

What Other Physical Effects Might Congenital Muscular Dystrophy Have on a Child?

As the muscles are weak and mobility is limited, the child may develop or be born with contractures, this means that the muscle tendons tighten up and the child is unable to move the limbs or joints as freely as a healthy child. Physiotherapy can help prevent this and a program of exercises should be worked out with a physiotherapist very soon after diagnosis. Even a very young baby can be helped to maintain suppleness. Hips are commonly affected, and if they are dislocated this may require treatment with a splint or sometimes surgery.

If the child sits awkwardly or has to twist his or her body in order to balance when walking, the spine may start to curve. This is called scoliosis. Passive and active stretching exercises help to keep the muscles flexible, prevent contractures, and stop the spine from curving.

Standing in standing frames and/or using night splints and braces can also help the child to stand symmetrically, and prevents or delays the onset of contractures and scoliosis. It is possible that a small operation which releases the Achilles tendon can help the child with congenital MD to stand more easily using braces or to continue walking after they would otherwise have had to start using a wheelchair. An operation on the spine is also sometimes advisable to help the child sit up straight.

Constipation, possibly due to the fact that a child is not very active or mobile, or possibly due to muscle weakness, is often an associated problem. This can be treated by a high fiber diet, drinking plenty of fluids, and very occasionally by laxatives.

What Is New in CMD?

Congenital muscular dystrophy is thought to be due to an abnormality in the muscle protein framework caused by deficiency in merosin (or laminin) a protein which normally helps connect the muscle framework to supportive structures outside the muscle membrane. Each laminin molecule is composed of a2, b1, and y1 chains.

A major advance in the understanding of CMD was the finding that the laminin a2 (or merosin M-chain) was found to be missing in the muscles of about half the patients diagnosed as having classical CMD. This led to the identification of a group of patients known as the merosin negative patients. These patients manifest a broad range of clinical symptoms and as a group are more severely affected than merosin positive patients. It is interesting to note that in the merosin negative CMD the nature of the genetic defect and the severity of the disorder do not always correlate.

The merosin protein (alpha 2 laminin chain) is composed of two protein fragments of different sizes (80kDa and 300kDa). It has been found that some people who have milder CMD than usual have minimal abnormality of the smallest fragment, but significantly reduced merosin levels in the larger fragment. This finding may help to explain the broad range of clinical symptoms associated with a merosin (alpha 2 laminin) deficiency, that is the type and severity of symptoms could be linked to which fragment is missing.

Genetic Advances

Most patients who lack merosin were found to have a genetic fault on chromosome 6 causing their condition. A different gene defect was localized on chromosome 9 causing the Japanese type of CMD otherwise known as Fukuyama congenital muscular dystrophy. In these patients merosin is present in reduced amounts, and it may be that the protein that helps to link merosin to the muscle structure is missing. The merosin positive patients probably lack another protein related to merosin which causes their type of CMD. It is likely that in the future the gene abnormality causing the classical merosin positive CMD will be localized.

Prenatal Diagnosis

Prenatal diagnosis is a promising development in the diagnosis of inherited conditions. It is based on being able to detect the abnormality in the developing fetus. This is useful in conditions associated with a specific protein deficiency or a recognized genetic defect. Unfortunately, at present no such test is available for the diagnosis of the merosin positive patients (no known protein deficiency or genetic fault). This picture is different in the merosin negative families. Merosin is normally expressed in fetal tissue; it is therefore theoretically feasible to detect its presence in chorionic villus samples (CVS) of at-risk pregnancies. The advent of a number of new genetic tests has enabled the experimental use of prenatal diagnosis in merosin negative families. Such tests include linkage analysis (a way of tracking genes inherited by different family members) and immunocytochemistry (examining tissue using specific tags which allow merosin to be detected visually). At present these tests may be suitable for some merosin negative families, but it is likely that they will become more widely available in the future. There may also be an option in merosin positive families if either the genetic fault or the protein abnormality is defined.

Future Areas of Research

At present there is no curative treatment for CMD, although the recent major genetic advances offer a number of possible treatments for the future. Some of these treatment possibilities include gene therapy and myoblast (muscle cell) transfer. Myoblast transplantations have been shown to restore the production of the extracellular merosin (alpha 2 laminin) chain, at least partially, in experiments done using the dy/dy mouse (mouse model for human congenital muscular dystrophy). However, at the moment it is unlikely that myoblast transfer will be helpful for children or adults with CMD. Finally, following the recent identification of merosin deficiency, it may be possible to try to compensate for this deficiency, particularly when the precise chemical consequences of merosin deficiency become clearer.

Chapter 6

Duchenne Muscular Dystrophy

Muscular dystrophies are genetic disorders characterized by progressive muscle wasting and weakness that begin with microscopic changes in the muscle. As muscles degenerate over time, the person's muscle strength declines.

Duchenne muscular dystrophy (DMD) was first described by the French neurologist Guillaume Benjamin Amand Duchenne in the 1860s. Becker muscular dystrophy (BMD) is named after the German doctor Peter Emil Becker, who first described this variant of DMD in the 1950s.

In DMD, boys begin to show signs of muscle weakness as early as age 3. The disease gradually weakens the skeletal or voluntary muscles,

This chapter includes excerpts from "Facts about Duchenne and Becker Muscular Dystrophies" with permission from the Muscular Dystrophy Association, www.mdausa.org. © 2002 The Muscular Dystrophy Association. For additional information, call the Muscular Dystrophy Association National Headquarters toll-free at (800) 572-1717. To find an MDA office in your area, look in your local telephone book, or click on "Clinics and Services" on the MDA website. "The Basics of Muscular Dystrophy and Beyond," is reprinted with permission from Parent Project Muscular Dystrophy. © 2003. All rights reserved. For additional information about Duchenne and Becker Muscular Dystrophy, visit the Parent Project website at www.parentprojectmd.org. "The Older Child with Duchenne Muscular Dystrophy," is reprinted with permission from the Muscular Dystrophy Campaign, a United Kingdom charity focusing on all muscular dystrophies and allied disorders. © 2003 Muscular Dystrophy Campaign. All rights reserved. Additional information is available at www.muscular-dystrophy.org.uk.

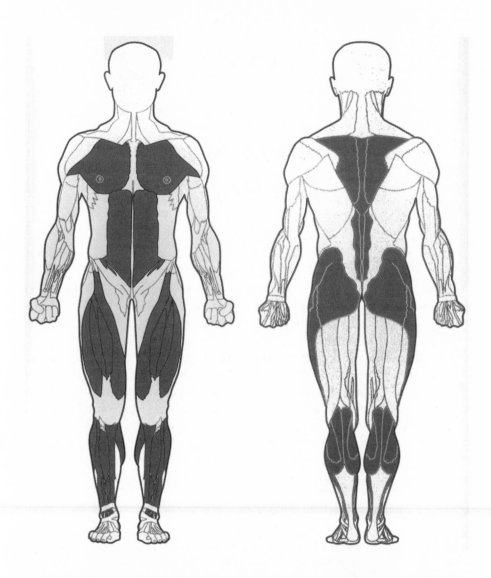

Figure 6.1. *Muscles Affected in Duchenne and Becker MD. In the early stages, Duchenne and Becker MD affect the pectoral muscles (which draw back the shoulders), the trunk, and the upper and lower legs. These weaknesses lead to difficulty in rising, climbing stairs, and maintaining balance.*

those in the arms, legs, and trunk. By the early teens or even earlier, the boy's heart and respiratory muscles may also be affected.

BMD is a much milder version of DMD. Its onset is usually in the teens or early adulthood, and the course is slower and far less predictable than that of DMD. Though DMD and BMD affect boys almost exclusively, in rare cases they can affect girls.

Causes of Duchenne Muscular Dystrophy

Until the 1980s, little was known about the cause of any kind of muscular dystrophy. In 1986, MDA-supported researchers identified the gene that, when flawed—a problem known as a mutation—causes DMD. In 1987, the protein associated with this gene was identified and named dystrophin.

Genes contain codes, or recipes, for proteins, which are very important biological components in all forms of life. DMD occurs when a particular gene on the X chromosome fails to make the protein dystrophin. BMD results from different mutations in the same gene. People with BMD have some dystrophin, but it's not enough or it's poor in quality. Having some dystrophin protects the muscles of those with Becker from degenerating as badly or as quickly as those of people with Duchenne. Eating or not eating food with protein cannot replace lost dystrophin.

Voluntary Muscles and DMD

The course of DMD is fairly predictable. Children with the disorder are often late in learning to walk. In toddlers, parents may notice enlarged calf muscles, or pseudohypertrophy. A preschooler with DMD may seem clumsy and fall often. Soon, he has trouble climbing stairs, getting up from the floor, or running.

By school age, the child may walk on his toes or the balls of his feet, with a slightly rolling gait. He has a waddling and unsteady gait and can easily fall over. To try to keep his balance, he sticks his belly out and puts his shoulders back. He also has difficulty raising his arms.

Nearly all children with DMD lose the ability to walk sometime between ages 7 and 12. In the teen years, activities involving the arms, legs, or trunk require assistance or mechanical support.

Diagnosing DMD

In diagnosing any form of muscular dystrophy, a doctor usually begins by taking a patient and family history and performing a physical

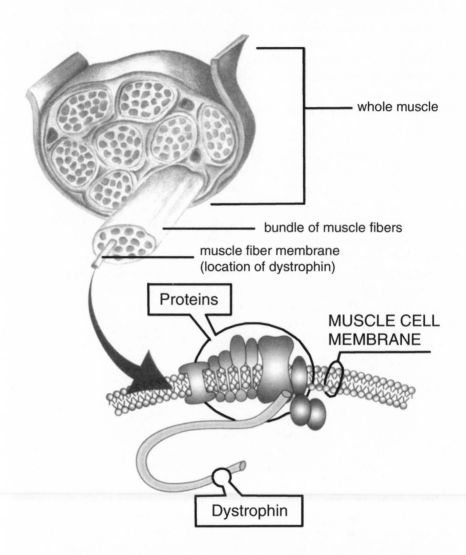

whole muscle

bundle of muscle fibers

muscle fiber membrane
(location of dystrophin)

Proteins

MUSCLE CELL
MEMBRANE

Dystrophin

Figure 6.2. *Cross Section of Muscle. Muscles are made up of bundles of fibers (cells). A group of independent proteins along the membrane surrounding each fiber helps to keep muscle cells working properly. When one of these proteins, dystrophin, is absent, the result is Duchenne muscular dystrophy; poor or inadequate dystrophin results in Becker muscular dystrophy.*

examination. Much can be learned from these, including the pattern of weakness. The history and physical go a long way toward making the diagnosis, even before any complicated diagnostic tests are done.

The doctor also wants to determine whether the patient's weakness results from a problem in the muscles themselves or in the nerves that control them. Muscle-controlling nerves, or motor neurons, originating in the spinal cord and brain and reaching out to all the muscles can cause weakness that looks like a muscle problem but really is not.

Usually, the origin of the weakness can be pinpointed by a physical exam. Occasionally, special tests called electromyography or nerve conduction studies are done. In these tests, the electrical activity of the muscles is measured and nerves are stimulated to see whether the problem lies in the muscles or the nerves.

Early in the diagnostic process doctors often order a special blood test called a CK level. CK stands for creatine kinase, an enzyme that leaks out of damaged muscle. When elevated CK levels are found in a blood sample, it usually means muscle is being destroyed by some abnormal process, such as a muscular dystrophy or an inflammation. Therefore, a high CK level suggests that the muscles themselves are the likely cause of the weakness, but it does not tell exactly what the muscle disorder might be.

To determine which disorder is causing a problem, a doctor may order a muscle biopsy, the surgical removal of a small sample of muscle from the patient. By examining this sample, doctors can tell a great deal about what is actually happening inside the muscles. Modern techniques can use the biopsy to distinguish muscular dystrophies from inflammatory and other disorders as well as between different forms of dystrophy.

Other tests on the biopsy sample can provide information about which muscle proteins are present in the muscle cells, and whether they are present in the normal amounts and in the right locations. This can determine whether the disease is DMD (with no dystrophin) or BMD (with some inadequate dystrophin). An MR (magnetic resonance) scan may also be ordered. These painless scans allow doctors to visualize what is going on inside weakening muscles.

The availability of DNA diagnostic tests, using either blood cells or muscle cells to get precise genetic information, is expanding rapidly. You can ask an MDA clinic physician or genetic counselor what tests are available. Since many men with BMD (and some with DMD) become fathers, it's important to know for certain which inherited disease an individual has. Sisters of people with DMD or BMD can also be tested to find out whether they are carriers of the disease, meaning they could have children with the disorder.

The Basics of Muscular Dystrophy and Beyond: Progression of Duchenne Muscular Dystrophy (MD)

Typically Duchenne MD is diagnosed between the ages of three and seven; however, the rate of progression and severity of each case is different. There are four stages that are usually associated with Duchenne MD.

Early Phase: Diagnosis through Age 7

Once a boy is diagnosed with Duchenne MD, it is often quite difficult to accept or believe that there is anything wrong with him. The onset of physical symptoms may be tough to recognize. Often times he will appear to be improving on the outside while his muscles are deteriorating on the inside. It is during this early phase that the calves may seem overdeveloped. He may appear clumsy and fall a lot. Jumping from a standing position may become nearly impossible.

Transitional Phase: 6–12 Years

Between the ages of 6 and 12, Duchenne MD has usually been diagnosed. The child will likely have trouble walking, mostly because his quadriceps (muscles in the front of the thighs) have grown weaker. This tends to keep him off balance as he attempts to shift his weight and walk. He may walk on the balls of his feet or on his toes with a slight, rolling gait. In order to compensate for a feeling of falling forward, boys with Duchenne MD will stick their bellies out and throw their shoulders back to keep their balance as they walk.

When asked to get up off of the floor, he will often put his rear end up in the air first and then walk his arms up his legs with his hands until he is standing using his arms for supports. The medical term for this is Gowers Maneuver.

Loss of Ambulation: 8–14 Years

By about age 12 years, boys with Duchenne MD will likely need a wheelchair for at least part of the time as mobility becomes more difficult. His weakened muscles will cause him to tire easily. In most cases, teen years are when the most significant loss of skeletal muscle strength takes place. It is at this point that activities involving the arms, legs, or trunk of the body will require assistance or mechanical support. Most boys will retain the use of their fingers through this phase so they can generally still write and use a computer.

Adult Stage: 15+ Years

During the teen years, in addition to skeletal muscle problems, boys with Duchenne MD will often develop heart muscle problems. Heart complications become the main threat to both health and life due to damage and loss of respiratory muscle. The muscle layer of the heart (called myocardium) begins to deteriorate, much like the skeletal muscles do. This puts the boys at risk of a heart attack. Major symptoms of myocardium include:

- shortness of breath,
- fluid in the lungs, or
- swelling in the feet and lower legs (caused by fluid retention).

When symptoms of Duchenne MD are managed conventionally, boys with the disorder usually die from respiratory failure before they turn 25. It has been estimated that anywhere from 9% to 50% of those with Duchenne MD die from cardiac failure.

The Older Child with Duchenne Muscular Dystrophy

Duchenne muscular dystrophy (DMD) is an incurable and inevitably progressive muscle disease affecting almost exclusively boys. This information is presented to help you appreciate the way the disease progresses and the timing of its complications. Please note all timings are approximate.

Ages Eight to Eleven

During the middle school years, the boy with DMD will usually deteriorate. He becomes unable to climb stairs and finds walking even short distances increasingly difficult. He falls more and more often hence at some stage during this period he will almost certainly lose the ability to walk independently. Walking may be prolonged through the use of aids such as leg braces, but these do not allow truly independent mobility.

Main Priority Areas

- Increasing need for support at school in lessons requiring any physical activity, or possibly full-time, according to needs.

- Maintenance of independent mobility through provision of an electric chair with appropriate seating to maintain good posture.

- Housing needs addressed and adaptations should have been completed before stair climbing becomes impossible to allow independent mobility in the home.

- Medical/orthopaedic surveillance of contractures and use of braces, etc.

- Consider needs for secondary education early (for example school adaptations, adapted toilet, and hoisting needs).

- Behavioral problems.

Ages Twelve to Fourteen

This is a relatively stable period in the life of a child with DMD. He is independently mobile in his electric chair and has home and school environments fully adapted to allow him maximum independence and dignity. He will be progressively losing upper limb function and should be provided with Internet technology and classroom support to compensate for progressive loss of writing skills. The major medical complication at this stage is the development of spinal curvature for which surgery may be needed. Medical surveillance for heart and breathing problems are also important now and there will be increasing hospital appointments in this period. On the whole however, the boy is unlikely to require hospitalization for these kinds of problems. Adolescent issues, including sexual frustration, will have the same importance to these boys as any others of this age.

Main Priority Area

- Full access to school in mainstream or special education as chosen by the family. This includes full access to toilets with appropriate hoisting arrangements as necessary.

- Medical surveillance for back, heart, and breathing especially.

- Respite arrangements for the boy and his family.

Fourteen and Older

The availability of surgical management for scoliosis and the medical management of cardiac and respiratory failure has allowed some boys with DMD to survive into their twenties.

As the young man with DMD approaches his late teens he is susceptible to chest infections and requires closer medical surveillance. Weight loss and fatigue may be a problem at this stage. His mobility may be restricted to hand movements only, and he may require adaptations to his wheelchair controls to maintain control.

Main Priority Areas

- Attention to post school education/employment.
- Medical surveillance.
- Respite care.

Chapter 7

Becker Muscular Dystrophy

What Is Becker Muscular Dystrophy (BMD)?

The muscular dystrophies are a group of genetic disorders which cause muscle weakness. The Becker type was first recognized in 1956 and is now known to be a much milder variant of the better known Duchenne type of MD. Becker MD is generally slowly progressive and affects only males.

What Causes It?

A fault in a particular gene (dystrophin) carried on the X chromosome leads to the formation of a faulty protein in muscle fibers. This protein, also called dystrophin, is absent or severely abnormal in Duchenne MD. In Becker MD, a milder fault makes the dystrophin molecule smaller (or occasionally larger) or less abundant than normal. When dystrophin is abnormal, the muscle fibers gradually break down and the muscles slowly become weaker. These dystrophin

This chapter contains "Becker MD," reprinted with permission from the Muscular Dystrophy Campaign, a United Kingdom charity focusing on all muscular dystrophies and allied disorders. © 2003 Muscular Dystrophy Campaign. All rights reserved. Additional information is available at www.muscular-dystrophy.org. And "Becker Muscular Dystrophy," © 2003 The Cleveland Clinic Foundation, 9500 Euclid Avenue, Cleveland, Oh 44195, 800-223-2273 ext. 48950, www.clevelandclinic.org. Additional information is available from the Cleveland Clinic Health Information Center, 216-444-3771, or www.clevelandclinic.org/health.

abnormalities in muscle provide a very good test for the diagnosis of Becker MD.

What Are the Symptoms?

The average age at diagnosis in BMD is 11 years, but the range is very wide—sometimes the diagnosis may be made in early childhood or well into adult life. Symptoms usually begin very mildly in childhood; often cramps on exercise are the only problem at first, but a few affected boys are late in learning to walk. Most people with BMD are not very athletic in childhood, and many struggle with school sports. Later, in the teens or twenties, muscle weakness becomes more evident causing difficulty in rapid walking, running, and climbing stairs. Later still, it may be difficult to lift heavy objects above waist level. Men with typical Becker muscular dystrophy may become unable to walk in their 40s or 50s or even later, but there are less frequent and more rapidly progressive variants of Becker muscular dystrophy in which this may happen in the 20s or 30s. Over a period of many years some muscles become weak and wasted, especially certain muscles of the shoulders, upper arms, and thighs, while others that are less weak are often enlarged—this is usually particularly noticeable in the calf muscles.

The muscles of facial expression, speech, swallowing, and the involuntary muscles (for example those of the bowel and bladder) are not affected in Becker MD. It is important to be aware that some people with BMD may have problems with their heart, and in the long term with the breathing muscles. These often do not cause any symptoms, and watching out for these problems which can often be treated, is an important reason to keep in touch with a specialist clinic.

Is There a Cure?

Unfortunately, there is no cure at present. Research is proceeding to try to find a way to induce the muscles to form dystrophin. Any treatment which may be found to be effective in Duchenne MD would theoretically be effective also in the Becker type MD.

What Can Be Done?

Active exercise strengthens normal muscle fibers (and the great majority are normal in the early years of Becker MD). It is important to try to keep as fit and active as possible. Regular daily exercise is better than occasional sudden bouts of exertion.

Cramps during exercise can bother people with Becker MD at some stage—especially as a teenager. If they are very troublesome, it may be worth experimenting with night splints (plastic splints to maintain a gentle stretch of the calf muscles overnight) with sessions of calf muscle massage, or compression with air-filled boots. There is not yet a properly tried and tested treatment for cramps.

In the later stages, a wheelchair is likely to be needed at least for getting about independently over long distances. There is a great deal of other equipment that may be useful to individuals, and much can be done to help both at home and at work to make certain tasks easier by careful choice of furniture, bathroom equipment, etc. Advice and help with these matters is increasingly available.

What about School?

Most young men with Becker MD leave school without having had any major muscle problems except that they are usually slow at running in their teens and not very successful at physical education or games. However, sometimes if cramps are a particular problem, keeping the school informed can be a good idea. In many cases the problem is recognized and diagnosed at around the age of 20.

A few boys with Becker MD also have learning problems, usually of a mild degree, but sufficient sometimes to limit their academic success at school. It is important to realize that this is not true of most affected boys, but when the problem does exist it is sensible to recognize and assess it early and to arrange the best possible plan to provide the right educational help. Unlike the muscle weakness, any learning problem will not get worse as the years go by. Despite the fact that to the outside observer BMD may cause relatively few problems in childhood, there is no doubt that some boys can find it a major psychological problem to be poor at sport in a society where boys are especially encouraged to pursue excellence at sport and where sporting heroes are so much in the news. Promoting self-worth in this period is a crucial factor.

What about Work?

People with Becker MD have been employed in a range of jobs from steel workers to research scientist. However, occupations requiring a considerable amount of physical activity are not feasible for most people who have Becker MD. It is clearly important for people to plan their careers on the basis that their existing physical capabilities are unlikely to improve and will eventually gradually decline. There is no reason why people with BMD should not work.

The important principles are to work for the best possible educational qualifications at school, to make good use of any opportunities for further education, and then either to plan a career that will depend as little as possible on physical strength and mobility, or to be prepared to re-train and change jobs appropriately as time goes on.

How Is Becker Muscular Dystrophy Inherited?

The disorder is inherited as an X-linked recessive trait, which means that it affects only males, but may be transmitted by unaffected female carriers of the gene to their sons.

The sons of carriers each have a 50:50 chance of being affected. The daughters of carriers each have a 50:50 chance of being carriers. The mothers and sisters of affected males may be carriers and may need to be tested. The sons of affected males do not carry the gene and will not be affected or transmit the gene. However, all the daughters of affected males are carriers of the gene and may transmit the disorder to the following generation.

How Early Can It Be Diagnosed?

Once Becker muscular dystrophy is known to affect one male in a family it is possible by simple blood tests to identify it or rule it out in any other boys at risk from birth onwards. In most families, but not in all, prenatal diagnosis is also possible, but this is more difficult. If at all possible, the situation needs to be fully assessed before a pregnancy is embarked upon.

Table 7.1. X-Linked Inheritance

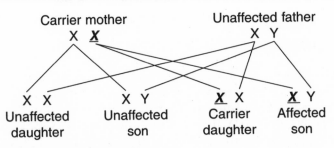

X = normal X-chromosome

$\underline{X}$ = defective gene on X-chromosome

Can Any Carriers in the Family Be Identified?

Using DNA analysis, most carriers can be detected if blood samples from their affected male relatives and certain other key members of the family are available for comparison. Although a simpler blood test for creatine kinase is positive in many carriers, only the DNA studies can rule out the carrier state in a woman at risk (for example in the sister of an affected man). However, in a few families, or if the key samples from relatives are not available, it may be possible only to calculate for each potential carrier her statistical risk of having an affected son.

Becker Muscular Dystrophy Information from Cleveland Clinic

Becker MD is very similar to Duchenne MD except it progresses much more slowly and affects primarily the legs and pelvis. It may also spread to the arms and neck, though its effects will not be as prominent as they are in the lower body. Becker MD is an X-linked recessive disease that affects approximately 3 out of every 100,000 boys. Its onset usually occurs between the ages of 7 and 26 years of age. Patients with Becker MD may have bones that develop abnormally or they may develop mental retardation. In almost all cases, a disease of the heart muscle known as cardiomyopathy develops, but congestive heart failure is rare. Some symptoms of Becker MD may include:

- Frequent falls
- Difficulty with leg muscle skills such as walking, running and jumping
- Skeletal and muscle deformities
- Muscle contractures (especially in the legs and heels)
- Fatigue
- Enlarged calf muscles (from compensating for other leg muscle loss)

Diagnosis

After carefully evaluating a patient's medical history, the doctor will perform a thorough physical exam to rule out other causes. If MD is suspected, there are a variety of laboratory tests that can be used to solidify a diagnosis. These tests may include:

Blood tests: When blood tests are performed to test for MD, the doctors are looking for an enzyme called creatine kinase (CK). This enzyme rises in the blood due to muscle damage or deterioration and may reveal some forms of MD before any physical symptoms appear.

Muscle biopsy: During a muscle biopsy, a small piece of muscle tissue is removed and then examined under a microscope. If MD is present, changes in the structure of muscle cells and other characteristics of the different forms of MD can be detected. The sample can also be stained to detect the presence or absence of particular proteins.

Electromyogram (EMG): An EMG is a test that measures the muscle's response to stimulation of its nerve supply (nerve conduction study) and the electrical activity in the muscle (needle electrode examination). Both components of the EMG are very useful in diagnosing MD.

Genetic tests: Several of the muscular dystrophies can be positively diagnosed by testing for the mutated gene involved. These include Duchenne, Becker, distal, and some forms of limb-girdle and Emery-Dreifuss dystrophies.

Treatment

There is no cure for muscular dystrophy, although some drugs still in the trial stage have shown promise in slowing or delaying the progression of the disease. For the time being, treatment is aimed at preventing complications due to the effects of weakness, decreased mobility, contractures, scoliosis, heart defects, and respiratory weakness.

Physical therapy: Physical therapy, especially regular stretching, is important in helping to maintain the range of motion for affected muscles and to prevent or delay contractures. Strengthening other muscles to compensate for weakness in affected muscles may be of benefit also, especially in earlier stages of milder MD. Regular exercise is important in maintaining good, overall health, but strenuous exercise may damage muscles further. For patients whose leg muscles are affected, braces may help lengthen the period of time that they can walk independently.

Surgery: If a patient's contractures have become more pronounced, surgery may be used to relieve the tension by cutting the tendon of the affected muscle then bracing it in a normal resting position while it regrows. Other surgeries are used to compensate for shoulder weakness in facioscapulohumeral MD, and to keep the breathing airway open for people with distal MD who sometimes experience sleep apnea. Surgery for scoliosis is often needed for patients with Duchenne MD.

Occupational therapy: Occupational therapy involves employing methods and tools to compensate for a patient's loss of strength and mobility. This may include modifications at home, dressing aids, wheelchair accessories, and communication aids.

Nutrition: Nutrition has not been shown to treat any conditions of MD, but it is essential to maintaining good health.

Cardiac care: Arrhythmias are often a symptom with Emery-Dreifuss and Becker MD and may need to be treated with special drugs. Pacemakers may also be needed in some cases and heart transplants are becoming more common for men with Becker MD.

Respiratory care: When the muscles of the diaphragm and other respiratory muscles become too weak to function on their own, a patient may require a ventilator to continue breathing deeply enough. Air may also be administered through a tube or mouthpiece. It is therefore very important to maintain healthy lungs to reduce the risk of respiratory complications.

Like many other disorders, understanding and education about muscular dystrophy is the most important tool with which to manage and prevent complications.

Additional Information

Muscular Dystrophy Association
3300 E. Sunrise Drive
Tucson, AZ 85718-3208
Toll-Free: 800-572-1717
Phone: 520-529-2000
Fax: 520-529-5300
Website: http://www.mdausa.org
E-mail: mda@mdausa.org

Muscular Dystrophy Family Foundation

2330 N. Meridian St.
Indianapolis IN 46208-5730
Toll-Free: 800-544-1213
Phone: 317-923-6333
Fax: 317-923-6334
Website: http://www.mdff.org
E-mail: mdff@mdff.org

Cleveland Clinic

Department of Patient Education and Health Information
9500 Euclid Ave. NA31
Cleveland, OH 44195
Toll-Free: 800-223-2273
Phone: 216-444-3771
Website: http://www.clevelandclinic.org

Contact for additional written health information.

Chapter 8

Emery-Dreifuss Muscular Dystrophy

What Is Emery-Dreifuss Muscular Dystrophy?

Like other muscular dystrophies it is a wasting disease of muscle. It usually begins in childhood or adolescence. The features, which make it unique and different from other muscular dystrophies, are the early development of muscle contractures, the distribution of muscle weakness, and the fact that the heart may be affected in a particular way.

What Are Muscle Contractures?

Muscle contractures are a tightening and shortening of certain muscle groups so that the joints, which are involved, become increasingly difficult to move. Such contractures are common at a late stage in most muscle wasting diseases and result from inactivity. In this disease muscle contractures develop very early or before there is any marked muscle weakness.

What Effect Do Contractures Have?

In this condition they limit elbow straightening so that the arms are often held in a semi-flexed way, they result in a tendency to walk on the toes, and they limit forward bending of the neck.

Reprinted with permission from the Muscular Dystrophy Campaign, a United Kingdom charity focusing on all muscular dystrophies and allied disorders. © 2003 Muscular Dystrophy Campaign. All rights reserved. Additional information is available at www.muscular-dystrophy.org.

Which Muscles Are Affected?

In the upper limbs weakness affects mainly the shoulders and upper arms. In the lower limbs, unlike most other dystrophies, weakness affects the lower legs first. This distribution of muscle weakness is sometimes referred to as scapulo-humero-peroneal.

At first there is difficulty in raising the arms above the head and lifting heavy objects, and a tendency to trip over carpets. Later the hip and thigh muscles also become affected so that climbing stairs becomes increasingly difficult, as does rising from a chair without assistance.

How Is the Heart Affected?

This is affected in a way that is unusual for muscular dystrophy, rather than affecting the heart muscle, it is the electrical wiring (called the cardiac conduction system) that controls the rate at which the heart beats that is mainly involved and is referred to as heart block. The heart rate is often abnormally slow, palpitations may occur (which feel like fluttering in the chest—this is not uncommon in normal individuals and alone would not be a cause for concern), as well as attacks of giddiness, and fainting spells. Increasing tiredness and breathlessness may also occur.

What Can Be Done If the Heart Is Affected?

If the heart becomes affected, and not every person is affected in this way, the doctor may recommend the insertion of a pacemaker. This small gadget is inserted just below the skin of the chest, and prevents further problems arising by ensuring that the heart thereafter beats normally.

How Severe Is the Disease?

In general, the condition is less severe than many other forms of muscular dystrophy and though life expectancy may be shortened, many affected individuals can expect to reach middle age or later. However, it is essential that affected individuals be checked at frequent intervals, say every 12 months, to ensure that the heart is not affected. There is evidence that a more severe recessive form also exists. Here weakness is present and progresses rapidly from early childhood, however, this is very rare.

Can Emery-Dreifuss Muscular Dystrophy Be Treated?

Unfortunately, there is as yet no cure or effective treatment apart from the insertion of a heart pacemaker when this is necessary. However, having an adequate diet and maintaining good general health are very important as in all muscular dystrophies.

Can I Improve Muscle Strength?

Regular, gentle exercise which is tolerated without causing stress is beneficial. But hard physical exercise (weight training for example) should be avoided. It is essential to eat a well balanced diet, to include plenty of roughage, and to avoid becoming overweight since this will only overburden the already weakened muscles.

Can Surgery Help?

Division of the heel cords can be useful in helping walking. Other operations can be indicated in individual cases where expert advice from a neurologist and orthopaedic surgeon should be sought. Because the heart may be affected and could complicate an operation, the anesthetist must be told of the diagnosis before any operation is undertaken.

Will I Become Disabled?

The condition progresses very slowly over the years (except for the very rare recessive form), and it may be that later in life a wheelchair may be required.

Job Prospects

As in other slowly progressive muscle diseases, in the early stages most occupations could be considered (a driving license however maybe subject to a medical examination). But since physical disability increases with age, some form of sedentary occupation is preferable in the long term.

Can It Affect My Children?

The condition is inherited and can therefore affect other members of the family. In many families it is inherited as a sex-linked (X-linked) trait, and therefore, only affects males and is carried by unaffected females. All the sons of an affected male will be unaffected, but all his daughters will be carriers. With regard to the offspring of a woman who is a carrier, on average each of her daughters has a 50:50 chance of also being a carrier, and on average each of her sons has a 50:50 chance of being affected.

Table 8.1. X-Linked Inheritance

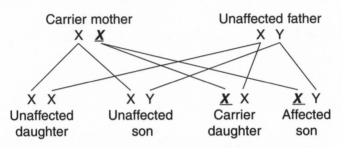

X = normal X-chromosome

_**X**_ = defective gene on X-chromosome

The condition can also be inherited as an autosomal dominant trait, which affects both males and females. Here the genetic risks are different. As in all autosomal dominant disorders, on average each son or daughter of an affected parent has a 50:50 chance of also becoming

Table 8.2. Autosomal Dominant Inheritance

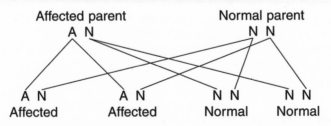

Both sexes are equally at risk.

X = Chromosome with defective gene

N = Chromosome with normal gene

affected. In the case of the recessive form, both parents are normal, but there is a 1 in 4 chance of any future children also being affected.

To make matters even more complicated, sometimes in X-linked and dominant cases there is no family history of the disorder, only one individual in the family being affected. In these cases the disease has arisen as the result of a new mutation in the affected individual, but who may then later transmit the disorder to his or her children.

For these various reasons it is very important to seek the professional advice of a neuromuscular specialist or medical geneticist if you are at all concerned about the risks to your children and other relatives.

What of the Future?

This is much more hopeful than in the past. Not only through the use of pacemakers in cases with heart disease, but the genes responsible both the autosomal dominant (codes for lamin A/C) and the X-linked forms of Emery-Dreifuss muscular dystrophy (codes for emerin) have been identified. This information is vital in the search for an effective treatment and also for prenatal diagnosis.

Some Other Similar Conditions

Rigid Spine Syndrome

In this disease, which begins in childhood, muscle weakness is usually slight, the main problem being contractures of the neck muscles, elbows, and knees. The heart is not affected. The condition is very heterogeneous being associated with various dystrophies. Expert advice is therefore necessary concerning the precise diagnosis and mode of inheritance in each case.

Rare Benign Sex-Linked Muscular Dystrophies

Apart from Becker muscular dystrophy and Emery-Dreifuss muscular dystrophy, other benign sex-linked dystrophies are very rare and have only been described in occasional families.

Limb-Girdle Dystrophies

In the late stages of Emery-Dreifuss muscular dystrophy the distribution of muscle weakness may resemble that in limb-girdle dystrophy. Again expert advice is required to confirm the precise diagnosis.

Part Three

Adult-Onset Muscular Dystrophies

Chapter 9

Distal Muscular Dystrophy

First described in 1902, distal muscular dystrophy (DD), or distal myopathy, is the name of a group of disorders that primarily affect distal muscles, those farthest away from the hips and shoulders such as muscles in the hands, feet, lower arms, or lower legs. Although muscle weakness is usually first detected in the distal muscles, with time, other muscle groups may become affected as well. Intellect is not affected in these diseases.

What Causes Distal Muscular Dystrophy (DD)?

The DDs are caused by many different genetic defects, not all of which are yet known. Also, some of the DDs have been given different names based on various symptoms, but may actually be caused by defects in the same gene.

Your own form of DD may or may not fit into one of these categories. Many of these diseases can vary from one person to the next, and in some cases researchers are still in the process of sorting out what symptoms are linked to a particular genetic defect.

Excerpted from "Facts About Rare Muscular Dystrophies" with permission from the Muscular Dystrophy Association, www.mdausa.org. © 2002 The Muscular Dystrophy Association. For additional information, call the Muscular Dystrophy Association National Headquarters toll-free at (800) 572-1717. To find an MDA office in your area, look in your local telephone book, or click on "Clinic and Services" on the MDA website.

What Are the Types of Distal Muscular Dystrophy?

Welander's Distal Myopathy

This form of distal muscular dystrophy follows a dominant pattern of inheritance and usually has an onset between 40 and 50 years of age. Upper extremities tend to be affected first, then lower ones. The degree of muscle weakness involved can range from benign to severe. Although its cause is not yet known, the disorder may be linked to the dysferlin gene, the same gene that is defective in Miyoshi myopathy and limb-girdle MD 2B.

Table 9.1. Classification of Distal Muscular Dystrophies (DDs)

Disease	Chromosome/ Gene	Inheritance Pattern
Welander's distal myopathy	chromosome 2	dominant
Finnish/Markesbery distal myopathy	chromosome 2	dominant
Miyoshi distal myopathy	dysferlin	recessive or sporadic
Nonaka distal myopathy	chromosome 9	recessive or sporadic
Gower's distal myopathy	chromosome 14	dominant
Hereditary inclusion-body myositis (HIBM)	GNE gene	recessive
Hereditary inclusion-body myositis (HIBM)	unknown	dominant
Distal myopathy with vocal cord and pharyngeal weakness	chromosome 5	dominant

Finnish/Markesbery Distal Myopathy

Markesbery muscular dystrophy follows a dominant pattern of inheritance with weakness starting after age 40 in the lower extremities and progressing slowly to the upper extremities and trunk muscles. Cardiac problems can be a feature.

Finnish muscular dystrophy (also called tibial MD) can be severe or benign, and typically affects only people of Finnish descent. Those with only one defective gene experience mild weakness of the tibial leg muscles (front of the calf) sometime after age 40. Those with two defective genes have progressive weakness starting in childhood and may lose the ability to walk by age 30.

Finnish and Markesbery distal myopathies may be caused by defects in the same gene.

Miyoshi Distal Myopathy

This disorder is inherited in a recessive pattern and involves weakness that begins in the lower extremities, especially in the calf muscle. It can progress to other muscles as well. Symptoms usually begin between 15 and 30 years of age.

The genetic defect that causes Miyoshi myopathy has been mapped to the gene for a protein of unknown function called dysferlin. Defects in the dysferlin gene can also cause limb-girdle muscular dystrophy 2B, which causes muscle weakness in and around the hips and shoulders. People with the same genetic defect in their dysferlin genes can have either disease, and it is not known what determines which pattern of symptoms a person gets.

Nonaka Distal Myopathy

Usually found in families of Japanese descent, this form of distal muscular dystrophy is inherited in a recessive pattern, and symptoms begin between ages 20 and 40. The anterior lower leg muscles (those in the front of the leg) are typically affected first, but the disease may progress to affect upper arm and leg muscles and neck muscles. The quadriceps muscles (in the thigh) tend to remain strong. The disease may be caused by a defect in the same gene that causes recessive hereditary inclusion-body myositis.

Gower's Distal Myopathy

This disorder is inherited in a dominant fashion and has its onset from childhood to 25 years of age. Weakness is first seen in the leg and neck muscles and progresses slowly to include upper leg muscles, hands, and more neck muscles.

Hereditary Inclusion-Body Myositis (HIBM)

This disorder can be inherited either as a dominant or a recessive disease. The recessive form appears in the teens or 20s, and muscle weakness appears in both the distal muscles (those farthest away from the shoulders and hips) and in the proximal muscles (the shoulder and hip muscles).

The dominant form has its onset at 25 to 40 years, and weakness occurs in the distal and proximal limb muscles with slow progression. In both forms of HIBM the muscle tissue, as seen in thin cross sections, is characterized by the presence of tiny holes in the muscle fibers called vacuoles.

Distal Myopathy with Vocal Cord and Pharyngeal Weakness

This disorder is inherited in a dominant pattern and has been linked to chromosome 5 in the same region as the gene that's defective in limb-girdle MD type 1A. Symptoms first appear between 35 and 60 years of age and include weakness of the hands, legs, or voice. Difficulty in swallowing, dysphagia, may be a feature.

Problems and Solutions in DD

- **Lower limb weakness:** Weakness of the lower limb muscles may make walking or standing from a sitting position difficult. In some cases, a type of brace called an orthosis that is worn over the shoe and lower or upper leg can help with leg weakness. Eventually, a wheelchair may be needed.

- **Arm weakness:** An MDA clinic can refer you to an therapist who will help you get the most out of your arm muscles in performing day-to-day activities. Often, the therapist can recommend devices that may improve grip strength or help you elevate your arms to better perform activities such as brushing your teeth or hair.

Additional Information

Muscular Dystrophy Association
National Headquarters
3300 E. Sunrise Drive
Tucson, AZ 85718
Toll-Free: 800-572-1717
Website: http://www.mda.org

Chapter 10

Facioscapulohumeral Muscular Dystrophy (FSHD)

Facioscapulohumeral Muscular Dystrophy: An Inheritable Muscle Disease

Facioscapulohumeral Disease (fa-she-o-skap-y-lo-hum-ral) adj.: relating to or affecting the muscles of the face, scapula, and arm (muscular dystrophies).

Facioscapulohumeral muscular dystrophy (Landouzy-Déjérine disease) is an inheritable muscle disease, commonly called FSH or FSHD. Progressive weakening and loss of skeletal muscle are its major effects. It has significant medical and health impacts on individuals, families, and society. Details about the nature of the disease and some basic knowledge of inheritance of genetic diseases are important to better understand FSHD. The FSH Society hopes this information more widely circulates understanding of FSHD, and that

This chapter includes "Facioscapulohumeral Disease," reprinted with permission from the FacioScapuloHumeral Society (FSH Society). © 2002 FSH Society, Inc. For additional information about facioscapulohumeral muscular dystrophy, visit www.fshsociety.org. Complete information about FSH Society is included at the end of this text. This chapter also contains "Effects of Facioscapulohumeral Muscular Dystrophy," reprinted with permission, from "Facioscapulohumeral Muscular Dystrophy," by the Muscular Dystrophy Association (MDA)–Australia, www.mda.org.au. © 2003 MDA–Australia. All rights reserved. "Scientists Identify a New Kind of Genetic Problem in Muscular Dystrophy," is from the National Institute of Neurological Disorders and Stroke (NINDS), August 8, 2002.

better understanding will help those who are living with and concerned about this unusual disease.

What is FSHD?

FSHD is a common form of muscular dystrophy, defined by a specific set of symptoms that collectively characterize the disease. Its major symptom is the progressive weakening and loss of skeletal muscles. The usual location of these weaknesses at onset is the origin of the name: face (facio), shoulder girdle (scapulo), and upper arms (humeral). Early weaknesses of the muscles of the eye (open and close) and mouth (smile, pucker, whistle) are distinctive for FSHD. These symptoms, in combination with weaknesses in the muscles that stabilize the scapulae (shoulder blades), are often the basis of the physician's diagnosis of FSHD. Other skeletal muscles invariably weaken. Involvement of muscles of the foot, hip girdle, and abdomen is common. Although the progression of FSHD is quite variable, it is usually slow. With FSHD, most affected people develop unbalanced (side to side) weaknesses. The reason for this asymmetry is unknown.

In more than half of FSHD cases, there are other symptoms like high-frequency hearing loss and/or abnormalities of blood vessels in the back of the eye. The vascular abnormalities in the back of the eye lead to visual problems in only about 1% of cases. Since these abnormalities are not exclusive of FSHD, one must be cautious of the fact that their presence alone, in an FSHD at-risk individual, is insufficient for a diagnosis of FSHD.

What causes FSHD?

By going from the large (muscle) to the small (DNA), one can partially understand the cause and origin of FSHD. DNA, short for deoxyribonucleic acid, is a long molecule found in the cells of our body. In association with some proteins, DNA makes up what we call our chromosomes. It holds the genetic instructions for our hereditary traits. Discrete segments of DNA, called genes, determine specific traits. Taken together, the combination of an estimated 100,000 genes makes each of us "an original."

A sudden structural change in DNA, a mutation, causes FSHD. The FSHD gene(s) is unknown, but its approximate location is toward the end of the DNA of the long arm of chromosome 4. The genetic location of this DNA region is 4q35. Nearly all cases of FSHD are associated with a deletion of DNA in this region. Researchers are investigating the molecular connection of this deletion and FSHD. It is not yet certain whether the deleted DNA contains an active gene or changes the regulation or activity of a nearby FSHD gene (a position effect).

Perhaps 2% of FSHD cases are not linked to chromosome 4. Their linkage to any other chromosome or genetic feature is under investigation.

How does a person inherit FSHD?

Most individuals with FSHD inherited that mutation from a parent with the disease. Inheritance is the means of transmission of DNA, and therefore inheritable traits, from parent to child. Chromosomes are the vehicles for those transmissions. Each chromosome contains a long, threadlike strand of DNA. Human cells usually contain 46 chromosomes. Forty-four of the chromosomes, also called autosomes, are homologous pairs and numbered from 1 though 22. The remaining chromosome pair consists of the nonhomologous chromosomes X and Y, the sex chromosomes. From each parent, children inherit one member of each pair of 46 chromosomes. A mother donates an X chromosome, and a father donates either an X or Y chromosome.

FSHD is the result of a DNA mutation on one member of the chromosome 4 pair. FSHD is highly penetrant. When a person inherits a chromosome 4 with the FSHD mutation, there is high probability that discernible muscle weaknesses will develop. Since weakness still occurs in the presence of the normal member of the chromosome 4 pair, the disease is considered dominant. FSHD is therefore an autosomal dominant inherited disease. Since each parent donates only one member of each chromosome pair to a child, the probability of passing the disease to an offspring is 50%.

What are sporadic cases of FSHD?

Sporadic FSHD cases are those resulting from a new mutation. Studies report 10% to as high as 33% of FSHD cases as sporadic. Approximately 20% of reported sporadic cases are those inherited from a seemingly unaffected parent who is a germline mosaic. Although the parent appears unaffected, the children are at risk. In the remaining sporadic cases, a new spontaneous mutation results in a chromosome 4 deletion that causes FSHD. When the 4q35 deletion fragment appears in a sporadic FSHD case, it is transmitted in an autosomal dominant manner to succeeding generations. The probability of passing the disease to an offspring is 50%.

How many people have FSHD?

It is difficult to calculate the exact incidence of FSHD. It may be under reported, but an accepted estimate of its occurrence in the general population is one in 20,000. FSHD occurs in all racial groups. It occurs with equal frequency in both sexes.

When do symptoms appear?

Although the FSHD gene is present at birth, weaknesses are generally noticeable during the second decade. A physician can usually recognize and diagnose FSHD beyond the age of 20. However, it is important to realize that the onset of FSHD is variable. Sometimes, muscle weaknesses are slight throughout adulthood. In perhaps 5% of cases of FSHD, a young child or an infant develops symptoms. In infantile FSHD (IFSHD) there are early facial weaknesses during the first two years of life, typical muscle weaknesses of FSHD, and in some of these children, early hearing losses and retinal abnormalities.

Early onset and infantile cases of FSHD often pose special problems arising from severity of the symptoms and schooling issues. The FSH Society provides helpful information that includes contact with a network of families with similar concerns.

What is the prognosis of FSHD?

Predicting the course and outcome of the disease, i.e., the prognosis, has its clinical certainties and uncertainties. There is certainty that some skeletal muscles will weaken and waste throughout life, and that this can and often does cause limitations on personal and occupational activities. FSHD appears not to diminish the intellect. The heart and internal (smooth) muscles seem spared and, with rare exceptions, those with FSHD have a normal life span.

There are uncertainties. The rapidity and extent of muscle loss differ considerably among FSHD patients, even among members of the same family. Some report few difficulties throughout life, while others may need a wheelchair as walking becomes too difficult or impossible. The degree of severity in an FSHD parent cannot accurately predict the extent of disability that may develop in that parent's child.

As a group, people with FSHD are well adjusted, educated, and motivated. They cope with a legion of adaptations. Muscle and motion are an important part of the full expression of much of life. Often, there are losses difficult to define in clinical terms. Interactions with family, friends, and associates may become limited. The accompanying losses often eclipse the clinical certainties and are an unspoken and significant part of the FSHD prognosis.

If a family member has FSHD, could I have the FSHD mutation?

Yes. If one has a blood parent, sibling, or other relative who has the FSHD mutation, there may be a risk of carrying that mutation. Professionals with knowledge of genetics and inheritance of FSHD can advise regarding that risk in individual circumstances. The FSH Society can provide answers and referrals about questions of risk.

Can a physician diagnose FSHD?

Yes. Even an adult at-risk, with no obvious symptoms, should avail themselves of a clinical diagnosis if they wish reassurance. Examinations by clinicians familiar with the disease are quite dependable when there are symptoms that follow an expected location and pattern of weakening muscles. By the age of 20, muscle weakness can be found approximately 95% of the time in affected individuals. Often the physician will supplement a physical examination with inquires about a possible family history of FSHD, measurement of specific enzyme levels in the blood, an electromyograph (EMG), and/or a muscle biopsy. An EMG records abnormal electrical activity of a functioning skeletal muscle. A biopsy consists of a small piece of muscle tissue, analyzed for visible abnormalities. A thorough examination will detect the disease in approximately 95% of affected individuals beyond the age of 20. However, the diagnosis may still be equivocal at younger ages and with some at-risk adults with mild or asymptomatic cases. This uncertainty can occur during years where there are important vocational, marital, and family planning choices at issue. This has created a real need in the FSHD population for a DNA test for the disease.

Is a DNA test for FSHD possible?

Yes. There is now a DNA test for FSHD in the clinical arsenal. It is highly reliable for many cases where diagnosis of FSHD is uncertain or impossible. The test detects the 4q35 DNA deletion described. Although several factors may occasionally complicate the test, confirmation of the 4q35 deletion is 98% reliable as a presumptive diagnosis of FSHD. The test requires no more than a small amount of blood that one's physician sends to a testing laboratory. The laboratory extracts sufficient DNA for the test from the cells present in the blood. The FSH Society can provide information regarding the test and laboratories that currently offer it. It does not, however, endorse any test or laboratory. An individual should consult their own physician and the laboratories about the DNA diagnostic test.

Currently, there is no DNA test available for those few cases where there is no linkage between FSHD and chromosome 4.

Is there a prenatal test for FSHD?

Yes. Using the same technology of the DNA test described, prenatal testing is possible. An individual who is interested in a prenatal test for FSHD should consult with their physician or contact the FSH Society. The Society can provide further information about this subject.

Are treatments and aids available for FSHD?

There is no treatment or cure for FSHD. There are, however, things that can alleviate its effects. Since muscles do their work through stimulation by nerves, neurologists are concerned with muscle and are often the primary physicians of muscle disease clinics. Physiatrists are physicians who work with chronic neuromuscular conditions. Periodic visits with a neurologist or physiatrist are useful to monitor the progress of FSHD and to obtain referrals to other professionals and services. An orthopedist, one concerned with the skeletal system and associated muscles, joints and ligaments, can advise about mobility issues and other functional problems of the muscular/skeletal system. Physical therapy, including light exercise, helps preserve flexibility. Swimming is especially helpful in this regard by making many movements easier. One should stay as active as possible, with rest breaks as needed during exercise and activities. Occupational therapy can help with suggestions for adaptations and physical aids that can often partially free an FSHD patient from some constrictions of the disease. Dietitians can help maintain a good diet and avoid unnecessary weight to reduce stress on already weakened muscles. In addition, speech and hearing therapists can help with limitations imposed by hearing loss and weakened facial musculature to improve speech and communication.

Sometimes a surgeon attaches the scapulae (shoulder blades) to the back to improve motion of the arms. An individual who is considering such surgery should consult with their neurologist or physiatrist and an orthopedic surgeon. Discussion of this procedure with individuals who have undergone the surgery is important. The FSH Society provides referrals to physicians and other professionals.

Pain is part of FSHD in many patients. No specific treatments are available. Pain medication and mild physiotherapy are often prescribed with moderate results.

Additional Information

Facioscapulohumeral Dystrophy (FSHD) Society
3 Westwood Rd.
Lexington, MA 02420
Phone: 781-860-0501
Fax: 781-860-0599
Website: http://www.fshsociety.org
E-mail: info@fshsociety.org

The FSH Society is a 501(c)(3) nonprofit, tax-exempt U.S. corporation. Established in 1991 by Daniel P. Perez, the Society solely addresses specific issues and needs regarding facioscapulohumeral muscular dystrophy (FSHD). It actively promotes research toward the prevention, cause, and treatment of FSHD. It also helps facilitate FSHD groups where individuals with like concerns have an opportunity to interact and receive helpful information concerning day-to-day life with FSHD. The Society publishes a newsletter with information about advances in research, political action effecting FSHD research, and profiles of people with FSHD living successful lives. The newsletter is one of several benefits of membership in the Society. The Society further offers assistance to physicians and other professionals interested in FSHD. Anyone with questions about FSHD should contact his or her physician(s), the FSH Society, or their local Muscular Dystrophy Association office.

Effects of Facioscapulohumeral Muscular Dystrophy

Which muscle groups are most affected in FSH?

The name facioscapulohumeral gives an indication of the distribution of muscle weakness, but not a complete one. "Facio" refers to the face, "scapulo" to the scapula or shoulder blade, "humeral" to the upper arm between shoulder and elbow.

The facial muscles are affected. The selective pattern of weakness often produces a recognizable facial appearance more noticeable when the muscles are in use, as in speaking or in producing facial expression. Weakness of eye closure may cause the affected person to sleep with the eyes slightly open. The face tends to become less than usually lined with age.

Muscles about the shoulder blades are affected. This leads to "winging of the scapulae," especially when the arms are held forward horizontally. "Winging" of the shoulder blades is a backward protrusion of their inner edges when the arms are held forward horizontally. The bulk of the muscles between the shoulder blades may be reduced.

The muscles which rotate the scapulae are affected. Looked at from behind, a normal person can be seen to raise the arms sideways to about horizontal with little or no change in the position of the scapulae, but to raise the arms above the head requires rotation of the scapulae. FSH dystrophy of more than very mild severity usually makes rotation of the scapulae, and therefore raising of the arms, difficult or impossible. The muscles around the humerus or upper arm bone are affected, causing weakness of bending (flexion) and straightening (extension) of the elbow. The forearm muscles are usually better developed than the upper arm muscles so that the strength of wrist and finger movements is relatively normal.

A feature of the weakness in FSH is that it is typically asymmetrical. Nearly always, in an affected person, some muscle groups are stronger on the left and others stronger on the right. The other muscular dystrophies tend to be symmetrical in their effects.

Are other muscles affected?

The name "facioscapulohumeral" gives an incomplete idea of the extent of weakness. In people who are more than slightly affected, there is nearly always some weakness of the back and the lower limbs. In some people, it is moderately severe and occasionally it is very severe.

How may the lower limbs be affected?

As with all muscular dystrophies, weakness is selective. Usually the calf muscles are strong and toe-walking is easy. Conversely the muscles in front of the lower leg are weak causing foot-drop, a tendency to trip and inability to walk on the heels with toes raised.

The big muscles which move the hips and knees may also be affected. Selective weakness may again be evident; some patients having very weak ability to extend (straighten) the hip joints, but very strong ability to straighten the knees.

114

How is the back affected?

The most noticeable effect is on posture. Not everyone with FSH has altered posture, but many do. The main effect is an exaggeration of the normal forward curvature of the spine above the pelvis. This exaggerated curve is called Lordosis. Occasionally it is very conspicuous and in that case the abdomen is excessively protuberant while the shoulders are held back excessively.

What difficulties are usually caused by FSH?

There is often difficulty raising the hands above shoulder level causing problems with combing the hair, reaching high shelves, or hanging out clothes to dry. Lifting heavy objects may be difficult, even below shoulder level. Some people first notice a problem in sport or recreation, as in swimming overarm or serving at tennis.

The effects on the lower limbs may cause foot-drop and a tendency to trip, an awkward gait with Lordosis, a tendency for one or both knees to give way, and difficulty with stairs and steps. Because weakness is asymmetrical, often the initial complaint is about trouble with one shoulder only, or one leg.

Are people with FSH all affected to about the same extent?

Severity varies greatly, even between affected members of one family. "Average severity" means becoming aware of disability in adolescence or early adulthood, being mildly to moderately handicapped through early and middle adult life, somewhat more severe in late middle age, retaining the ability to walk and having a normal lifespan.

At one end of the spectrum of severity, affected people are handicapped in infancy or early childhood and are unable to walk by adolescence or early adulthood. At the other end of the spectrum, an affected person might never experience any handicap at all and even an experienced physician would find it difficult to be sure that he or she was affected.

The heart is a muscle. Is the heart affected?

The heart is not affected in FSH dystrophy.

Are other tissues or organs affected?

Recent research has shown changes in the eyes of people with FSH dystrophy. Changes in the blood vessels at the back of the eye have been reported and researchers have questioned whether there might be similar changes in the blood vessels in the muscles. These changes seldom cause trouble with vision, nevertheless it has been suggested that people with FSH dystrophy should have periodic examination by an eye specialist.

In children who are affected by severe FSH dystrophy of early onset, deafness is frequent. Since this was first observed, deafness has been looked for in more mildly affected people, and it has been found that it is more frequent than in the general population.

Is FSH dystrophy always progressive?

In very mild cases, it may not be possible to detect progression of weakness. In the average case, progression is evident but slow, and severity sometimes seems to level off and to progress no more—to plateau. Compared with other muscular dystrophies, FSH dystrophy is described as relatively benign and relatively slowly progressive.

Scientists Identify a New Kind of Genetic Problem in Muscular Dystrophy

A newly identified genetic problem underlies a common neuromuscular disorder called facioscapulohumeral muscular dystrophy (FSHD), scientists say. In a new study, they show that deletion of repetitive DNA sequences in people with this disorder allows nearby genes to go into overdrive. The finding solves a decade-old riddle about the cause of this disorder and may ultimately lead to the first effective treatments.

The study found that abnormally short strings of repeated DNA sequences on chromosome 4 interfere with the function of a protein complex that controls nearby genes. This leads to over-activity of several genes that may play a role in the disorder. This type of genetic problem has never before been identified in a human disease. The study was funded in part by the National Institute of Neurological Disorders and Stroke (NINDS) and appeared in the August 9, 2002, issue of *Cell*.[1]

Scientists first linked the short strings of DNA in this region to FSHD in 1992. People with FSHD typically have fewer than 11 copies of this nucleic acid sequence, called D4Z4, due to a deletion of part of the chromosome. In contrast, people without the disorder usually carry between 11 and 150 copies of the sequence. People with a very small number of copies (three or fewer) have severe disease symptoms that begin in childhood, while those with several more copies typically have milder symptoms that begin in the teens or early adulthood. However, until now, researchers have been unable to determine exactly how the number of DNA sequences influences the disease.

FSHD is the third most common inherited neuromuscular disorder, affecting one in every 20,000 people (only Duchenne muscular dystrophy and myotonic dystrophy are more common). People with FSHD have progressive muscle degeneration that primarily affects the face, shoulder blades, and upper arms, although other muscles also deteriorate. Despite intensive efforts, researchers have been unable to identify any genes that are altered in this disorder.

In the new study, Rossella Tupler, M.D., Ph.D., of the University of Massachusetts Medical School in Worcester and the Universita' degli Studi di Pavia in Pavia, Italy, and colleagues studied human muscle tissue from healthy individuals and from people with FSHD as well as several other types of muscular dystrophy. They analyzed the expression of three genes located near the D4Z4 region and found that activity of all three genes was elevated in the muscle from FSHD patients compared to that of other people.

The researchers also analyzed the interaction between the D4Z4 sequence and proteins present in the nucleus of the cell. They found that one part of the sequence binds to a protein complex that normally suppresses gene activity. Having fewer than 11 copies of D4Z4 reduced the number of functional protein complexes, which in turn reduced control of genes from nearby parts of the chromosome.

"This breakthrough is important scientifically, as it teaches us about novel ways genes can influence disease, which will someday help not only those people who suffer from FSHD, but hopefully, others as well," says Katrina Gwinn-Hardy, M.D., a program director at NINDS.

The researchers do not know which of the overactive chromosome 4 genes is responsible for the symptoms of FSHD. One of the genes they considered, called ANT1, triggers cell death when it is too active. Therefore, it may be responsible for the progressive loss of muscle cells in this disorder. However, FSHD is a complex disease, and other genes or environmental factors also may play a role.

"These findings have specific implications for the disease, and general implications for genetic research," says Dr. Tupler. Knowing how the D4Z4 deletions affect nearby genes points to new strategies for treating the disorder. For example, researchers might be able to find a way to mimic the effect of the protein complex that goes awry in this disorder, thereby reducing the activity of all the affected genes. If a specific gene that causes the disorder can be identified, researchers also might be able to slow or halt that gene's activity with drugs or other treatments.

While most people with FSHD have D4Z4 deletions, about 5 to 10 percent do not. These people may have mutations that affect the protein complex, Dr. Tupler says. Researchers have also identified people without FSHD who are missing the entire D4Z4 region and several nearby genes. This suggests that an abnormal D4Z4 region somehow creates havoc in muscle cells and/or that the nearby genes are necessary for development of the disease.

The findings also suggest that repetitive DNA sequences play a previously unsuspected role in human disease by influencing gene activity, Dr. Tupler says. About 40 percent of the human genome is comprised of these repetitive sequences, and they might play a role in several other human disorders. For example, certain variations in repetitive DNA sequences near the insulin gene in Type 1 diabetes have been linked to insulin levels and birth size. Other DNA repeats have been associated with bladder cancer. Studies of sequences like these could lead to a much better understanding of how gene activity is regulated, Dr. Tupler suggests.

Scientists can now focus on identifying which genes on chromosome 4 contribute to FSHD and how to regulate the gene activity, says Dr. Tupler. "Hopefully, other researchers will help with that," she adds.

Reference

1. Gabellini D, Green MR, Tupler R. "Inappropriate gene activation in FSHD: A repressor complex binds a chromosomal repeat deleted in dystrophic muscle." *Cell,* Vol. 110, No. 3, August 9, 2002, pp. 339-348.

Additional Information

National Registry of Myotonic Dystrophy and FSHD Patients and Family Members
University of Rochester
Box 673
601 Elmwood Ave.
Rochester, NY 14642
Toll-Free: 888-925-4302
Phone: 585-506-0004
Fax: 585-273-1255
Website: http://www.dystrophyregistry.org
E-mail: dystrophy_registry@urmc.rochester.edu

Molecular Genetics Testing Laboratory
NYU School of Medicine
550 First Ave. Rm. MSB136
New York, NY 10016
Phone: 212-263-7621
Fax: 212-562-2642
Website: http://www.med.nyu.edu/genetics/lab/index.html

Provides mutation analysis genetic test for FSHD.

Prenatal, Presymptomatic, and Diagnostic Testing for FSHD Chromosome 4-Linked Families

Children's Hospital of Eastern Ontario
Molecular Genetics Diagnostic Laboratory
401 Smyth Road
Ottawa, Ontario
Canada K1H8L1
Phone: 613-737-7600
Fax: 613-738-4822
Website: http://www.cheo.on.ca
E-mail: webmaster@cheo.on.ca

Alberta Children's Hospital
Molecular Diagnostic Laboratory
Calgary, Alberta
Canada T2T 5C7
Phone: 403-943-7026
Fax: 403-943-7624

Chapter 11

Limb-Girdle
Muscular Dystrophy

Limb-girdle muscular dystrophy (LGMD) is a diverse group of disorders affecting the voluntary muscles, mainly around the pelvic (hip) and shoulder regions. Occasionally, the cardiac (heart) and respiratory (breathing) muscles may be involved. Different types of LGMD vary in severity, age of onset (when symptoms are first noticed), and how they are inherited. The variation seen in the LGMDs is caused by the differences in the type of gene alteration. Our genetic blueprint is made up of thousands of different genes that contain the information needed to produce specific proteins. Genes can be become altered by changes (mutations) that occur in the sequence of chemical structures known as basic pairs (represented by the four letters A,T,C, and G) that make up the gene in question. Mutations in different genes can cause different forms of LGMD, as can different changes within the same gene. These differences can lead to more severe or milder forms of LGMD. Presently, scientists have identified 14 different genes that can be altered to cause LGMD and are working on locating others.

What are the symptoms of Limb-Girdle muscular dystrophy?

The onset of LGMD may involve the pelvis, the shoulder area, or both. Early symptoms can include difficulty walking, running, and

121

rising from the floor. Usually, and eventually, affected individuals will find it hard to climb stairs, stand up from a squatting position, and walk. Weak shoulder muscles can make it difficult to raise arms above the head, hold the arms outstretched, or carry heavy objects. The brain, the intellect, and the senses are not impaired. Rarely, certain forms of LGMD can involve the heart muscle, causing symptoms of heart failure or rhythm disturbance. Uncommon forms of LGMD can also affect breathing, which can result in sleepiness, headaches, and lack of energy. As heart and breathing symptoms may be difficult to recognize, the heart and respiratory system of affected individuals should be monitored to detect changes.

How does Limb-Girdle muscular dystrophy progress?

Limb-girdle muscular dystrophy is progressive, which means that the affected person's muscles continue to get weaker throughout their lifetime. There is a wide range of severity for all limb-girdle disorders, so the rate of progression is extremely variable. Generally, over time, a person with LGMD loses muscle bulk and strength. The muscles involved may show different levels of weakness between right and left sides (i.e. the left shoulder may be weaker than the right). Weakness can also extend to the neighboring muscles. When the rate of progression is slow and unnoticeable, the disorder may seem to suddenly get worse when a loss of function occurs. For example, a person may not notice the rate of progression until they find it impossible to rise from a chair, or raise an arm to brush his or her hair. When the muscle strength falls below the minimum level needed to accomplish a task, it makes the disease appear to progress rapidly. This is called the "stair step" phenomenon in which progression seems to stop for a while, then suddenly worsen.

When the onset of LGMD begins in childhood, the increases in body weight and size from natural growth, combined with the increase in muscle weakness caused by the disease, can make the progression seem very rapid. As an adult, body growth stops. Therefore, weakness only increases as the body's muscles break down. LGMD is so variable that it is not yet possible to predict the course of the disease in most people.

How do you get LGMD?

LGMD is inherited when a faulty gene is passed on from one or both parents to a child. There are two ways a person can inherit the disorder: autosomal dominant and autosomal recessive. The term autosomal refers to the fact that genetic error can occur on any one of the 46 chromosomes in each cell of the human body, except for the two sex chromosomes. There are always two copies of a gene—one from the person's mother and one from the father. When a single copy of a gene mutation causes LGMD, it is referred to as dominant. A recessive form of LGMD occurs when it is necessary for both parents to pass on an altered gene, and thus no normal gene copy is present.

Dominant forms of LGMD can arise by a new mutation in the affected individual, or it can be inherited from an affected parent. Inherited autosomal dominant traits need only one affected parent to transmit the gene mutation. There is a 50% chance that a child of either sex, born to an affected parent, will inherit the disorder.

Inherited autosomal recessive traits, on the other hand, involve children who receive the altered gene from both parents. In most cases, each parent is a carrier. This means they have one copy of the altered gene, but are not affected and do not show any symptoms because the other copy of the gene in question is normal. Each child of either sex born to parents who are both carriers has a 25% chance of having the disorder, a 50% chance of being a carrier, and a 25% chance of having two normal gene copies.

In a recessive disorder, if one parent is affected and shows the symptoms, it means that both of his or her gene copies are altered. Therefore, an affected parent has a 100% chance of passing on the gene. However, except in very rare cases, the other parent has two normal copies of the gene. Therefore, the children of these parents will be carriers (through the gene passed from the affected parent), but not affected.

How is LGMD diagnosed?

Better tests to diagnose LGMD are now being developed. Because the physical symptoms are similar to other neuromuscular disorders such as Becker MD, a diagnosis for LGMD is often reached after eliminating other possible causes for the weakness around the hips and shoulders. Before any laboratory tests, a medical history of the person's family and a physical exam are taken to determine the pattern of weakness in the individual. Early in the diagnostic process, a special blood test called a CK Test is performed. CK stands for creatine kinase, an enzyme that leaks out of damaged muscles. If a blood sample shows high levels of CK, it suggests that the muscles themselves are the likely cause of the weakness. This test cannot identify the specific type of disorder affecting the muscle.

To obtain more information, laboratory exams may be conducted to find evidence of general changes in muscle weakness and other muscle changes. Sometimes a special test called electromyography is done to discover the location of the weakness. This test measures the electrical activity of muscle cells. A muscle biopsy may be performed by surgically removing a sample of the affected muscle for examination, to find the underlying cause of the weakness. DNA testing may be done to determine specific types of LGMD, and muscle stains may be used in some cases, to look for the precise protein that is missing.

These techniques have not yet been perfected to provide 100% accurate information about the exact type of LGMD, but progress is being made in diagnosing problems in the muscle cells.

How disabling is LGMD?

LGMD is not normally a fatal disease. The greatest danger comes from weakening heart muscles or respiratory muscles. Monitoring for heart or breathing complications is recommended for the later stages of the disorder, but these cases are rare. Affected individuals may require a wheelchair after several years, but some remain mobile throughout their lives.

What is the age of onset?

Because there is so much variability in the disorder, the onset of a specific LGMD is difficult to determine. Often people with LGMD first notice problems when they begin to walk with a waddling gait because of weakness in hip and leg muscles.

Research

Researchers in the US, Canada, and throughout the world are focusing on finding ways to defeat limb-girdle muscular dystrophy. Currently, gene therapy is one technique being tested, as a potential treatment for LGMD. In this research, the genes of a virus are removed, and replaced by healthy human genes. They are then injected into the affected person's body. The outer shell of the virus is used as a vehicle or carrier to deliver the healthy genetic material to cells. The virus itself is disarmed, so that it is no longer infectious. Most of the virus's genes are replaced with human DNA, ensuring that the virus is unable to divide and cause harm. There are many other areas of research in both mainstream and alternative medicine, and researchers are vigorously pursuing every potential direction.

Symptom Management

Maintaining good health is beneficial to everyone. For individuals affected by LGMD, it is a good way to preserve strength. A well-balanced diet and moderate exercise can help reduce or control weight. Intense workout is impractical and sometimes dangerous, but activities like swimming, water aerobics, and low resistance exercise may facilitate greater mobility. Physical and occupational therapy, as well as assistive devices, may also help to maintain mobility and flexibility. Affected individuals should keep walking as long as they can. This may mean using a wheelchair or scooter for long distances, thus preserving strength for short walks.

In some cases, joint deformities may be prevented through exercises, physiotherapy, orthoses, and surgery. To avoid spinal instability, proper seating and back support should be maintained.

These techniques can alleviate stress from weak muscles and from joints, but they cannot reverse the symptoms of LGMD or strengthen already weakened muscles.

Known Types of LGMD

Note: Chromosomes have two arms, a short *p* and a long *q*, in which genes are located.

LGMD1–Dominant

1A:

- Onset: young adults
- Progression: slow, late loss of ambulation
- Gene location: Chromosome 5q31
- Gene product: Myotolin

1B:

- Onset: 4 to 38 years
- Progression: slow
- Gene location: Chromosome 1q11-q21
- Gene product: LaminA/C

1C:

- Onset: usually childhood
- Progression: variable
- Gene location: Chromosome 3p25
- Gene product: Caveolin

1D:
- Onset: early adulthood
- Progression: slow
- Gene location: Chromosome 7q
- Gene product: unknown

1E:
- Onset: early adulthood
- Progression: slow
- Gene location: Chromosome 6q
- Gene product: unknown

LGMD2–Recessive

2A:
- Onset: 3 to 30 years
- Progression: the earlier the onset the more rapid the progression
- Loss of walking in 20 years
- Gene location: Chromosome 15q15-21
- Gene product: Calpain 3

2B:
- Onset: late teens
- Progression: generally slow, some more rapid
- Gene location: Chromosome 2p13
- Gene product: Dysferlin—same gene responsible for the distal Miyoshi myopathy

2C:
- Also known as: severe childhood autosomal recessive muscular dystrophy
- Onset: variable, generally during first decade
- Progression: very variable, even within families
- Gene location: Chromosome 13q12-13
- Gene product: gamma-sarcoglycan

2D:
- Onset: most variable, generally during first decade
- Progression: very variable
- Gene location: Chromosome 17q12-21
- Gene product: alpha-sarcoglycan, formerly called adhalin

2E:
- Onset: variable, generally during first decade
- Progressions: very variable, often in wheelchair by 10–15 years
- Gene location: Chromosome 4q12
- Gene product: beta-sarcoglycan

2F:
- Onset: variable, generally during first decade
- Progression: variable
- Gene location: Chromosome 5q33-34
- Gene product: delta-sarcoglycan

2G:
- Onset: childhood
- Progression: moderate
- Gene location: Chromosome 17q11-12
- Gene product: telethonin

2H:
- Onset: 8 to 27 years so far reported
- Progression: slow
- Chromosome 9p31-33
- Gene product: unknown

2I:
- Onset: not known
- Progression: not confirmed
- Gene Location: Chromosome 19q13
- Gene Product: not known

Genetics and Limb-Girdle Muscular Dystrophy (LGMD)

The limb-girdle muscular dystrophies are known to be genetically heterogeneous, with both dominant and recessive forms reported.

Autosomal Dominant Limb-Girdle Muscular Dystrophies

The dominant LGMDs usually show adult onset. In addition to muscle weakness, the creatine kinase (CK) values are elevated in affected individuals usually 4–10 times the normal laboratory values. Currently, neither presymptomatic nor prenatal testing is available for any form of dominantly inherited limb-girdle muscular dystrophy.

LGMD1A: A single large family has been localized to a region approximately 7 cm in size at 5q22.3-313. More than 50% of affected family members have a nasal quality to their speech and this particular speech pattern has not been seen in any other autosomal dominant families studied to date. The average age of onset is 27 years. All other families investigated for linkage to date have been shown to be unlinked to this area of 5q. Subsequently, the gene which codes for the protein myotilin was found to be located on chromosome 5q in the same region as LGMD 1A. Recently, the Center for Human Genetics at the Duke University Medical Center reported the identification of the mutation in the myotilin gene, causing a change in the amino acid sequence, which is responsible for the production of the abnormal form of the protein. This finding allows the next phase of research to begin, which is to understand why abnormalities in myotilin lead to LGMD.

LGMD 1B: The gene for LGMD 1B has been linked to chromosome 1q11-q21. This form of LGMD was linked in several families in 1997. The clinical characteristics of this form of LGMD are the age of onset is less than 20 with slow progression, beginning in the lower extremities, and progressing to involve the upper extremities by age 20–30. Individuals with this form of LGMD do not develop significant contractures. The feature which separates LGMD 1B from the other forms is the association of cardiac involvement in a high percentage of individuals in the families studied. The cardiac abnormalities reported have been atrioventricular (AV) conduction disturbances and abnormal cardiac rhythms with individuals developing symptoms of abnormally slow heart rates, fainting, and sometimes death. Presymptomatic treatment has necessitated the placement of a cardiac pacemaker in some individuals. The mutation for LGMD 1B has been identified in the Lamin A/C gene on chromosome 1q. Two other syndromes which also have mutations in this gene are familial partial lipodystrophy (Köbberling-Dunnigan syndrome) and Emery-Dreifuss muscular dystrophy, type 2.

LGMD 1C: The gene for this form of LGMD has been localized to chromosome 3p25 and is known as the Caveolin-3 gene. This is a childhood onset disorder (mean 5 years) which results in moderate weakness of the hip and shoulder girdle muscles. Often there is enlargement (hypertrophy) of the calf muscles which may cause confusion with another myopathy which commonly causes calf hypertrophy, Duchenne muscular dystrophy. A common feature is the development of muscle cramps after exercise. The creatine kinase (CK) level in individuals with this disorder may be elevated from 4–25 times normal, a much higher CK range than in any of the other dominantly inherited LGMD forms.

LGMD 1D: In 1999 the Center for Human Genetics lab reported the identification of a new locus for autosomal dominant LGMD which maps to 7q in two families. The clinical characteristics in these families are similar to other dominantly inherited LGMD forms, namely, the hip girdle muscles more involved than shoulder girdle, slow progression, but no associated findings such as unusual speech patterns, contractures, or cardiac effects. About 20% of patients have swallowing difficulties. The mean age of onset is 38 in these 2 families. Currently, the lab is trying to narrow the region of disease gene location.

Familial Dilated Cardiomyopathy with Conduction Defect and Muscular Dystrophy: Only 1 family of French Canadian ethnicity has been described with these clinical features and linkage to chromosome 6q23. The age of onset is teens and later. A few individuals have been reported to have calf hypertrophy. The progression is quite slow with no one yet reported to become wheelchair dependent. The cardiac manifestations which begin in the early to mid-twenties are the development of abnormal heart rhythms. From the twenties to the forties family members have been reported to develop congestive heart failure including the enlargement of all four chambers of the heart. Sudden death has occurred in some individuals who had no previous history of cardiac symptoms.

Other LGMD 1 forms: There are now 5 genes which can lead to autosomal dominant LGMD, but there are still a large number of other families with autosomal dominant transmission which do not link to any of the previously mentioned loci. Given the number of unlinked families, one must assume there are chromosomal loci that are yet to be determined This once again underscores the significant heterogeneity within the LGMD1 diagnostic classification.

Autosomal Recessive Limb-Girdle Muscular Dystrophies

The recessive LGMDs are more frequent than the dominant forms, and usually have childhood or teen-age onset. Currently, genes for nine different forms of recessive LGMD have been localized and/or identified. Additional loci have yet to be identified as there are families which are unlinked to any of the known loci. Genes responsible for LGMD2B, LGMD2C, LGMD2D, LGMD2E, and LGMD 2F have been shown to be a part of the sarcoglycan complex, intimately related to the dystroglycan complex and important for muscle integrity. You will note that the clinical descriptions of many of the recessive LGMD families are very similar. What distinguishes one form from the other, besides the genetic location, are the ethnic differences, the involvement of other body systems, and the rates of progression.

LGMD2A: Individuals with this form have been shown to have a defect in the calpain-3 gene on chromosome 15q. To date, at least 100 different mutations have been identified including single base pair deletions, small insertions and deletions, and a large genomic deletion. The gene for LGMD2A was originally identified in families of French descent on LaRéunion Island and subsequently in the northern Indiana Amish families, Basque country, Spain, and in Russia. The age of onset is between 2 and 40 years, with the mean being 14 years. The weakness pattern involves the hip girdle and abdominal muscles more than upper extremities with loss of ambulation occurring at a mean age of 17. There is no cardiac involvement but some individuals with mild mental retardation. CK elevations range from 7–80 times normal.

LGMD2B: The second recessive LGMD locus to be identified was on 2p12-14. The gene for this form of LGMD produces the protein dysferlin which is found primarily in skeletal muscle, but also the heart. Mutations including missense, deletions, and insertions have been identified. Attempts at correlating the type of mutation with the clinical presentation have not been successful. Interestingly, a different form of muscular dystrophy called Miyoshi myopathy, which affects distal muscles (lower leg and forearm) instead of proximal (upper arm, hip girdle, shoulder) muscles, has also been shown to be localized to this area. It is anticipated that different changes in the identical gene may lead to these different forms of muscular dystrophy. The onset age for LGMD 2B is 12 to 39 years, beginning with leg weakness. It is more slowly progressive than 2A as individuals do not become wheelchair dependent until at least their mid-30s. CKs are very high, like 2A, 10–72 times normal.

LGMD2C: Patients affected with this form of recessive LGMD are usually more severely affected than patients with the other types of LGMD with onset in childhood. Formerly called Duchenne-like muscular dystrophy or severe childhood autosomal recessive muscular dystrophy (SCARMD), the gene responsible for this disorder was localized to chromosome 13 and the gene later identified as a defect in sarcoglycan. Only a small proportion of American recessive LGMD families are felt to be LGMD2C, although this type of muscular dystrophy is more common in different parts of the world such as northern Africa. The mean age of onset is 5 years with loss of ambulation from 10–13 years. Both calf and tongue hypertrophy have been reported. Respiratory failure occurs in the 20s and cardiac involvement in the late stages of the disease.

LGMD2D: The gene responsible for LGMD2D, also called primary adhalinopathy, has been localized to 17q21 and found to be a defect in a-sarcoglycan. The age of onset is 2 to 15 years. This form of the disorder has been associated with a variable severity: earlier onset with rapidly progressive weakness, and the later onset with ambulation preserved throughout life. The original description of this disorder was in Algerian families, with subsequent identification in Brazilian families. The thigh muscles (quadriceps) are severely affected as are the muscles of the shoulder blades, especially in the early onset form. Only rare reports of cardiac involvement. CK is often >5000.

LGMD2E: Defects in the ß-sarcoglycan gene on chromosome 4q12 are responsible for LGMD2E. This mutation was originally described in the southern Indiana Amish families, where all families segregating for this mutation have been found to be homozygous for the same mutation. Other populations now known to have this mutation are in northern Indiana Amish and Bern, Switzerland. The age of onset is < 3 years to teens. Calf hypertrophy and winging of the shoulder blades is common. Wheelchair dependency occurs by age 25, but may occur as early as age 10–15. CK is >5000.

LGMD 2F: This gene, d-sarcoglycan, is located on chromosome 5q33-34, interestingly very close to the gene for LGMD 1A. It was identified in families with African-Brazilian ancestry. The mutations identified are frameshift, missense, and nonsense. The clinical course is quite severe with onset at 2–10 years and death at 9–19 years. Almost all patients are wheelchair bound by age 16. Calf hypertrophy and muscle cramps are frequent. Only rare cardiac abnormalities have been reported with no affect on intelligence. The CK range is 10–50 times normal.

LGMD 2G: This gene, known as Telethonin, like LGMD 2F was identified in Brazilian families. It is located on chromosome 17q11-12. Point mutations and small deletions in the gene have been reported as the cause of the disorder. The mean age of onset is 12 years with a range of 9–15 years. This disorder not only affects hip and shoulder girdle, but causes foot drop as well. About 2 in 5 individuals will not be ambulatory by their 20–30s. More than half have cardiac involvement. CK range is 3–30 times normal.

LGMD 2H: This recessively inherited LGMD is also known as the Manitoba (Canada) Hutterite Dystrophy and is located on chromosome 9q31-33. The Hutterites are a religious group which originated in 1530, reside in primarily rural areas in North America, and generally do not marry outside their religion. The age of onset is 8 to 27. In addition to weakness of the hip and shoulder girdles and back pain, weakness of the facial muscles is also a feature. This is unusual among the LGMD types since facial weakness is found is a number of the non-LGMDs; e.g., facioscapulohumeral dystrophy and myotonic dystrophy. Progression is slow as many affected individuals are still ambulatory in their 50s. The CK range is 250–4500.

LGMD 2I: This form of LGMD has been identified in a Tunisian family and is located on chromosome 19q13.3. The age of onset is from 2–27 years. Again, lower extremities are affected before and more severely than upper extremities. More than three-quarters of the affected individuals have calf hypertrophy. No cardiac or intellectual involvement has been reported. The progression is slow with only one quarter of the individuals being wheelchair dependent in their 50s. CKs range up to 5700.

Chapter 12

Myotonic Muscular Dystrophy

Myotonic muscular dystrophy (MMD) is a form of muscular dystrophy that affects muscles and many other organs in the body. Unlike some forms of muscular dystrophy, MMD often does not become a problem until adulthood and usually allows people to walk and be pretty independent throughout their lives. However, the infant form of MMD is more severe. Unfortunately, it can occur in babies born to parents who have the adult form, even if they have very mild cases.

The word myotonic is the adjective for the word myotonia, an inability to relax muscles at will. In MMD, the myotonia is usually mild. In fact, many people attribute it to stiffness or think they have arthritis. If anything is noticeable, it is usually difficulty with one's grip, for example when using a tool or writing instrument.

Reprinted from "Facts about Myotonic Muscular Dystrophy," with permission from the Muscular Dystrophy Association, www.mdausa.org. © 2000 The Muscular Dystrophy Association. For additional information, call the Muscular Dystrophy Association National Headquarters toll-free at (800) 572-1717. To find an MDA office in your area, look in your local telephone book, or click on "Clinics and Services" on the MDA website. And, reprinted with permission from, "Excessive Daytime Sleeping and Myotonic Dystrophy" by Mrs. M. A. Bowler, S.R.N., S.C.M., National Coordinator, Myotonic Dystrophy Support Group, Nottingham, England, May 2001. © Myotonic Dystrophy Support Group. All rights reserved. For additional information, visit www.mdsguk.org. Also, "Faulty Gene is Key to Understanding Myotonic Dystrophy," by Katie Lai, *Spotlight on Research*, November 2002, National Institute of Arthritis and Musculoskeletal and Skin Diseases (NIAMS).

Myotonia is not a feature of any other form of muscular dystrophy (although it occurs in other kinds of muscle diseases, where it can be severe). When a person suspected of having muscular dystrophy has myotonia, the diagnosis is likely to be MMD.

The term muscular dystrophy means slowly progressive muscle degeneration, with increasing weakness and wasting (loss of bulk) of muscles. The weakness and wasting of muscles generally presents much more of a problem to people with MMD than does the myotonia. However, they usually are not as severe as in some other types of muscular dystrophy.

MMD symptoms sometimes begin at birth. Infants with this disorder, congenital MMD, have severe muscle weakness, including weakening of muscles that control breathing and swallowing. These problems can be life-threatening and need intensive care. Myotonia is not part of the picture in infants with MMD.

MMD symptoms can also begin in children past infancy but not yet adolescents, although this is unusual. Generally, the earlier MMD begins, the more severe the disease is. Myotonic muscular dystrophy is often known simply as myotonic dystrophy and is occasionally called Steinert's disease, after a doctor who originally described the disorder in 1909. It is also called *dystrophia myotonica*, a Latin name, and therefore often abbreviated DM. MMD varies greatly in severity, even within the same family. Not everyone has all the symptoms and not everyone has them to the same degree. There is, however, a distinct difference between the type that affects newborn infants—congenital MMD—and the type that begins in adolescence or adulthood—adult-onset MMD.

What causes myotonic muscular dystrophy?

Myotonic muscular dystrophy is caused when a portion of a particular gene is larger than it should be.

What Happens in Adult-Onset MMD?

It is reassuring to know that when MMD begins in the teen years or during adulthood, it is often only a moderately disabling condition with very slow progression. As one doctor put it, "Some people with MMD go through much of their lives without troubling or being troubled by the medical profession."

There can be troubling symptoms, however, for many people. Although many different parts of the body can be affected by MMD, most

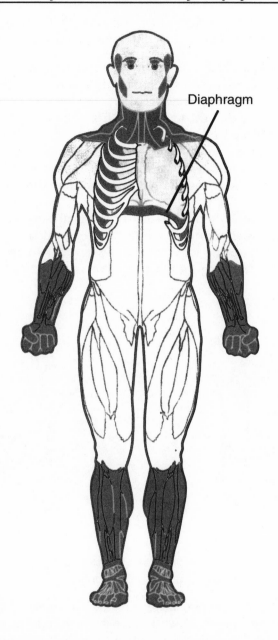

Diaphragm

Figure 12.1. *Weakness and wasting of voluntary muscles in the face, neck, and lower arms and legs are common in myotonic muscular dystrophy. Muscles between the ribs and those of the diaphragm, which moves up and down to allow inhalation and exhalation of air, can also be weakened.*

people with the disease have only some of the following symptoms. Most of the problems can be lessened with medical treatment.

Limb muscles. Weakness of the voluntary muscles, such as those that control the arms and legs, is usually the most noticeable symptom for people with adult-onset MMD.

The distal muscles—those farthest from the center of the body— are usually the first, and sometimes the only, limb muscles affected. The forearms, hands, lower legs, and feet are the parts of the body that have these distal muscles. Over time, these muscles get smaller, so the lower legs and arms may appear thinner than the upper legs and arms.

People with MMD often notice that their grip is weak and that they have trouble using their wrist or hand muscles. At the same time, the muscles that pick up the foot when walking weaken, so the foot flops down, leading to tripping and falling. This is called foot drop.

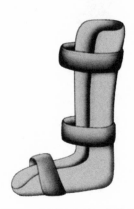

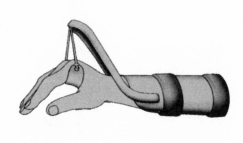

Figure 12.2. Ankle-Foot Orthosis (AFO)

Figure 12.3. Wrist Support

Some people can compensate for weak foot muscles by picking up the foot from the knee and walking with a marching step. Eventually, though, many people with MMD find that a cane or walker is helpful to compensate for foot and leg weakness.

A lower leg brace, called an ankle-foot orthosis or AFO, may be needed. A few people with MMD use a wheelchair or a power scooter for convenience when covering long distances.

Various devices that hold the hand in a good position for using a keyboard or writing or drawing can help compensate for weak wrist and hand muscles.

Head, neck, and face muscles. The muscles of the neck, jaw, and parts of the head and face may weaken in MMD. Weakness and loss of bulk in these muscles leads to a characteristic appearance doctors and experienced family members recognize as MMD. In men, early balding in the front part of the scalp is very common, adding to the distinct appearance of MMD. Eyelids may droop (called ptosis, but the *p* is silent), the temples appear hollow, and the face looks long and thin.

Severe ptosis can be troubling. It may be hard to hold the eyes open for reading, watching television, or driving. Special glasses with eyelid crutches can hold the eyes open. You cannot buy these off the shelf, but a skilled optician can make them for you. Surgery can be done, but weakness often comes back, making it necessary to repeat the operation. Weak neck muscles can make it hard to sit up quickly or lift one's head straight up off a bed or couch. The stronger trunk muscles have to be used for these actions.

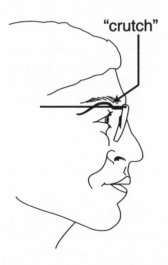

"crutch"

Figure 12.4. Special glasses with crutches to hold skin away from the eyes can help when muscles in this area are weak.

Breathing and swallowing muscles. Respiratory muscles can become weak in MMD, affecting lung function and depriving the body of needed oxygen. This is probably at least part of the reason many people with MMD feel sleepy much of the time.

The respiratory problems are further aggravated, many experts believe, by an abnormality in the brain's breathing control center. This abnormality can also lead to a condition known as sleep apnea, in which people stop breathing for several seconds or even a minute many times a night while they are sleeping.

A good way to treat respiratory muscle weakness is with a small, portable ventilator that pumps air into the lungs during the night. It is usually used with a face mask that can easily be taken on and off. (This kind of breathing assistance can also be used during the day, but that is usually not convenient or necessary.)

Devices and techniques to assist with coughing up secretions can be used, too, especially when the person with MMD has a cold or chest infection. An MDA clinic doctor, respiratory therapist, or a specialist called a pulmonologist can help advise you about these devices and how to use them.

Swallowing muscles, if weakened, can lead to choking, or "swallowing the wrong way," with food or liquid going down the trachea (windpipe) instead of the esophagus (tube from the throat to the stomach). Swallowing is partly voluntary and partly involuntary, and both sets of muscles can be affected.

Vomiting can be very dangerous for a person with MMD whose swallowing muscles are weak. A head-down position is crucial to prevent inhaling the vomit—a possibly fatal problem.

A swallowing specialist can help people learn to swallow more safely, and if needed, how to change the consistencies of foods and liquids so they can be swallowed more easily. It is important to watch for swallowing problems, such as a tendency to choke on food or drinks, and mention them to the doctor.

If swallowing difficulties are extreme (more common in congenital MMD than in adults with MMD), a feeding tube can be inserted into the stomach. It can later be removed if the problem resolves itself.

Myotonia. The myotonia of voluntary muscles can make it hard for someone with MMD to relax their grip, especially in cold temperatures. Door handles, cups, and tools may pose a problem, although many people never notice it.

Myotonia can affect other muscles, but usually it is not noticeable. After sneezing, it can be hard to relax the muscles around the eyes. This can pose a driving hazard. If myotonia becomes troublesome, drugs can be used to treat it.

Heart problems. The heart can be affected in adult MMD. Oddly, since MMD is mostly a muscle disease, it is not the muscle part of the heart (which pumps blood) that is most affected, but rather the part that sets the rate and rhythm of the heartbeat—the heart's conduction system. It is common in MMD, especially after many years, to develop a conduction block, a block in the electricity-like signal that keeps the heart beating at a safe rate.

Fainting, near fainting, or dizzy spells are the usual symptoms of conduction block, and these should never be ignored! Such problems can be fatal. In the early stages, a partial conduction block may cause no symptoms, but can be detected by an electrocardiogram (EKG), a painless test of how the heart is beating. The doctor will likely order regular EKGs. Conduction blocks can usually be corrected by a cardiac pacemaker, an electronic device that is surgically inserted near the heart to regulate the heartbeat. Not everyone with MMD needs treatment for heart problems, but everyone should be checked for them.

Internal organs. Most of the internal organs in the body are hollow tubes (such as the intestines) or sacs (such as the stomach). The walls of these tubes and sacs contain involuntary muscles that squeeze the organs and move things (food, liquids, a baby during childbirth, and so forth) through them. In MMD, many of the involuntary muscles that surround the hollow organs can weaken and can also have myotonia. These include the muscles of the digestive tract, the uterus, and the blood vessels.

Abnormal action of the upper digestive tract can impair swallowing. Once food is swallowed, the involuntary muscles of the esophagus take over. These can have spasms and weakness, causing a feeling of food getting stuck and sometimes leading to inhaling food into the lungs. Care in swallowing, sometimes with the advice of a specialist, may be needed.

The lower digestive tract—large intestine (colon), rectum, and anus—can also be affected by weakness and spasm in MMD. Crampy pain, constipation, and diarrhea can occur. Your doctor can advise you about setting up a bowel routine and using diet and other treatments to help manage this kind of problem.

The gallbladder—a sac under the liver that squeezes bile into the intestines after meals—can weaken in MMD. People with MMD are probably more likely than the general population to develop gallstones. Symptoms are difficulty digesting fatty foods and pain in the upper right part of the abdomen. Surgery can be done if necessary. Drugs such as metoclopramide (Reglan) help move things along the

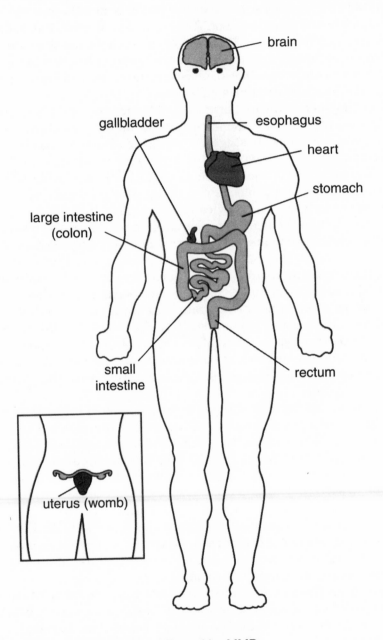

Figure 12.5. *Internal Organs Affected by MMD*

digestive tract and are sometimes used to treat problems in this area in MMD. Fortunately, most people do not have problems in urinating or holding urine in MMD.

Because of weakness and uncoordinated action of the muscle wall of the uterus, women with MMD often have complications in childbirth that can be serious for both mother and baby. These may involve excessive bleeding or ineffective labor. Sometimes a Caesarean section is advised, but surgery can also be a problem in MMD. A pregnant woman with MMD has to be certain that all her doctors, including any who will manage the delivery, are well informed about her neuromuscular condition. Disasters can result if this step is missing.

Blood pressure in MMD tends to be low. This is probably due to low tone of the smooth muscles in the blood vessels. It usually poses no problem and may even be one beneficial effect in MMD.

The brain. Some people with MMD have been labeled slow, dull, uncaring, unenthusiastic, or depressed by doctors and family members. Only recently have researchers tried to get at the truth or untruth of these descriptions.

First, as with other aspects of MMD, there is a wide range in severity of the mental and emotional symptoms of the disorder. Some people function very well, others poorly, many somewhere in between.

Children born with the severe, congenital form of MMD have a lot of learning problems and may even be mentally retarded. They often need special education because of these disabilities.

In adults, severe mental impairment is less common, but an overall inability to settle down to something, apply oneself to work or family life, concentrate, or become engrossed in a task is often reported.

Adults with MMD often find they need much more sleep than do other people and may feel at the beginning of the day the way most people feel at the end of a long workday. This can be very hard for others to understand.

Recent research suggests that in MMD there may be abnormalities in the parts of the brain that determine the rhythm of sleeping and waking. Respiratory regulation and weakness of the respiratory muscles, along with irregular breathing during sleep, all combine to make this problem severe in some people (though not in everyone).

Weakness of the facial muscles, with drooping eyes, can add to an outsider's impression that the person with MMD is apathetic or dull. Facial expression can be misleading in this disorder.

Daytime sleepiness can sometimes be helped with medication. One drug that can be used is methylphenidate (Ritalin). A newer drug is modafinil (Provigil). These drugs may work on the sleep-wake cycle in the brain.

Another approach that can be tried is to coax the body into a better rhythm of sleeping and waking by going to bed and getting up at the same time every day no matter what the requirements of the day may be. It may be possible to train the body to stay awake and sleep on a better schedule.

The eyes. Cataracts—cloudy areas of the lens of the eye that can eventually interfere with vision—are extremely common in MMD. Cataracts are caused by a chemical change in the lens, which gradually goes from clear to cloudy the way the clear part of an egg changes to white when cooked. Exactly why cataracts occur in MMD is not known.

The person with a cataract may notice that things start to look blurry, hazy, or dim, and that this worsens gradually over time. It often happens in both eyes, but not necessarily at the same time or at the same rate. Surgery can remove a lens that contains a cataract.

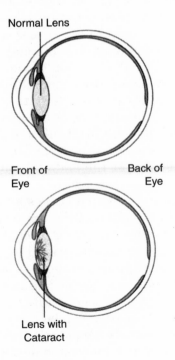

Figure 12.6. Eye Lens without and with Cataract

Normal Lens

Front of Eye

Back of Eye

Lens with Cataract

Then, the surgeon either puts in an artificial lens, or the patient can wear special contact lenses or eyeglasses.

Vision correction with cataract surgery is quite good. However, with this operation or any procedure requiring anesthesia, the medical team must be informed about the underlying MMD. Anesthesia can pose special problems for the patient with MMD.

The muscles that move the eyes, as well as those that open and close them, can also be affected in MMD, and other eye problems can sometimes occur. Your primary care provider or MDA clinic physician can refer you to an eye doctor (ophthalmologist) when eye problems need attention or for regular checkups.

Diabetes. If you read about MMD in books or on the Internet, you may find diabetes listed among the problems in this disorder. Fortunately, most people with MMD do not have severe diabetes, but they may develop a mild type sometimes referred to as insulin resistance with high blood sugar. This means the body makes insulin (a hormone needed for the cells to take up and use sugars), but for some reason, the insulin is not quite doing its job.

Your doctor may order blood and/or urine tests to see if you have insulin resistance or diabetes. If you do, you may be advised to change your diet or exercise habits or to take medication. Your doctor may refer you to a specialist or primary care physician for further treatment for diabetes.

Anesthesia. An unusually high rate of complications and even deaths associated with general anesthesia (given during any surgery) have been reported in people with MMD. This can occur even if the MMD is mild. In fact, these cases can be particularly dangerous, because the surgeon, anesthesiologist, and patient may be less likely to pay much attention to the MMD when planning the surgery.

Surgery can usually be safely undertaken these days with careful monitoring of cardiac and respiratory functions before, during, and after the surgery. Be sure to tell the entire medical team, especially those responsible for the anesthesia, that you or your family member has MMD. Have the anesthesiologist and the neurologist communicate long before the surgery if at all possible.

What happens in congenital MMD?

The most serious form of MMD is the congenital (at birth) form of the disease. When a child with congenital MMD is born, it is almost always found that the mother has adult-onset MMD—even though her symptoms may be so mild that she does not even know she has the disorder.

Mothers with MMD can also pass on the adult-onset form. When fathers with MMD have children, the child can also inherit the disease, but it is almost always the adult-onset form. These unusual features of MMD are not seen in other genetic disorders.

Weak muscles. Babies born with congenital MMD have very weak muscles and a lack of muscle tone (hypotonia). They appear floppy, have trouble breathing, and suck and swallow poorly. In the past, many of these infants did not survive. Today, with special care in neonatal intensive care units, such children have a much better chance of survival, but they enter childhood with multiple problems.

Respiratory support, such as artificial ventilation, will probably be needed, at least at first. Voluntary and involuntary aspects of respiration are probably affected in congenital MMD. Because swallowing muscles are affected, special feeding techniques or a feeding tube that goes into the stomach may be needed to provide adequate nutrition and prevent choking on foods during infancy.

Children with congenital MMD have severe facial weakness, leading to a lack of facial expression and an upper lip that comes to a point—known as a tented upper lip. Babies with congenital MMD are often born with clubfeet—a curvature of the feet and lower legs. Clubfeet need surgical correction for the child to be able to walk. The problem may be due to abnormal muscle development in the lower legs and feet during fetal life. Infants with MMD do not have myotonia. If they survive, however, they will develop it later in life.

Mental retardation. Infants born with congenital MMD are likely to be mentally retarded, although this is not always the case. This seems to be related to maldevelopment of parts of the brain, presumably caused by genetic abnormalities.

Some experts have suggested that the very high incidence of labor and delivery complications in mothers with MMD could also be a contributing factor to the mental problems seen in these babies. For this reason, it is very important to make doubly sure that everyone on the medical team is aware of and can work to minimize the risks surrounding labor and delivery to the mother and child with MMD.

Speech and hearing difficulties. The muscles involved in talking are often affected in congenital MMD. Hearing can also be impaired.

Therapy from a speech-language pathologist (in a medical center) or speech therapist (in a school) can help. Even before a child enters school, early intervention programs are vital. Talk to your pediatrician, MDA clinic physician, or medical social worker about such programs in your area.

Vision problems. The eye muscles in congenital MMD are affected and can cause the eyes not to work together; this condition is called strabismus. If severe, it can be corrected with surgery.

Cataracts, common in adult-onset MMD, are not a feature of congenital MMD during early childhood. However, children with MMD are likely to develop them later.

Outgrowing congenital MMD. Infants and children with MMD symptoms may outgrow many of the muscle-related aspects of the disorder as they mature. The mental retardation does not improve, but these children can learn if given the right tools and environment. Unfortunately, despite early gains during childhood, all children with congenital MMD go on to develop the adult form of MMD when they reach adolescence or adulthood.

How is MMD diagnosed?

Doctors who have experience with neuromuscular disorders find it easy to diagnose MMD. They can usually just look at a person, examine him, and ask a few questions to make the diagnosis. Teenagers and adults with MMD usually have a characteristic long face with hollow temples and, in men, early balding.

Many people tell the doctor about recurring abdominal pain or constipation. If they have had children, there may have been obstetrical complications, and the children may have serious physical and mental difficulties. Others say their parents had some muscle problems.

Sometimes, an eye doctor will notice the particular type of cataract found in MMD and suspect the diagnosis, referring the patient to a neurologist.

Many people may not realize they have any trouble relaxing their grip, but others say they have had trouble letting go of a shovel, screwdriver, or some other device, especially in cold weather.

The doctor may check for myotonia by lightly tapping the area just under the thumb with a rubber hammer. In most people, there is little or no response. In people with myotonia, there is a swift contraction of the muscle, which takes several seconds to relax.

The doctor may want to do electrical testing of the muscles and nerves, using an examination called an electromyogram, or EMG. In this exam, small needles are inserted into muscles to measure their electrical activity.

In a few cases, a muscle biopsy may be considered. In this test, a small piece of muscle is surgically removed for examination.

Since DNA testing has become available, the doctor may move from the history and physical exam to a DNA test to confirm a diagnosis of MMD. The DNA test involves only a blood sample and, in almost all cases, can determine whether the family has MMD.

How is MMD treated?

At this time, there is no specific treatment that gets at the root of MMD. Treatment is aimed at managing symptoms and minimizing disability as much as possible. For example, canes, braces, walkers, and scooters can help with mobility problems. Careful monitoring of cardiac and respiratory functions can lead to early treatment of these problems with a cardiac pacemaker or a portable ventilator.

Medications and other treatments for constipation and other digestive tract complaints can be employed. Surgery for cataracts and either surgery or special eye crutches for drooping eyelids can markedly improve vision. New medications to treat excessive sleepiness can make life more enjoyable for the person with MMD and his or her family.

In children with the congenital form of MMD, early intervention is crucial. Hearing and vision abnormalities should be diagnosed and treated as soon as possible. Surgery for uncoordinated eye muscles and special education are among the interventions that can greatly influence a child's later success in life.

If you have a child with congenital MMD, it is very important to seek out an early intervention program in your area through your MDA clinic, pediatrician, medical social worker, school system, or other community resources.

Information about Excessive Daytime Sleeping and Myotonic Dystrophy from the Myotonic Dystrophy Support Group

The Myotonic Dystrophy Support Group receives many comments and inquiries about excessive daytime sleepiness. It is clearly an area of concern which can affect all members of the family; partner, parent, extended family, caregiver, or friend.

Some people may not be aware that falling asleep during the day-time can be caused by myotonic dystrophy. Others may blame getting older or find different reasons for the sleepiness, but the fact is that myotonic dystrophy does cause people to fall asleep more often, and at inappropriate and inconvenient times.

One lady described the sleep as if she was having a cloak pulled over her. Once the sleepiness began she could not prevent herself from falling asleep. She knew she could not fight it. This cannot be very pleasant for the person to experience.

This type of sleeping affects many myotonic dystrophy families. Extreme tiredness can make it difficult to time a discussion so that you can examine the issues properly, resolve some of the problems, and accept some compromise if changes cannot be made.

It is always important to remember that this type of sleepiness is a symptom of an illness, myotonic dystrophy, but it can and does often appear to change a person's personality. You may only hear part of a conversation before you fall asleep, or miss the view or part of the enjoyment of an outing with family or friends. Perhaps you have been looking forward to seeing a television program or film, only to fall asleep and miss the ending.

Information for caregivers. This sleepiness affects the person you live with or are closest to. You know that the sleep problem is part of the illness, yet still may find it difficult to live with. There are some households where there are several people with myotonic dystrophy, and only one person does not have the condition. This one person can appear to be very impatient. This is a normal reaction. It can be extremely irritating and frustrating to be busy with all the jobs, large and small, that need to be done if other members of the household are asleep.

Several people have experienced a split in the family because these irritations and frustrations are not explained and spoken about. Families do not always recognize that the sleepiness, lethargy, and apparent apathy are the result of myotonic dystrophy.

People will often deny being asleep in the daytime or it can be variously described as just resting or closing my eyes. The caregiver will probably be more aware of these unwelcome naps than the person with myotonic dystrophy. A person my fall asleep several times a day, sometimes for seconds or minutes, sometimes for hours at a time. The sleeping inhibits the flow of conversation or prevents the opportunity to take part in discussions or conversation. Messages are not communicated and generally less and less stimulating conversation takes place between members of the household. Decisions are made without consultation or discussion, and patience is tried for everyone.

People with myotonic dystrophy are extra tired, but everyone needs stimulation and encouragement. On a practical note, it might be helpful to have a dry erase board for daily use. A list of jobs for the home and garden could be written on the board, to be erased when completed. Encouragement to take on even a few light tasks will help to reduce the sleepiness at least for some part of the day. Family tensions may be reduced as a result.

Many people with myotonic dystrophy are offered sleep tests which include an overnight stay in the hospital. In some instances these investigations result in being given a machine to use at home each night. In very simple terms, this machine enables the body to do its job more efficiently, thereby providing the lungs with a better supply of air. The result of this can be an improved quality of life, as the person is more alert and less inclined to sleep during the day.

Faulty Gene is Key to Understanding Myotonic Dystrophy

After much mystery, researchers funded by the National Institute of Arthritis and Musculoskeletal and Skin Diseases have succeeded in linking the gene defect in myotonic dystrophy (DM) to its biological malfunction. Their findings emphasize how misreading of a gene can lead to improper conduction of electrical impulses in skeletal muscle.

Two different studies were completed. Thomas A. Cooper, M.D., and his team of scientists at Baylor College of Medicine in Texas examined tissue samples from skeletal muscle in patients with myotonic dystrophy. The results revealed that extra genetic material caused by the defect in the DNA sequence affects the chloride channels that control muscle relaxation.

In New York, at the University of Rochester, Charles A. Thornton, M.D. and his colleagues, measured electrochemical muscle impulses in a mouse model of the disease. The results indicated that the genetic defect affects the conductance of electrical signals, resulting in delayed muscle control. People with DM have the normal gene with additional information that interferes with the translation of proteins. While further study still needs to be done, these findings are a key step in understanding the causes of muscular dystrophies.

Myotonic dystrophy belongs to a group of genetic diseases called muscular dystrophies characterized by progressive weakness and degeneration of the skeletal or voluntary muscles that control movement. Tens of thousands of people in the United States are affected. An early sign of DM is delayed skeletal muscle relaxation following voluntary contraction.

References

Charlet NB, Savkur RS, Singh G, Philips AV, Grice EA, Cooper TA. Loss of the muscle-specific chloride channel in type 1 myotonic dystrophy due to misregulated alternative splicing. *Molecular Cell* 2002;10:45-53.

Mankodi A, Takahashi MP, Jiang H, Beck CL, Bowers WJ, Moxely RT, Cannon SC, Thorton CA. Expanded CUG repeats trigger aberrant splicing of CIC-1 chloride channel pre-mRNA and hyperexcitability of skeletal muscle in myotonic dystrophy. *Molecular Cell* 2002;10:35-43.

Additional Information

International Myotonic Dystrophy Organization, Inc.
P.O. Box 1121
Sunland, CA 91041-1121
Toll-Free: 866-679-7954
Phone: 818-951-2311
Website: http://
www.myotonicdystrophy.org
E-mail:
info@myotonicdystrophy.org

Muscular Dystrophy Association
3300 E. Sunrise Dr.
Tucson, AZ 85718-3208
Toll-Free: 800-572-1717
Phone: 520-529-2000
Fax: 520-529-5300
Website: http://www.mdausa.org
E-mail: mda@mdausa.org

Athena Diagnostics, Inc.
Four Biotech Park
377 Plantation St.
Wochester, MA 01605
Toll-Free: 800-394-4493
Phone: 508-756-2886
Fax: 508-753-5601
Website: http://
www.athenadiagnostics.com
E-mail: genetic.counselor@
athenadiagnostics.com

Performs testing on both Type 1 and Type 2 Myotonic Dystrophy, DM1 and DM2.

Chapter 13

Ophthalmoplegic Muscular Dystrophy

It has been recognized for many years that some patients with muscle disease have particular problems with the muscles around the eyes, although other parts of the body can also be involved. While research is continuing, it appears that most of these patients have either oculopharyngeal muscular dystrophy (OPMD) or mitochondrial chronic progressive external ophthalmoplegia (CPEO). The main features of these disorders are discussed in this chapter. Some of the symptoms and signs are common to both disorders.

Frequent Medical Terms

Ptosis: describes drooping of the eyelids due to weakness of the muscle that normally lifts up the eyelid.

External ophthalmoplegia: weakness and restriction of muscle movement around the eye (external to the eye). It shows as slowness and incomplete range of movement of the eyes, and includes the eyelid muscle weakness that causes ptosis. These problems typically progress very slowly, hence the term chronic progressive external ophthalmoplegia.

"Ocular Myopathies," is reprinted with permission from the Muscular Dystrophy Campaign, a United Kingdom charity focusing on all muscular dystrophies and allied disorders. © 2003 Muscular Dystrophy Campaign. All rights reserved. Additional information is available at www.muscular-dystrophy.org.uk.

Diplopia: means double vision and occurs when the eye muscles on each side are not affected equally, so that the eyes point in slightly different directions.

Dysphagia: difficulty in swallowing. When mild, it may simply be a feeling of food sticking in the throat, but patients with severe dysphagia may not be able to swallow at all and can even choke on their own saliva.

Oculopharyngeal Muscular Dystrophy (OPMD)

Muscular dystrophy is a term used to describe a number of conditions in which there is progressive muscle weakness, caused by the patient having a faulty gene. In OPMD the weakness mainly affects the ocular (eye) and pharyngeal (throat) muscles.

Symptoms and Signs

Although the abnormal gene is present from birth, patients do not usually develop symptoms until the fifth or sixth decade of life. The first sign of the disorder is usually ptosis, but occasionally it is dysphagia. Very slowly, over many years, these problems progress. There is progressive restriction of eye movements and in rare cases this can lead to diplopia. The increasing ptosis may lead to the eyelid covering the pupil and impairing vision, and in an effort to compensate for this the forehead muscle becomes overactive, trying to help to lift up the eyelids, giving a frowning appearance, and the patient adopts a rather characteristic posture with the head tilted backwards.

Dysphagia, which is initially mainly for solid and dry foods, progresses slowly and eventually even swallowing fluids, including saliva, may become a problem. If dysphagia is severe, then there is a danger of aspiration of food and saliva.

After many years the patient may become aware of mild limb weakness, first around the shoulders and later around the hips and of facial weakness, but marked weakness is uncommon. Life expectancy is little, if at all, altered.

Management

There is no specific treatment for OPMD, but much that can be done to help the main symptoms of ptosis and dysphagia.

Glasses can be fitted with fine metal bars (ptosis props) that lift up the drooping eyelids. If these are unacceptable, and if the ptosis is severe, surgical elevation of the eyelids can be very successful.

Mild dysphagia can be helped by suitable attention to the consistency of the diet (with a dietitian's advice) and by exercises taught by a speech therapist. Occasionally drugs (e.g., Cisapride) can be of value. In more severe cases, a relatively minor operation called cricopharyngeal myotomy, which cuts one of the throat muscles internally, can be valuable. If the dysphagia is preventing adequate nutrition or there is a risk of aspiration pneumonia, then alternative methods of feeding can be used. The most acceptable, in the long term, is gastrostomy. A minor operation is used to pass a tube through the front of the abdomen directly into the stomach. Patients and their relatives find this easy to manage at home.

Physiotherapy may be useful to help patients cope with limb weakness, although this is usually mild, and to reduce the risk of chest problems.

How Is OPMD Inherited?

In most cases the condition is inherited as an autosomal dominant disorder, which means that each child of an affected individual has a 50% risk of inheriting the same condition. It is now possible, through a blood test, to determine whether somebody has inherited the abnormal gene, but that is not always terribly helpful. Even if somebody has inherited the abnormal gene, it is impossible to predict when, if ever, they will develop symptoms. Such testing should only be performed after detailed discussion with a genetic counselor.

Table 13.1. Autosomal Dominant Inheritance

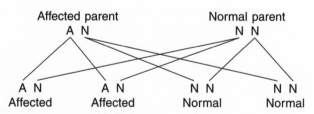

A = Chromosome with defective gene

N = Chromosome with normal gene

Both sexes are equally at risk.

Diagnosis

The diagnosis can be confirmed by a blood test that identifies the underlying genetic abnormality. Electrical tests (EMG) and muscle biopsy are now rarely necessary.

Research of OPMD

The genetic fault that causes OPMD was identified in 1998. Although this was a very important discovery, which has given us a simple diagnostic test, it is likely to be some time before the research allows us to identify a specific treatment for this condition. In the meantime, there is a great deal of research trying to identify how the genetic fault causes the physical problem.

Mitochondrial Chronic External Ophthalmoplegia (CPEO)

Mitochondria are very small structures that are present within every cell in the body. They are vitally important for the chemical processes that generate the energy required to keep the cell alive and functioning normally. They contain many hundreds of proteins, most of which are generated as a result of the DNA (the genetic material) contained within the nucleus of the cell. However, mitochondria are unique in that they also have a small amount of their own DNA, which is responsible for producing some of the mitochondrial proteins.

Another unique feature is that this mitochondrial DNA is always inherited from the mother, not the father. Disorders of mitochondrial structure and function have been associated with a wide range of clinical problems, but one of the commonest features is chronic progressive external ophthalmoplegia (CPEO).

Symptoms and Signs

The clinical features of the eye muscle involvement (the CPEO) are very similar to those described for oculopharyngeal muscular dystrophy (OPMD), and indeed in older patients it is not always easy to distinguish between the two conditions. Ptosis is the first feature, followed by progressive limitation of the range of eye movements. This is more severe than in OPMD and sometimes all eye movements are lost, with the eyes fixed in the mid-position so that the patient has to turn his/her head to see in different directions. Diplopia is uncommon. Overactivity of the forehead muscle occurs, as in OPMD.

Many other abnormalities have been described in patients with mitochondrial CPEO. Particularly common, but rarely causing symptoms, is a pigmentary retinopathy. At the back of the eye, over the outer edges of the retina, dark spots can be seen. Rarely, this can cause impairment of night vision or more troublesome visual problems.

Mild facial, neck, and limb weakness may be apparent, and other common associated symptoms include mild dysphagia, deafness, and short stature. Less commonly, there is clumsiness of limb movement (ataxia), epilepsy, mental subnormality, heart involvement, and diabetes.

The pattern of symptoms varies with age of onset. In childhood, the combination of CPEO, pigmentary retinopathy and heart problems is referred to as the Kearns Sayre syndrome. In older patients heart involvement is uncommon and the main feature is the progressive external ophthalmoplegia. Virtually all possible combinations of the symptoms and signs mentioned have been reported.

In children with Kearns Sayre syndrome, the main concern is the heart involvement, but this can be treated successfully with a pacemaker. In adults, the ophthalmoplegia progresses slowly and although limb weakness and tiring on exercise may develop, they are rarely major problems.

Management

Although a number of drugs have been tried, none is of proven benefit. Management of the ophthalmoplegia and dysphagia is as described for OPMD, but dysphagia is less frequently a significant problem. Because of the occasional involvement of the heart, tests such as an electrocardiogram (ECG) and echocardiogram may be required. If the heart rhythm is disturbed a pacemaker may be needed.

How Is CPEO Inherited?

In the majority of cases no other family members are affected and there is little risk of patients passing the condition on to their children. However, there are exceptions and genetic counseling is required. In some cases the condition can be passed from an affected mother to her children, but not from an affected father because of the maternal inheritance of mitochondrial DNA.

Diagnosis

Most patients require a muscle biopsy. Under the microscope a rather typical pattern of abnormalities can be seen. In many patients, it can be shown that there is a piece missing (a deletion) from the mitochondrial DNA extracted from the muscle biopsy specimen, which confirms the diagnosis. In other patients there is not a piece missing, but one of the 16,500 components (known as bases) of the DNA has been changed (mutated) to a different type.

Sometimes, more detailed tests are required, including exercising the patient and looking at chemical changes in the blood.

Laboratories Offering Diagnostic Testing for OPMD

University of Tennessee Medical Center
Molecular Diagnostics Laboratory
1924 Alcoa Highway
Knoxville, TN 37920-6969
Phone: 865-544-9030
Fax: 865-544-8580
Website: http://www.utmedicalcenter.org

Method: Mutation analysis.

Athena Diagnostics, Inc.
Four Biotech Park
377 Plantation St.
Worcester, MA 01605
Toll-Free: 800-394-4493
Phone: 508-756-2886
Fax: 508-753-5601
Website: http://www.athenadiagnostics.com
E-mail: genetic.counselor@athenadiagnostics.com

Methods: Mutation analysis and Southern blot analysis.

Children's Hospital of Eastern Ontario
Molecular Genetics Diagnostic Laboratory
401 Smyth Road
Ottawa, Ontario
Canada K1H 8L1
Phone: 613-737-7600
Fax: 613-738-4822
Website: http://www.cheo.on.ca
E-mail: webmaster@cheo.on.ca

Method: Mutation analysis.

Prenatal diagnosis is also offered.

Part Four

Diagnostic Tests

Chapter 14

Accurate and Affordable Diagnosis of Duchenne Muscular Dystrophy

Researchers have developed a simple and affordable blood test that detects the most common form of muscular dystrophy (MD) in more than 95 percent of cases. Until now, gene mutations causing Duchenne muscular dystrophy (DMD) went undetected in roughly 35 percent of children with the disease, in spite of extensive and sometimes invasive tests that cause great discomfort and stress for patients, says study author Kevin Flanigan, M.D., of the University of Utah. "Before, many DMD diagnoses required a muscle biopsy, which is invasive and involves some risks," Dr. Flanigan says. "Even then, some mutations were missed because of limitations with previous tests." Now, a simple blood test can detect almost all DMD cases.

The published study was funded in part by the National Institute of Neurological Disorders and Stroke and appears in the April 2003 issue of the *American Journal of Human Genetics*.[1]

Muscular dystrophy is a group of genetic diseases characterized by progressive weakness and degeneration of the muscles that generate movement. Duchenne MD is the most common fatal X-linked recessive disorder, which means that the disease is carried by mothers but usually appears only in boys. DMD occurs once in every 3,500 live male births. Those with the devastating disease have difficulty walking, an abnormal gait, and severe limb weakness. Most are

"Accurate and Affordable Diagnosis of Duchenne Muscular Dystrophy," by Tania Zeigler, National Institute of Neurological Disorders and Stroke (NINDS), April 18, 2003.

wheelchair-bound by age 7 or 8 and die by their early twenties due to respiratory or cardiac complications. To date, there is no cure.

Particular mutations in the dystrophin gene on the X chromosome cause DMD. The dystrophin gene is the largest human gene that we know of, and several different types of mutations can cause DMD.

The new test, called Single Condition Amplification/Internal Primer sequencing (SCAIP), allows clinicians and geneticists to sequence the entire dystrophin gene to find mutations that confirm DMD. "With the currently available genetic tests, we could look for only one type of mutation. Now, we can rapidly look at genetic variations in the entire gene. That's very exciting," says Dr. Flanigan.

A big hope is that the new DMD test will soon be widely available in various clinical settings. In the meantime, the SCAIP test is available to the public at the University of Utah.

The commonly used DMD test looks for missing portions of the dystrophin gene, called exons. An exon is the region within a gene that contains important parts of the genetic code. About 60 percent of DMD cases are caused by deletions in one or more exons within the dystrophin gene.

Until now, the enormous size of the dystrophin gene made it prohibitively expensive to test for mutations in the entire gene. Instead, the old test would just check exon hotspots, catching about 98 percent of exon deletions. Other available tests detect exon duplications, which account for about 5 percent of DMD cases. But before the development of SCAIP, geneticists could not find the 35 percent of mutations that were not exon deletions or duplications unless they obtained RNA from an invasive muscle biopsy, or used intermediate screening tests of variable sensitivity to determine specific regions of the gene to sequence from blood DNA samples.

This is a very important development, not only for diagnosing DMD, but also for finding female carriers of the disease before they pass it on to their male children. Since so many DMD mutations have been missed with previous tests, genetic counseling for the disease has been extremely difficult.

The new test will also aid researchers who are developing more effective treatments for DMD. "If we're going to treat this disease successfully, we need to be able to identify specific mutations and then tailor therapies to correct defects caused by each mutation," says Dr. Flanigan. "This test is an important first step, but there is much work that remains to be done."

Dr. Flanigan and his colleagues are coordinating with three research centers to develop an extensive patient database containing careful clinical and genetic evaluations of large groups of DMD patients. They hope that detailed genetic information about those patients will help researchers generate new hypotheses and eventually new treatments for the disease. "As a researcher, I'm very excited about where this new method will lead us, and as a clinician, I am very happy to find a way to speed up the diagnosis of DMD and minimize the degree of uncertainty that parents face because they can't get a correct diagnosis," Dr. Flanigan says.

Reference

1. Flanigan KM, von Niederhausern A, Dunn DM, Alder J, Mendell J, Weiss, RB. "Rapid Direct Sequence Analysis of the Dystrophin Gene." *American Journal of Human Genetics*, April 2003, vol. 72, no. 4, pp. 931-939.

Chapter 15

New Test for Myotonic Muscular Dystrophy

Researchers have developed a genetic test that detects a common form of muscular dystrophy with 99 percent accuracy. The accurate diagnosis of myotonic muscular dystrophy type 2 (DM2) allows researchers to fully describe its clinical features for the first time.

"So many DM2 patients have been undiagnosed or misdiagnosed," says John W. Day, M.D., Ph.D., of the University of Minnesota Department of Neurology and Institute of Human Genetics in Minneapolis. "By establishing a correct diagnosis, we can start to treat people much more effectively and estimate risks in families with a history of the disease."

The study, co-authored by Dr. Day and Laura Ranum, Ph.D., and their colleagues in the University of Minnesota Department of Genetics, Cell Biology, and Development and the Institute of Human Genetics, was funded in part by the National Institute of Neurological Disorders and Stroke and appeared in the February 2003 issue of *Neurology*.[1]

The muscular dystrophies (MD) are a group of genetic diseases characterized by progressive weakness and degeneration of the muscles that control movement. Myotonic dystrophy, the most common type of MD in adults, affects the eyes, heart, hormonal systems, blood, and muscles.

"A New Test for Myotonic Dystrophy: Exposing an Enemy That's Too Big to See," by Tania Zeigler, National Institute of Neurological Disorders and Stroke (NINDS), March 26, 2003.

DM2 has been difficult to diagnose for two main reasons. First, DM2 affects many different parts of the body, so people with the disease often visit several specialists to treat different symptoms and rarely get a diagnosis of DM2. Second, there has been no simple and reliable test for the disease. Although the DM2 mutation was identified by this group in 2001, the mutation is so large and unstable that standard methods of genetic testing do not reliably detect the abnormality.

Drs. Day and Ranum designed an improved method for detecting the DM2 mutation and then characterized the clinical features of the disease in 379 individuals with genetically confirmed DM2. The new test, dubbed the DM2 repeat assay, uses a two-step procedure that allows the detection of large mutations missed with standard testing. The researchers basically combined a genomic test called Southern analysis with a modified version of the polymerase chain reaction (PCR) test. This repeat assay successfully detected the DM2 mutation in 99 percent of cases, compared to 80 percent by genomic Southern analysis alone.

"Now that we have the ability to genetically diagnose the disorder, we're realizing that DM2 is much more common than was previously recognized," says Dr. Day. Before this study, only 2 percent of myotonic dystrophy cases were thought to be DM2.

Dr. Day says DM2 may turn out to be as common as the more severe form, DM1, which was thought to account for about 98 percent of myotonic dystrophy cases before this study. DM1 occurs in about one of every 7,000 people worldwide. DM1 is found in all ethnic groups, but DM2 had previously been found only in people of European origin, particularly those of German descent.

Among DM2 patients with a genetically confirmed diagnosis, the researchers found that the clinical features of DM2 closely resemble those of adult-onset DM1, with common features including progressive weakness, difficulty relaxing muscles after voluntary contraction has stopped, muscle and cardiac problems, cataracts, and insulin insensitivity.

Despite the striking similarities between the two diseases, Dr. Ranum notes that there are important differences, namely that DM1 has a broader range of ages of onset and sometimes presents with significant symptoms at birth, while DM2 usually starts in early adulthood.

"We wanted to define the clinical features of DM2 not only to compare it to DM1, but also to gain a better understanding of the molecular mechanisms of the disease," says Dr. Ranum. "The clinical

similarities between DM1 and DM2 tell us that the mutations causing them have similar effects at the cellular level." Both forms of the
disease are caused by large, unstable repetitive DNA sequences in genetic regions that lack instructions for proteins.

The researchers plan to continue studying the biological mechanisms of DM2. "We're excited about this new test and this new information about myotonic dystrophies," says Dr. Ranum. "Our research
efforts are now focused on understanding the biology of the mutations
that lead to these diseases." The new DM2 test is available to the general public from Athena Diagnostics of Worcester, Massachusetts.

Reference

1. Day JW, Ricker K, Jacobsen JF, Rasmussen LJ, Dick KA,
    Kress W, Schneider C, Koch MC, Beilman GJ, Harrison AR,
    Dalton JC, Ranum LPW. "Myotonic dystrophy type 2: molecu-
    lar, diagnostic and clinical spectrum." *Neurology*, February
    2003, pp. 657-664.

Additional Information

Athena Diagnostics, Inc.
Four Biotech Park
377 Plantation St.
Worcester, MA 01605
Toll-Free: 800-394-4493
Phone: 508-756-2886
Fax: 508-753-5601
Website: http://www.athenadiagnostics.com
E-mail: genetic.counselor@athenadiagnostics.com

Chapter 16

Creatine Kinase Test

Almost everyone with a neuromuscular disorder has had, or will have, a creatine kinase test. But what exactly is creatine kinase (CK), and why are its levels measured in neuromuscular diseases?

CK, also known as phosphocreatine kinase, or CPK, is a type of protein called an enzyme. It catalyzes, or encourages, a biochemical reaction to occur. The normal function of CK in our cells is to add a phosphate group to creatine, turning it into the high-energy molecule phosphocreatine. Phosphocreatine is burned as a quick source of energy by our cells.

However, the normal function of CK is not as relevant, in this case, as what happens to CK when muscle is damaged. During the process of muscle degeneration, muscle cells break open and their contents find their way into the bloodstream. Because most of the CK in the body normally exists in muscle, a rise in the amount of CK in the blood indicates that muscle damage has occurred, or is occurring.

To measure CK levels, a blood sample is taken and separated into fractions that contain cells and a fraction that does not—the serum.

Reprinted from "Simply Stated...The Creatine Kinase Test," *QUEST*, Volume7, Number 1, February 2000. Reprinted with permission from the Muscular Dystrophy Association, www.mdausa.org. © The Muscular Dystrophy Association. For additional information, call the Muscular Dystrophy Association National Headquarters toll-free at (800) 572-1717. To find an MDA office in your area, look in your local telephone book, or click on "Clinics and Services" on the MDA website. And, "Creatine Kinase (Total) Test," reprinted from Clinical Reference Systems Senior Health Advisor, 2002.1 with permission from McKesson Health Solutions. Copyright 2003 McKesson Health Solutions LLC.

The amount of CK in the serum is reported in units (U) of enzyme activity per liter (L) of serum. In a healthy adult, the serum CK level varies with a number of factors (gender, race, and activity), but normal range is 22 to 198 U/L (units per liter).

Higher amounts of serum CK can indicate muscle damage due to chronic disease or acute muscle injury. For this reason, if you are scheduled to have blood drawn for a CK test to diagnose a potential muscle disorder, you should limit your exercise to normal activities before the test.

CK tests are used to evaluate neuromuscular diseases in five basic ways:

1. To confirm a suspected muscle problem before other symptoms occur.

2. To determine whether symptoms of muscle weakness are caused by a muscle or a nerve problem.

3. To differentiate between some types of disorders such as dystrophies versus congenital myopathies.

4. To detect carriers of neuromuscular disorders, particularly in Duchenne muscular dystrophy. A carrier has a genetic defect, but does not get the full-blown disease. A carrier's child may have the full disease.

5. To follow the course of a disease that fluctuates (primarily the inflammatory myopathies), or to document episodes of acute muscle injury, as might occur in some metabolic myopathies.

Because elevated CK levels indicate muscle damage, many parents wonder why their children with Duchenne muscular dystrophy (DMD) had higher CK levels when they were younger and had more muscle function. This seeming paradox occurs because muscle degeneration is more rapid at the earlier stages, and possibly because there is more muscle bulk available to release CK into the circulation at this time.

CK levels can be slightly elevated (500 U/L) in nerve disorders like Charcot-Marie-Tooth disease, amyotrophic lateral sclerosis, or spinal muscular atrophy, or grossly elevated (3,000 to 3,500 U/L) in DMD or inflammatory myopathies.

During episodes of acute muscle breakdown (rhabdomyolysis), CK levels can temporarily go off the scale, topping out at 50,000 to 200,000 U/L. At the same time, some neuromuscular disorders, such as the congenital myopathies (nemaline, central core disease, and others) and myasthenia gravis, may not trigger any elevation of CK levels. CK levels do not always reflect the level of functional impact on the individual.

What Is the Total Creatine Kinase Test?

This test measures an enzyme in the blood. The enzyme is called creatine kinase (CK). Muscle cells make this enzyme. When muscle cells are injured or diseased, enzymes leak out of the cells and enter the bloodstream.

Why is this test done?

The CK test can show if muscles have been injured. It also gives an idea of how bad the injury is, when it happened, and whether it is healing. The test may be done to:

- Find out if you have had a heart attack (myocardial infarction).

- Diagnose chest pain.

- Look for other muscle injuries or disease, such as muscular dystrophy or rhabdomyolysis.

- Check blood flow to the heart after heart surgery or other treatments that affect the heart muscle.

If this test shows that some muscle has been injured, other tests may also be done to see which muscles are injured.

How do I prepare for this test?

- If you are being checked for problems with your skeletal muscles, do not exercise for 24 hours before the test.

- You may need to avoid taking certain medicines before the test because they might affect the test result. Make sure your health care provider knows about any medicines, herbs, or supplements that you are taking.

- Talk to your health care provider if you have any other questions.

How is the test done?

A small amount of blood is taken from your arm with a needle. The blood is collected in tubes and sent to a lab. Having this test will take just a few minutes of your time. There is no risk of getting AIDS, hepatitis, or any other blood-borne disease from this test.

How will I get the test result?

Ask your health care provider when and how you will get the result of your test.

What does the test result mean?

The normal range for CK is 32 to 267 units per liter. The normal range may vary slightly from lab to lab. Normal ranges are usually shown next to your result in the lab report. Your CK level may be higher than normal because:

- You have had a heart attack.
- You have recently had surgery.
- You have recently had a shot in one of your muscles.
- You have recently been in an accident or hurt one of your muscles.
- You have a muscle disease.

If your CK level is high, the test may be repeated (as often as every 8 hours) to see if the injury is healing or getting worse.

What if my test result is not normal?

Test results are only one part of a larger picture that takes into account your medical history and current health. Sometimes a test needs to be repeated to check the first result. Talk to your health care provider about the results and ask questions. If your test result is not normal, ask your health care provider:

- if you need additional tests,
- what you can do to work toward a normal value, and
- when you need to be tested again.

Chapter 17

Muscle Biopsy

Muscle biopsies often play a crucial part in the accurate diagnosis of muscle wasting conditions. But what happens to the sliver of muscle when it is removed from a patient? Where does it go, and when scientists examine it under the microscope, what do they find?

Accurate diagnosis is extremely important. Without one, the patient may not know how the condition is likely to progress. If the diagnosis is of an inherited disorder, then the patient can be told about the risks of passing it on to his or her children, and the diagnosis may help identify other members of the patient's family who unknowingly carry the same genetic abnormality. Muscle biopsy can be very useful in achieving a specific diagnosis. Other tests are also important including blood tests and electrical studies of the muscles and nerves.

A muscle biopsy is a small sample of muscle measuring only a few millimeters in diameter. It is usually taken from the thigh, calf, shoulder, or upper arm. All these muscles are safe to sample as the major nerves and blood vessels are deep in the bulk of the muscle. It is important to sample a muscle that is affected, but not so badly wasted that there is little muscle to examine.

Muscle biopsies are usually performed on an out-patient basis, and in most hospitals they are taken under a local anesthetic, similar to that used by dentists. Children may be given some premedication to

171

make them drowsy, and in some hospitals may have a brief general anesthetic. As always with neuromuscular conditions, anesthetics have to be very carefully chosen and their effects closely monitored.

A small incision is made in the skin, the length being dependent on the method; if a needle technique is used, the incision is a few millimeters long, but if an open method is used it is several centimeters long. The needle is about 5mm in diameter and is quickly inserted through the incision and the sample obtained in a matter of seconds. After the biopsy the small incision is held together with a plaster and no stitches are required; the scar left is very small. An open biopsy takes a little longer as the sample has to be cut from the muscle and requires stitches afterwards which leave a scar. Both methods have disadvantages and advantages and hospitals vary as to their preferred method.

Rapid and efficient handling of the biopsy is essential for good results. Usually a small piece is cut off the sample and put into a preservative to be processed for electron microscopy to look at the fine structure of each muscle fiber. The remainder is then rapidly frozen at about negative 160 degrees. A separate small piece may also be frozen in liquid nitrogen if specific proteins are going to be examined biochemically. Freezing the tissue not only gives the rigidity needed to cut very thin slices, but also preserves the activity of the enzymes and other proteins within the muscle fibers. Sections a fraction of a millimeter thick are cut from the frozen block. They are collected on small pieces of glass and then stained with dyes to reveal the structure of the tissue.

Normal Appearance

Healthy muscle is made of closely packed fibers, more or less evenly sized. Connective tissue surrounds bundles of fibers, but rarely appears between the fibers. Each fiber has several nuclei around its edges; they contain DNA, our genes. Blood vessels carrying nutrients and oxygen to the muscle fibers can be seen between them, and occasionally a small peripheral nerve that provides the impulse for muscle contraction is visible.

Appearance in Disease

In dystrophic muscle the fibers vary in size. Some fibers may be more intensively stained indicating that they are damaged while others may be very pale and have died. New fibers, however, can regenerate and these appear as clusters of smaller fibers with different staining properties. Unlike healthy muscle, dystrophic fibers are separated by connective tissue and fat often appears as patches between the fibers. Some nuclei may be inside the fiber instead of on the edge, and some fibers may be split or disrupted.

Fiber Types

Muscle is composed of two main types of fibers that have different functions and biochemical properties. This difference is easily observed in some animals like chickens that have pale breast muscles, but dark muscles on the drumstick. In humans most muscles are more mixed than this. The pattern can be observed under the microscope by staining the enzymes contained by each type. In normal muscle this produces a checkered pattern of light and dark fibers, but in neuromuscular disorders deviations occur.

In dystrophic muscle, there are more fibers for posture than for fast actions like sprinting. This is also seen in several other muscle disorders. In spinal muscular atrophy the large fibers are all of one type while the small ones are mixed or mostly of the other type. Wasting of only one type of fiber tends to be seen in disorders such as myotonic dystrophy and some of the congenital myopathies such as centronuclear myopathy, named after the centrally placed nuclei in many fibers.

Structural Changes

Some disorders show specific structural defects in muscle fibers, only visible under the microscope. In nemaline myopathy clusters of small rod-like bodies occur in many fibers. In mitochondrial disorders the mitochondria that provide the energy for the fiber may be of abnormal shape, size, and structure. Other changes occur in the myofibrils, the components of the fibers that slide together to make them contract. In central core disease the central part of most fibers is disrupted and also lacks mitochondria, while in mini-core disease these disruptions are smaller and occur throughout the fiber.

Checking for Enzymes and Accumulation of Storage Products

In some disorders an enzyme essential for a chemical reaction may be absent. For example, in McArdle's disease the enzyme phosphorylase which is involved in the breakdown of sugar molecules is totally absent. This results in the accumulation of glycogen, a starch-like molecule. Glycogen or fat storage can be seen in other metabolic disorders. In some mitochondrial disorders the enzyme cytochrome oxidase is missing in a few fibers.

Abnormalities in Specific Proteins

One major advance in our ability to assess muscle biopsies has been provided by antibodies. These are produced in the laboratory. They stick to a particular protein when put on a section of muscle. By marking the antibodies with a label that is visible under the microscope, scientists can see where they bind thus identifying where specific proteins are and where they are absent.

Antibodies to many muscle proteins are now available and some of them enable us to distinguish between disorders that have a very similar pathology and symptoms. This is well illustrated by Duchenne and Becker muscular dystrophy and the limb-girdle dystrophies. In Duchenne MD the defective protein, dystrophin, is missing or only present in very reduced amounts, while in the Becker form some dystrophin is present, but there is less of it or it is unevenly distributed. Antibodies can sometimes be useful in identifying carriers of Duchenne MD. Although most carriers do not have symptoms, minor changes in the amount and distribution of dystrophin can occur. Sometimes an isolated fiber may have no dystrophin. Occasionally there are several fibers without dystrophin, and in these rare cases a carrier may have muscle weakness. This helps to distinguish carriers with manifestations of Duchenne MD from patients with a limb-girdle form of dystrophy. In a manifesting carrier, a mosaic of dystrophin positive and dystrophin negative fibers is seen, but in limb-girdle patients the dystrophin is normal.

In some forms of limb-girdle dystrophy a deficiency of another protein, adhalin, can be seen in the muscle using antibodies. Adhalin also lies at the periphery of fibers and is one component of a group of proteins associated with dystrophin. The reason for the deficiency of adhalin is not the same in all cases and defects in at least three different genes can cause it. But examination of adhalin in biopsies gives a starting point for the molecular analysis and for differentiating between the different types of limb-girdle dystrophy.

The complex of proteins associated with dystrophin is linked on the outside of the fiber to a matrix that coats the fiber. A deficiency in one component of this outer coat, the protein known as merosin, occurs in about half the cases of congenital muscular dystrophy. Its absence, revealed in a muscle biopsy, can be used for prenatal diagnosis.

It is therefore apparent that muscle fibers need this complex of dystrophin, its associated proteins, and the outer coat to be complete for normal function, and that defects in just one component can cause a neuromuscular disorder. It is likely that there are other disorders associated with one of the other proteins of this complex.

In addition to specific protein defects, other abnormalities can be detected with antibodies. In polymyositis and dermatomyositis, it is common to find many fibers have abnormal amounts of a protein associated with the body's immune system called the class 1 major histocompatibility complex. This tricks the body into thinking that muscle is foreign and makes the body react against itself, and may be an important factor in the inflammatory reaction.

Chapter 18

Electromyography (EMG)

Your doctor has just ordered a test called an EMG. EMG stands for electromyogram which loosely translated means electrical testing of muscles, but in fact has come to mean electrical testing of nerves and muscles. The EMG is performed by a specialist, the electromyographer, who is usually a neurologist or a physiatrist. Parts of the test (the nerve conductions) may be performed by a specially trained technician. It is an in-office procedure and does not require hospitalization. On average, an EMG takes anywhere between 30 minutes and 2 hours, depending on how extensive a testing your doctor orders. It can be done at any time during the day, and with few exceptions, does not require any special preparation.

Sometimes EMGs are thought to be a treatment of some sort, or a type of acupuncture. This is not true; an EMG is only a test, much like an EKG or an x-ray is a test and not a treatment.

What are some problems for which EMGs are ordered?

EMGs are usually ordered when patients are having problems with their muscles or nerves. They test the nerves and muscles of the body's extremities, looking for a problem in either one of these areas. An EMG

---

may be ordered to see if you have a pinched nerve in the back or the neck. If you have tingling or numbness in your arms or legs, an EMG may show if you have a nerve entrapment somewhere or a nerve injury. Weakness of the muscles or fatigue (tiredness) may be indicative of nerve or muscle disease and require an EMG. There are many other medical problems that might suggest the need for an EMG. If you have any doubts as to why you need this test, ask your doctor.

What happens during an EMG?

During this test, you will be lying on an examination table, next to an EMG machine (which looks like a desktop or laptop computer). The test consists of two parts, though at times one may be done without the other. The first part is called a nerve conduction study. In this part some brief electrical shocks are delivered to your arm or leg in an effort to determine how fast or slowly your nerves are conducting the electrical current, and therefore in what state of health or disease they may be. A nerve works something like an electrical wire. If you want to see if the wire is functioning properly, the easiest thing to do is to run electricity through it. If there are any problems along its length, you will know it by a failure of the current to go through. To do this, the doctor will attach small recording electrodes to the surface of one part of your limb, and will touch your skin at another point with a pair of electrodes delivering the shock. When this happens, you will feel a tingling sensation that may or may not be painful. Between the brief shocks, you will not feel pain. As there are several nerves in each extremity which need to be tested, the procedure is repeated 3 or 4 times or more per extremity studied. The amount of current delivered is always kept at a safe level. Patients wearing pacemakers or other electrical devices need not worry since this current will rarely interfere with such devices. During the nerve conduction study, the doctor or the technician performing the study will occasionally pause to make calculations and measurements.

The second part of the test is called needle examination and as the name implies, involves some needle sticking. The needles used are thin, fine, and about one and a quarter inches long. This part tests the muscle to see if there has been any damage to it as a result of the nerve problem, or if the disease involves the muscle itself rather than the nerve. Usually 5 to 6 muscles are sampled in one extremity, but occasionally, if you have problems in more than one area, additional muscles may need to be studied. The needle is usually inserted in the relaxed muscle and moved inside gently in order to record the muscle activity. When this is done, you will be able to hear the sound of the muscle activity amplified by the EMG machine; it will sound something like radio static. The painful part of this section is when the needle is first inserted through the skin since all of the pain receptors are located in this area. Once inside the muscle, the sensation is usually perceived as discomfort or pressure rather than pain. During the needle exam, no electrical shocks are delivered. Also, since the needle probe is used here only as a recording device, no injections are given through the needle into the muscle. On the average, a muscle can be sampled in 2 to 5 minutes though this may vary with the type of problem being investigated.

How long does an EMG take?

The nerve conduction part of the test usually takes longer than the needle exam because one needs to make calculations and measurements during it. On average, if one extremity is studied, the nerve conductions take anywhere between 15 and 30 minutes. The needle exam for one extremity usually takes 15 to 20 minutes. You can count on being in the examination room for about one hour if only one extremity is requested; longer if more extremities need to be tested.

What kind of preparations are necessary for an EMG?

Few preparations are needed on the day you have an EMG. You do not need to fast, or eat any particular kinds of food before the test. You can drive yourself to and from the test, so you do not need to bring a friend or a relative with you, any more than you would if you went to the dentist. You can count on resuming your regular activity after the test is completed. As for clothing, it is not as much what you wear as it is what you do not wear. Since in a great majority of cases the low back and buttocks area may need to be studied or in cases of neck problems, the back of the neck and shoulder areas studied, it is best not to wear clothes which will interfere with access to these areas.

With few exceptions, you may continue taking medication prescribed by your physician as ordered without this interfering with the EMG. However, if you are taking a blood thinner, you should notify the lab where your EMG is being done, since in that case the needle part of the test may cause bleeding inside the muscle. Also, if you are on any medication for Myasthenia Gravis such as Mestinon or other, your medication may interfere with the test, so you should also notify the lab. If you have any doubts about other medications you are taking, it is best to check with the lab to be on the safe side.

Can I ask for some pain medication?

Different labs have different policies about pain medication. Some physicians may recommend you take two aspirin or Tylenol before the test. Others may mail you a prescription drug to take an hour before the test. Sometimes you may be given an injection prior to the test. It is common however, that no sedation is given in any form since in most instances, patients wish to return to work or other regular activity after the test is completed. Another reason for not giving sedation is that you should always have someone accompany you to drive you home after receiving sedation and this is not always easy to arrange.

How soon will I find out the results?

Though the physician performing the test has a general idea of what the findings are during the test, the full results are only arrived at after more calculations and measurements are performed after the end of the test. The results are therefore usually not ready until later that day or even the next in complicated cases. They are usually not released directly to the patient. Instead they will be conveyed to the referring physician since he or she has to assess the results in light of the patient's other findings.

How much will an EMG cost?

As a rule the more areas you need studied, the more the test will cost. However, cost may vary from one physician to another and is different in different states. It is always best to inquire about cost with your physician.

Most insurance policies cover EMGs, though frequently the coverage is not 100% and the primary care or insurance physician will have to approve it before it can be ordered. It is best to have your doctor's office find out what kind of coverage you have for an EMG.

Chapter 19

Gene Testing

What Is Gene Testing? How Does It Work?

Gene tests (also called DNA-based tests), the newest and most sophisticated of the techniques used to test for genetic disorders, involve direct examination of the DNA molecule itself. Other genetic tests include biochemical tests for such gene products as enzymes and other proteins and for microscopic examination of stained or fluorescent chromosomes. Genetic tests are used for several reasons, including:

- carrier screening, which involves identifying unaffected individuals who carry one copy of a gene for a disease that requires two copies for the disease to be expressed,

- preimplantation genetic diagnosis,

- prenatal diagnostic testing,

- newborn screening,

- presymptomatic testing for predicting adult-onset disorders such as Huntington's disease,

- presymptomatic testing for estimating the risk of developing adult-onset cancers and Alzheimer's disease,

- confirm a diagnosis of a symptomatic individual, and

U.S. Department of Energy Human Genome Program and the Human Genome Management Information System, Oak Ridge National Laboratory, 2003. For additional information visit www.oml.gov/hgmis.

- forensic/identity testing.

In gene tests, scientists scan a patient's DNA sample for mutated sequences. A DNA sample can be obtained from any tissue, including blood. For some types of gene tests, researchers design short pieces of DNA called probes, whose sequences are complementary to the mutated sequences. These probes will seek their complement among the three billion base pairs of an individual's genome. If the mutated sequence is present in the patient's genome, the probe will bind to it and flag the mutation. Another type of DNA testing involves comparing the sequence of DNA bases in a patient's gene to a normal version of the gene. Cost of testing can range from hundreds to thousands of dollars, depending on the sizes of the genes and the numbers of mutations tested.

Screening Embryos for Disease

Preimplantation genetic diagnosis (PGD) is a test that screens for genetic flaws among embryos used in in-vitro fertilization. With PGD, DNA samples from embryos created in-vitro by the combination of a mother's egg and a father's sperm are analyzed for gene abnormalities that can cause disorders. Fertility specialists can use the results of this analysis to select only mutation-free embryos for implantation into the mother's uterus.

Before PGD, couples at higher risks for conceiving a child with a particular disorder would have to initiate the pregnancy and then undergo chorionic villus sampling in the first trimester or amniocentesis in the second trimester to test the fetus for the presence of disease. If the fetus tested positive for the disorder, the couple would be faced with the dilemma of whether or not to terminate the pregnancy.

With PGD, couples are much more likely to have healthy babies. Although PGD has been practiced for years, only a few specialized centers worldwide offer this procedure.

What Are Some of the Pros and Cons of Gene Testing?

Gene testing already has dramatically improved lives. Some tests are used to clarify a diagnosis and direct a physician toward appropriate treatments, while others allow families to avoid having children with devastating diseases or identify people at high risk for conditions that may be preventable. Aggressive monitoring for and removal of colon growths in those inheriting a gene for familial adenomatous polyposis, for example, has saved many lives. On the horizon is a gene test that will provide doctors with a simple diagnostic test for a common iron-storage disease, transforming it from a usually fatal condition to a treatable one.

Commercialized gene tests for adult-onset disorders such as Alzheimer's disease and some cancers are the subject of most of the debate over gene testing. These tests are targeted to healthy (presymptomatic) people who are identified as being at high risk because of a strong family medical history for the disorder. The tests give only a probability for developing the disorder. One of the most serious limitations of these susceptibility tests is the difficulty in interpreting a positive result because some people who carry a disease-associated mutation never develop the disease. Scientists believe that these mutations may work together with other, unknown mutations or with environmental factors to cause disease.

A limitation of all medical testing is the possibility for laboratory errors. These might be due to sample misidentification, contamination of the chemicals used for testing, or other factors. Many in the medical establishment feel that uncertainties surrounding test interpretation, the current lack of available medical options for these diseases, the tests' potential for provoking anxiety, and risks for discrimination and social stigmatization could outweigh the benefits of testing.

For What Diseases Are Gene Tests Available?

Currently, more than 900 genetic tests are available from testing laboratories. Some gene tests available in the past few years from clinical genetics laboratories are listed. Test names and a description of the diseases or symptoms are in parentheses. Susceptibility tests, noted by an asterisk, provide only an estimated risk for developing the disorder.

Some Currently Available DNA-Based Gene Tests

- Alpha-1-antitrypsin deficiency (AAT; emphysema and liver disease)

- Amyotrophic lateral sclerosis (ALS; Lou Gehrig disease; progressive motor function loss leading to paralysis and death)

- Alzheimer's disease* (APOE; late-onset variety of senile dementia)

- Ataxia telangiectasia (AT; progressive brain disorder resulting in loss of muscle control and cancers)

183

- Gaucher disease (GD; enlarged liver and spleen, bone degeneration)

- Inherited breast and ovarian cancer* (BRCA 1 and 2; early-onset tumors of breasts and ovaries)

- Hereditary nonpolyposis colon cancer* (CA; early-onset tumors of colon and sometimes other organs)

- Charcot-Marie-Tooth (CMT; loss of feeling in ends of limbs)

- Congenital adrenal hyperplasia (CAH; hormone deficiency; ambiguous genitalia and male pseudohermaphroditism)

- Cystic fibrosis (CF; disease of lung and pancreas resulting in thick mucous accumulations and chronic infections)

- Duchenne muscular dystrophy/Becker muscular dystrophy (DMD; severe to mild muscle wasting, deterioration, weakness)

- Dystonia (DYT; muscle rigidity, repetitive twisting movements)

- Fanconi anemia, group C (FA; anemia, leukemia, skeletal deformities)

- Factor V-Leiden (FVL; blood-clotting disorder)

- Fragile X syndrome (FRAX; leading cause of inherited mental retardation)

- Hemophilia A and B (HEMA and HEMB; bleeding disorders)

- Hereditary hemochromatosis (HFE; excess iron storage disorder)

- Huntington's disease (HD; usually midlife onset; progressive, lethal, degenerative neurological disease)

- Myotonic dystrophy (MD; progressive muscle weakness; most common form of adult muscular dystrophy)

- Neurofibromatosis type 1 (NF1; multiple benign nervous system tumors that can be disfiguring; cancers)

- Phenylketonuria (PKU; progressive mental retardation due to missing enzyme; correctable by diet)

- Adult polycystic kidney disease (APKD; kidney failure and liver disease)

- Prader Willi/Angelman syndromes (PW/A; decreased motor skills, cognitive impairment, early death)

- Sickle cell disease (SS; blood cell disorder; chronic pain and infections)

- Spinocerebellar ataxia, type 1 (SCA1; involuntary muscle movements, reflex disorders, explosive speech)

- Spinal muscular atrophy (SMA; severe, usually lethal progressive muscle-wasting disorder in children)

- Thalassemias (THAL; anemias—reduced red blood cell levels)

- Tay-Sachs disease (TS; fatal neurological disease of early childhood; seizures, paralysis)

Is Genetic Testing Regulated?

Currently in the United States, no regulations are in place for evaluating the accuracy and reliability of genetic testing. Most genetic tests developed by laboratories are categorized as services, which the Food and Drug Administration (FDA) does not regulate. Only a few states have established some regulatory guidelines. This lack of government oversight is particularly troublesome in light of the fact that a handful of companies have started marketing test kits directly to the public. Some of these companies make dubious claims about how the kits not only test for disease, but also serve as tools for customizing medicine, vitamins, and foods to each individual's genetic makeup. Another fear is that individuals who purchase such kits will not seek out genetic counseling to help them interpret results and make the best possible decisions regarding their personal welfare.

Does Insurance Cover Genetic Testing?

In most cases, an individual will have to contact his or her insurance provider to see if genetic tests, which cost between $200 and $3000, are covered. Usually insurance companies do not cover genetic tests, those that do will have access to the results. Insured persons would need to decide whether they would want the insurance company to have this information. States have a patchwork of genetic-information nondiscrimination laws, none of them comprehensive. Existing state laws differ in coverage, protections afforded, and enforcement schemes. The National Conference of State Legislatures provides a listing of current legislation regarding genetic information and health insurance. The recent marketing of genetic test kits directly to consumers, may lead to an increase in demand for insurance coverage.

Additional Information

Gene Tests
Children's Hospital and Regional Medical Center
P.O. Box 5371
4800 Sand Point Way N.E.
Seattle, WA 98105-3594
Phone: 206-524-6398
Fax: 206-522-3594
Website: http://www.genetests.org
E-mail: genetests@genetests.org

Quackwatch
Website: http://www.quackwatch.org/index.html

More information on questionable test kits is available from Dubious Genetic Testing, an online report provided by Quackwatch.

Part Five

Treatment and Management of Muscular Dystrophies and Related Concerns

Chapter 20

Osteoporosis: A Serious, but Manageable Effect of Muscular Dystrophy

A 27-year-old woman with limb-girdle muscular dystrophy breaks a hip after tripping over a pair of shoes and falling onto a carpeted floor.

A 6-year-old boy with Duchenne muscular dystrophy is found to have low bone density while undergoing routine testing to enter a clinical trial.

A middle-aged woman who's been taking medication for an inflammatory myopathy for many years steps off a curb and fractures her ankle.

In addition to having neuromuscular disorders, these three people have something else in common: osteoporosis (OP), an invisible, progressive loss of bone that, if left untreated, can lead to further disability.

Although OP is not rare in people with neuromuscular disorders, especially if they are taking certain medications; it is one of the more treatable—and even preventable—complications of these conditions. Unfortunately, some people have misconceptions about what OP is and what can and cannot be done about it. Getting the facts is the first step in solving most problems, and OP is no exception.

Reprinted from "Sticks and Stones Break Fragile Bones" by Margaret Wahl, *QUEST*, Volume 8, Number 6, December 2001. Reprinted with permission from the Muscular Dystrophy Association, www.mdausa.org. © The Muscular Dystrophy Association. For additional information, call the Muscular Dystrophy Association National Headquarters toll-free at (800) 572-1717. To find an MDA office in your area, look in your local telephone book, or click on "Clinic and Services" on the MDA website.

Myth: Osteoporosis means a curved back or dowager's hump.

Fact: The hump on the backs of many elderly women and some elderly men is the result of OP, but is not the disorder itself.

The curved back that sometimes goes along with OP results from the destruction of the vertebrae in the spine, as they thin and collapse, tipping the spine forward. The word osteoporosis comes from two Greek words meaning *passages in bones*, a fairly accurate description of what happens in the disorder as the framework inside bones is gradually eaten away. The process leaves gaps in the structure that weaken it, allows fractures to occur with little force, and changes the shape of the vertebrae.

Two kinds of cells are always at work in bones—the osteoblasts, the bones' construction crew, which works to lay down new bone; and the osteoclasts, the demolition crew, which works in the opposite direction, to destroy old bone. Osteoporosis happens when the demolition cells get ahead of the construction cells, which can occur for a variety of reasons.

As bone weakens under the influence of the demolition cells, fractures occur. Hot spots for fractures are the wrists, hips, and vertebrae.

Myth: Osteoporosis only affects elderly women.

Fact: Osteoporosis can affect people of both sexes and all ages. Major risk factors for people with neuromuscular disorders include prolonged lack of weight-bearing exercise and taking corticosteroid medications. These are added to the usual risk factors, such as menopause and aging.

Don't Like Milk?

There are a lot of high-calcium choices.

1. Calcium-fortified orange juice, 1 cup, 350 milligrams (mg) calcium.

2. Cheddar cheese, 1 ounce, 204 mg calcium.

3. Low-fat yogurt with fruit, 1 cup, 345 mg calcium; 6 ounces, 259 mg calcium.

4. Nonfat (skim) milk, 1 cup, 302 mg calcium; low-fat (1 percent fat) milk, 1 cup, 300 mg calcium.

5. Canned salmon with bones, 3 ounces, 167 mg calcium.

6. Vanilla ice cream, 1 cup, 176 mg calcium.

7. Kale, cooked from raw and drained, 1 cup, 94 mg calcium.

8. Turnip greens, cooked from raw and drained, 1 cup, 197 mg calcium.

9. Collard greens, cooked from raw and drained, 1 cup, 148 mg calcium.

10. Broccoli, cooked from raw and drained, 1 cup, 177 mg calcium.

Menopause

We think of middle-aged and elderly women as the prime candidates for osteoporosis, and this is certainly true in the general population—although beyond about age 65, OP affects both sexes. Women in their late 40s to early 60s, unless they take preventive steps, usually develop OP associated with menopause. (African-American women, for reasons that are not completely understood, have an advantage over white women when it comes to OP associated with menopause. The extent to which this advantage persists in other bone-destructive situations is not clear.)

For those with neuromuscular disorders, aging adds another OP risk factor. At menopause, the production by the ovaries of a group of female hormones known as estrogens (usually just called estrogen) and another group, the progestins (usually referred to by the main one, progesterone), ceases. It is the lack of estrogen at menopause that tips the balance of bone building and bone destruction toward the latter. When women with neuromuscular disorders experience menopause, this risk factor for OP is added to other factors they may already have.

Aging

Aging itself seems to contribute to OP in both sexes beginning in the late 60s. Complex biochemical processes again tip the balance toward bone destruction. For those with neuromuscular disorders, aging adds another OP risk factor.

Lack of Weight Bearing

Weight-bearing exercise—specifically, standing, walking, running, jumping, and probably lifting—puts stress on the bones that helps them stay strong. For those whose muscle weakness has greatly limited these activities, OP is always a risk. Standing, even while leaning on something, such as a walker, can help slow the course of bone loss.

Corticosteroid Drugs

Of all the risks for OP to which people with neuromuscular disorders are exposed, taking corticosteroid medications is perhaps the most serious.

These drugs have names like prednisone (brand names Deltasone, Orasone, and others); prednisolone (Prelone); dexamethasone (Decadron); deflazacort (Calcort); and triamcinolone (Aristocort). They are used to treat inflammatory myopathies, such as polymyositis, dermatomyositis, and sometimes inclusion-body myositis; myasthenia gravis and Lambert-Eaton myasthenic syndrome; and often Duchenne muscular dystrophy.

"With patients on prednisone [probably the most commonly prescribed oral corticosteroid in the United States], osteoporosis is a huge problem," says neurologist Richard Barohn, who treats patients at the MDA clinic at the University of Kansas Medical Center in Kansas City, Kansas. If steps are not taken to prevent bone loss, Barohn says, fractured vertebrae are too often the result.

"Every time I put a patient on prednisone, I put them on a prophylactic regimen for osteoporosis," he says. "Prednisone is a great drug for some of these diseases. It is still the best drug we have, and it works more quickly than other drugs, but it has so many side effects. Doctors using prednisone have to become experts on the side effects, because they are putting patients at risk."

Duchenne Muscular Dystrophy

Until recently, most doctors did not think diseases of the nerves or muscles directly caused bone loss, assuming that OP associated with these disorders came from immobility or drug treatment. But now, says Richard Henderson, a pediatric orthopedist at the University of North Carolina School of Medicine in Chapel Hill, that concept has been challenged. In a recent study conducted at Henderson's medical center, boys with DMD who were still active and not on corticosteroids were found to have low density in their thigh bones, despite predictions to the contrary.

"What we expected to find was that bone density would be good early on and then would drop when they stopped walking," Henderson says. "But that's not really what we found. When we looked at bone density, it was already very poor when the children were still walking and playing, and then it went down from there." Bone density in the femur (thigh bone) was low long before immobility became a factor.

Henderson's group found that bone density in the lumbar (lower) spine was (as expected) normal during the children's active years and then deteriorated as they became less mobile. The surprise was that bone density in the femur (thigh bone) was low long before lack of mobility became a factor.

"What it tells me is that poor bone in Duchenne dystrophy is not as simple as lack of weight bearing," says Henderson, who plans to do further studies on these findings.

Myth: If you don't have any symptoms, and x-rays show normal bones, you probably do not have to worry about osteoporosis.

Fact: By the time osteoporosis is visible on an ordinary x-ray, the problem is well advanced. Better tests are now available to detect OP earlier, when treatment can make a real difference. There are few warning signs of osteoporosis, other than broken bones or collapsed vertebrae, which occur when bone loss is well advanced.

OP does not usually hurt, although chronic back pain can be a warning sign that vertebrae are collapsing from within.

Ordinary x-rays usually are not reliable indicators of bone density, but other tests, which are often covered by insurance, are much better. The standard test for OP now is the dual-energy x-ray absorptiometry test, or DEXA, which is painless and noninvasive and scans the body at the hip or lumbar spine. It is usually done in the radiology department of a hospital or in a specialized clinic.

Newer tests use ultrasound (sound waves) to measure bone density at the heel. The device for the heel test is small and portable and fits nicely into a doctor's office or clinic, so these tests are gaining in popularity. Whether they will prove to be as reliable as the DEXA scan remains to be seen.

Myth: You cannot do anything about osteoporosis.

Fact: There is a great deal you can do to treat or prevent OP, ranging from dietary changes and adapted exercises to new, highly effective medications.

Calcium and Vitamin D

A first step in preventing or treating OP is a dietary evaluation to see whether you are taking in enough calcium and vitamin D. A dietitian or nutritionist associated with an MDA clinic can help with this.

People usually get enough vitamin D, which is needed to absorb calcium from the intestines into the bones and to prevent excess excretion of it in the urine. Our bodies manufacture it from a previtamin hormone that, when exposed to sunlight through the skin, makes vitamin D. The vitamin is also added to almost all milk sold in the United States, and to other products, including some cereals.

The National Academy of Sciences, through its National Institute of Medicine/Food and Nutrition Board, recommends that children and young adults take in 200 international units (IU) of vitamin D per day; adults age 51 and older, 400 IU; and adults 71 and older, 600 IU. Most people can meet this standard. But residents of sunlight-poor areas, and people who keep their bodies completely covered at all times (for example, for religious reasons), or who almost never go outside, are at risk of vitamin D deficiency, as are people taking corticosteroids.

Many diets do not provide enough calcium to prevent OP, especially for people who are on corticosteroids. However, the vitamin is easily taken as a supplement in a variety of preparations. In fact, most major calcium preparations on the market are now sold either with or without added vitamin D.

Dietary calcium deficiency, by contrast, is a common problem. The academy says an adequate intake of calcium for adults is 1,000 to 1,200 milligrams a day; for children and teens ages 9 to 18, 1,300 milligrams; for children ages 4 to 8, it is 800 milligrams. Some experts recommend an intake of 1,500 milligrams a day for men and women over 65 and for postmenopausal women after age 50 who are not taking estrogen.

These guidelines are not so easy to meet. Many diets do not provide enough calcium to prevent OP, especially for people who are on corticosteroids or have other risk factors. There are plenty of supplements to choose from, but it is also possible (and, some say, preferable) to increase calcium intake through the diet. Many types of calcium supplements, some with added vitamin D, are sold over the counter. Ask your doctor, nutritionist, and digestive system what works best for you.

"The first thing is to point out how to increase the dietary intake of foods high in calcium," says registered dietitian Judith Trautlein, a nutritionist at Children's Clinics for Rehabilitative Services in Tucson, Arizona, where she sees many children with neuromuscular disorders. About risk factors for OP, Trautlein says, "When they're not weight bearing, that's a big one. The other thing is, once they're in a wheelchair, calorie needs go down, so it's harder to get all the nutrients you need in your diet. A lot of times they want to eat plenty, but to keep their weight under control, they can't." It's hard enough to get adequate calcium when calories are plentiful, Trautlein says, but when calories are severely restricted to avoid weight gain, getting calcium from the diet can be a real problem.

Then, too, not everybody likes calcium-rich foods. "Some kids are really into milk, so it's not a problem," Trautlein says. "But once they're in their teenage years, very often they'd rather have soda. Some eat yogurt, but not very many."

That's where supplements come in. "We use Tums a lot," she says. "They're cheap, and kids will chew Tums. They come in mint and fruit flavors. But they're not the best absorbed. Calcium citrate gives the best absorption."

When calories are severely restricted to avoid weight gain, getting calcium from the diet can be a real problem. Neurologist Richard Barohn routinely prescribes vitamin D and calcium for patients taking corticosteroids. "Everybody on prednisone gets supplemental calcium, either calcium citrate or calcium carbonate," he says. "Calcium citrate is a little better absorbed. Those are over the counter. "Then I put patients on an additional tablet that's a vitamin D supplement. It's usually not enough to put them on calcium tablets with vitamin D. It's not enough if you're on prednisone. You have to use a separate vitamin D pill."

He often prescribes calcifediol (Calderol), an activated form of vitamin D that is available by prescription. This compound has gone through additional chemical processing during its manufacture that allows the body to use it more quickly and easily. When other drugs for OP are prescribed, calcium and sometimes vitamin D are usually recommended, too.

Hormones and Related Drugs

Until recently, most women experiencing menopause-related problems, including bone loss, were reassured by their doctors that taking hormones to replace those that were lost was a safe and reliable strategy. But new evidence has shown that taking estrogens alone increases the risk of cancer of the lining of the uterus (endometrial cancer), and taking estrogen in combination with a progestin greatly reduces that risk. For women who have had a hysterectomy, the progestin is not necessary.

However, even more recent evidence complicates the picture. Estrogen taken alone poses a small increase in a woman's risk of breast cancer, but estrogen taken with a progestin—the combination prescribed to reduce the risk of endometrial cancer—significantly increases a woman's risk of developing breast cancer. At this time, the solution to postmenopausal therapy in general is still uncertain. Postmenopausal women with neuromuscular diseases should discuss all risk factors with their doctors before deciding on a course.

There are dozens of hormone replacement preparations on the market. Fortunately, when it comes to treating and preventing osteoporosis, there are an increasing number of choices in addition to hormone therapy with estrogens and progestins.

A new class of medications called selective estrogen receptor modulators, or SERMs, has been developed to act the way estrogen does with respect to bone, but not to have estrogen-like effects on other tissues, such as the breasts or uterus. The drug raloxifene (brand name Evista) is a SERM that is on the market to prevent and treat osteoporosis in women past menopause. It has to be taken with adequate amounts of calcium and vitamin D. For men with low testosterone, replacement preparations of this hormone can be prescribed to treat or prevent osteoporosis.

Another medication that is technically a hormone, but is not a sex hormone is calcitonin (Miacalcin). The calcitonin that is marketed for osteoporosis treatment (but not prevention) is derived from salmon. It interferes with the work of osteoclasts, the cells that break down bone.

Bisphosphonates

A new class of medications called bisphosphonates shows great promise in preventing and treating OP. These medications actually become part of the bone tissue and in so doing interfere with the efforts of the osteoclasts to break down bone. Alendronate (Fosamax) and risedronate (Actonel) are examples of bisphosphonates that have U.S. Food and Drug Administration approval to treat and prevent postmenopausal osteoporosis, and to treat osteoporosis in patients taking corticosteroid medications.

One problem with these drugs is that they can severely irritate the esophagus, the tube that goes from the mouth to the stomach. To minimize this risk, the drugs have to be taken in an upright position (sitting or standing), and the person taking them has to remain sitting or standing for at least 30 minutes. They cannot be taken by people who have trouble swallowing or who cannot remain in a sitting or standing position for at least 30 minutes.

Despite these concerns, these drugs show great promise in treating osteoporosis without the use of hormones. "These drugs work," says Chester Oddis, a rheumatologist at the University of Pittsburgh who treats patients with inflammatory myopathies, which often require corticosteroids. "Steroid therapy weakens the framework [of bone]," Oddis says. "It reduces new bone formation, increases bone loss, and decreases calcium absorption—everything you don't want." Oddis likes to start treating patients with a bisphosphonate early in their corticosteroid therapy course.

"With many patients, if they're young and starting on steroids, I give them 70 milligrams of Fosamax once a week or 5 milligrams a day. I'm treating them earlier than I did before." He says he thinks he is seeing fewer bone fractures in these patients, but he does not yet have the data to prove it.

Myth: If you cannot do strenuous, weight-bearing exercise, you might as well forget about trying to exercise to prevent osteoporosis.

Fact: Standing a few times a day, even while leaning on something, provides bones with at least some stress that is probably helpful.

"Weight bearing generally means standing up," says Robert McMichael, a neurologist and MDA clinic director in Arlington, Texas, who has limb-girdle muscular dystrophy and occasionally uses a wheelchair. Not standing or bearing weight is a risk factor for osteoporosis, McMichael says. "When you put stress on the long bones by standing, that helps to maintain their strength." McMichael does not see many arm fractures in his neuromuscular disease patients and suspects that daily arm use may be adequate to prevent these.

"Some people can't walk, but can stay supported on a piece of furniture," McMichael says. "Some people get a standing frame to stand in, and that's good, too."

McMichael is all for standing and weight bearing where practical, but he doesn't think people should become fanatical about it when weakness prevents much exercise. Medications, he says, can compensate for lack of weight bearing when it comes to osteoporosis.

Carol Marulic, a physical therapist at University of Arizona Medical Center in Tucson, who has had a long association with the MDA clinic there, says weight-bearing activities help strengthen bones. But compromises and alternatives to full weight bearing also help bones stay strong.

For those unable to stand independently, leaning on something, such as a kitchen counter or walker, can help put pressure on joints in the spine, legs, and arms. Being on the hands and knees can also put some pressure on the bones in a way that strengthens them.

Table 20.1. Drugs to Prevent or Treat Osteoporosis (continued on next page)

Drug or Supplement: Generic Name (Brand Name)	How It Works
Calcium (Tums, Os-Cal, Citracal, CalBurst, others)	Calcium can be used by the body to build bone.
Vitamin D; also called ergocalciferol and cholecalciferol	Vitamin D helps the body absorb calcium from intestines and prevents its excessive excretion in urine.
Activated forms of vitamin D, such as calcitriol (Rocaltrol) and calcifediol (Calderol)	Vitamin D has to be activated by enzymes in the liver and kidneys. Some experts believe the activated forms may be better than "plain" vitamin D.
Combined calcium and Vitamin D (Citracal + D, Os-Cal 500 + D, others)	Vitamin D is often combined with calcium because it helps with the absorption of calcium and prevents excessive excretion of the mineral.
Estrogens (Cenestin, Estinyl, Estrace, Premarin, and others are pills; Alora, Estraderm, FemPatch, and others are patches applied to the skin; Estrace and others are skin creams; and Estring is a vaginal ring)	Estrogens help to keep bone destruction from outpacing bone formation.
Progestins (Amen, Cycrin, Prometrium and Provera are pills or capsules; Crinone is a vaginal gel)	Adding a progestin to estrogen protects against the development of cancer of the endometrium (uterine lining).

Even standing and exercising in a pool, although it doesn't allow for as much weight bearing as being on land, is better than nothing, Marulic says. "For those who are somewhat unstable on their feet, it's a great way to exercise," Marulic says. "This still allows the weight bearing but in a safer medium."

If weakness prevents much exertion of any kind, Marulic recommends passive exercise—in which the work is performed by another person. A therapist or other helper (after being instructed by a professional) can apply intermittent, gentle pressure to compress joints and simulate weight bearing.

Table 20.1. Drugs to Prevent or Treat Osteoporosis (continued from previous page)

Drug or Supplement: Generic Name (Brand Name)	How It Works
Combinations of estrogens and progestins (Estratest, FemHRT, and others are pills; CombiPatch is a skin patch)	Adding a progestin to estrogen protects against development of cancer of the endometrium.
Raloxifene (Evista)	Raloxifene, a selective estrogen receptor modulator, or SERM, is used by post-menopausal women because it has positive effects on bone with minimal effects on the breasts or uterus.
Testosterone (Androderm, Testoderm skin patches)	Testosterone is a male hormone that works to build and maintain bone in men much the way estrogen does in women.
Calcitonin (Miacalcin, others)	Calcitonin is a hormone derived from salmon that is similar to a hormone made in the human thyroid gland. Calcitonin impairs the activity of the bone-destroying osteoclasts. It is usually taken as a nasal spray but can also be given by injection.
Alendronate (Fosamax)	Alendronate is a bisphosphonate that interferes with the activity of osteoclasts, the bone-destroying cells.
Risedronate (Actonel)	Risedronate is a bisphosphonate that interferes with the activity of osteoclasts, the bone-destroying cells.

Additional Information

National Osteoporosis Foundation
1232 22nd Street N.W.
Washington, DC 20037-1292
Phone: 202-223-2226
Website: http://www.nof.org
E-mail: communications@nof.org

Chapter 21

The Heart Is a Muscle, Too: Cardiac Problems in Muscular Diseases

Cardiac problems are common in several neuromuscular disorders. They can be quite serious, particularly in Duchenne and Becker muscular dystrophy (DMD and BMD).

The heart has an electrical system and a mechanical (muscular) system. When electrical impulses travel, they cause heart muscle cells to contract rhythmically. When something goes wrong with these electrical impulses, the result is an arrhythmia, an irregularity in the heart's pacing system. When something goes wrong with the muscle layer of the heart, the result is a cardiomyopathy, a problem with the heart's mechanical pump.

Which neuromuscular disorders involve the heart?

The heart is a muscle that responds to the nervous system and contains special nerve-like tissue, so it is not surprising that it is affected in many neuromuscular disorders. What actually is surprising is that there are some disorders in which the heart is not affected, and that there is a lot of variation in the type and degree of cardiac involvement in the same disease.

Reprinted from "The Heart is a Muscle, Too—Frequently Asked Questions about Cardiac Problems," by Margaret Wahl, *QUEST*, Volume 6, Number 2, April 1999. Reprinted with permission from the Muscular Dystrophy Association, www.mdausa.org. © The Muscular Dystrophy Association. For additional information, call the Muscular Dystrophy Association National Headquarters toll-free at (800) 572-1717. To find an MDA office in your area, look in your local telephone book, or click on "Clinic and Services" on the MDA website.

Heart problems have been reported in nearly all the neuromuscular disorders, but they are much more common and severe in some of these than in others. Most muscular dystrophies can involve the heart, but heart problems of one type are particularly common and serious in Duchenne and Becker MD, while problems of another type are common and serious in myotonic (MMD) and Emery-Dreifuss (EDMD) MD. Heart complications are not common in limb-girdle MD (LGMD), facioscapulohumeral MD, or congenital MD, although there are reports of them in all of these conditions in some patients.

Diseases that primarily involve the nervous system or the neuromuscular junction are not likely to involve the heart. Heart complications are rare, for example, in spinal muscular atrophy and amyotrophic lateral sclerosis and in myasthenias. However, Friedreich's ataxia (FRDA), a disease that mostly affects peripheral nerves, is a notable exception, where heart problems are common and can be serious.

Heart complications occur in various other types of neuromuscular disorders, such as the metabolic muscle disorders, and they are sometimes seen in inflammatory myopathies (polymyositis and dermatomyositis). They have been reported in central core disease and occasionally in periodic paralysis.

What actually happens to the heart in neuromuscular disorders? Are the problems the same as heart problems in general?

Most of the heart disease we hear about in the newspaper or on television is a type of heart problem known as coronary artery disease, a plugging of the blood vessels that supply the heart. This is the kind of problem that appears to result from a diet rich in fat and calories, being overweight, being sedentary, and smoking (although it is possible to have coronary artery disease in the absence of these risk factors). It is the type of heart disease most often associated with heart attack, a total blocking of one or more of these vessels.

People with neuromuscular disorders are in no way immune to coronary artery disease, or to any other common ailment of modern life. However, coronary artery disease is not the problem most often associated with neuromuscular disorders.

Two types of heart problems are closely associated with various neuromuscular disorders. They are cardiomyopathy, a problem with the muscle layer of the heart, and cardiac arrhythmias, abnormalities in the electrical pacing system of the heart. (It may sound strange to talk about the heart having an electrical system, but it does. Electricity is a form of energy that results from the interaction of charged particles. It is the same energy, whether in a biological or man-made system.)

Cardiomyopathy, the heart muscle problem, is the kind of abnormality most often seen in DMD and BMD, while arrhythmias, the pacing system problems, are the ones more commonly seen in myotonic and Emery-Dreifuss MD. When there are heart complications in other forms of MD, the main problem is usually cardiomyopathy, although arrhythmias can also occur. Both cardiomyopathy and arrhythmias occur often in metabolic muscle disorders. In FRDA, both types of problem are also common.

Cardiomyopathy and cardiac arrhythmias are common disorders in the general population (though not as common as coronary artery disease), and cardiologists are familiar with them. Their diagnosis and treatment are not markedly different when the underlying cause is a neuromuscular disease. However, the patient's ability to exercise, his respiratory status, and the possible effects of cardiac drugs on other muscles (particularly the respiratory ones) must be taken into account by the cardiologist when there is a neuromuscular disorder in addition to the cardiac problem.

What actually causes cardiomyopathy in MD?

The primary cause of cardiomyopathy in DMD and BMD is probably a lack of the protein dystrophin, the same protein deficiency that exists in the skeletal muscles and leads to generalized weakness, wasting, and respiratory complications. Dystrophin is also needed by cardiac muscle, and its lack (complete in DMD and partial in BMD) probably leads to the loss of cardiac muscle cells under the stress of constant contraction.

When heart problems do occur in other forms of MD, such as LGMD or congenital, it is likely that the underlying cause is also a lack of a muscle protein. For example, in four forms of LGMD the sarcoglycan proteins are known to lie near dystrophin in the muscle cell membrane, and their absence could be a factor in any heart problem in those disorders.

But the story is a little more complicated. For instance, most people with DMD and BMD have heart involvement, but some do not. And, in the sarcoglycan-deficient forms of LGMD, heart involvement is unusual, despite the probable role of the sarcoglycan in heart muscle.

The answers to these puzzles may lie in the heart muscle's differences from skeletal muscle. Heart muscle has a slightly different structure, and its proteins often come in a slightly different form from their cousins in skeletal muscle. These slightly differing proteins, known as isoforms, come from the same gene. (Each gene is a recipe for a protein.) Some genetic mutations, such as those in Duchenne, Becker, and limb-girdle MD, probably have a preference for the skeletal or cardiac form of the protein, leading to more or less heart involvement.

Then, too, protein deficiencies are probably not the whole story in cardiac dysfunction in neuromuscular disease. For example, blood flow through the tissues and the return of blood to the heart are compromised in a person who cannot exercise, so varying exercise capabilities may also be a factor in the degree of cardiac involvement.

What happens to someone with cardiomyopathy?

Cardiomyopathy (something wrong with the muscle layer, or myocardium, of the heart), usually takes one of two forms.

In one form, a portion of the heart muscle enlarges, a condition known as hypertrophic cardiomyopathy. As the heart muscle wall enlarges and overgrows, the heart itself may be slightly enlarged, but the main pumping chambers—the ventricles—have less room to fill with blood because of the thickened muscle layer. If the thickened part includes the divider between the ventricles (septum), ejection of blood from the heart to the rest of the body can be impaired.

In the second form, dilated cardiomyopathy, the myocardium dilates and expands. The ventricles thin out and become floppy. The heart is enlarged, sometimes markedly, but its function is compromised by the abnormal, thinned muscle layer. In some people, hypertrophic cardiomyopathy becomes dilated cardiomyopathy after a time.

In either type of cardiomyopathy, if the problem is bad enough, a condition known as heart failure (also sometimes called congestive heart failure) is the end result. Heart failure can develop quickly, but more often, it develops gradually, over several years.

What is heart failure?

The term heart failure sounds scary, and it is in fact a very serious disorder. However, heart failure does not mean that the heart stops. It means that the heart can no longer meet the demands of the body's tissues for blood and its nutrients—mainly, oxygen. Heart failure can be treated and its progress slowed with medications and other approaches. In some people with severe heart failure, however, only a heart transplant can permit survival.

Are there degrees of heart failure?

Yes. Heart failure can be mild, moderate, or severe and can change over time. There are many different causes of heart failure, muscular dystrophy being only one of many, but the results and the progression are generally the same.

What does a person experience as the heart fails?

The heart has enormous reserves of energy, so that, even under adverse conditions, such as a weakening muscle structure, it can usually adapt and keep up an adequate blood supply to the body for some time, often years. By the time symptoms start to show up, usually quite a bit of damage has already occurred.

In a person who is not exercising, such as an older boy with DMD, there may be no symptoms that would indicate heart failure until the problem is quite far advanced. The heart problems can, however, be detected with diagnostic tests.

In someone who is able to exercise, symptoms of heart failure are likely to occur as he exerts himself. He is likely to feel short of breath and fatigued with exertion. (An often used medical term for this shortness of breath is dyspnea.) These symptoms arise because, when the blood's pump begins to fail, the body's tissues do not receive enough blood to support the demands of exercise, particularly with respect to oxygen.

Later, as the heart fails further, dyspnea will occur even at rest, because the blood supply to the tissues becomes inadequate even under these circumstances. Usually, heart failure is quite advanced by the time dyspnea at rest is detected.

As heart failure progresses, blood backs up behind the failing ventricle, just as fluid backs up behind any pump that is not moving it forward. Usually, the left ventricle fails first. Blood normally returns to the left ventricle after picking up oxygen and dropping off carbon dioxide in the lungs. If the left ventricle is not pumping normally, blood begins to accumulate in the large veins that lead back from the lungs to the heart (pulmonary veins).

Blood pressure rises in the pulmonary blood vessels, and fluid (mostly water) starts to leak out across the small capillaries that supply the lung tissue. Fluid begins to build up in the air sacs of the lung, a serious condition known as pulmonary edema. Breathing can become difficult, especially when the person lies down. He may develop a cough, sometimes tinged with slightly bloody (pink) sputum.

205

The right ventricle can also fail, especially if the left ventricle is already weakened, causing more stress on the right side. Blood returning to the right ventricle comes from the general circulation via two major veins that return blood to the right side of the heart. If the right ventricle is too weak to pump the blood forward into the lungs, or if pressures in the pulmonary vessels are too high for it to push against, blood will start to back up as it enters the right side of the heart. As this blood accumulates, it raises blood pressure in the general circulation. Eventually, pressure builds in the capillaries of the general circulation, and fluid starts to leak out across the capillary walls into the tissues.

The person with right heart failure starts to show edema (swelling, or fluid retention) in the parts of the body that are most affected by gravity. So, if he's standing or sitting most of the time, the ankles and feet will show the most edema. The first inkling of the problem may be that the shoes or socks are too tight. If he's lying down, the area around the lower spine may be most affected.

As right heart failure progresses, generalized edema may occur, including fluid retention in the abdominal organs, with abdominal distention and possibly nausea and vomiting. The person with generalized edema gains weight and finds his clothes and rings are too tight. At night, if he tries to lie flat, fluid from the periphery of the body will move by gravity to the lungs, compounding any pulmonary edema that is already there and causing an urgent sensation of needing to sit upright.

Fortunately, all these symptoms can be controlled, at least for a long time, with medications and other treatments.

Why does heart failure get worse?

Heart failure almost always worsens over time, partly because of progressive deterioration in the myocardium (particularly true in muscular dystrophy), but also, ironically, because of the body's misguided attempts to remedy the situation.

As the myocardium weakens and blood flow to the tissues decreases, the body's strategically placed pressure sensors send out urgent signals to the nervous system and kidneys indicating that pressure is down. The nervous system sends out chemicals that constrict blood vessels, raise blood pressure, and make the heart beat harder and faster. At the same time, the kidneys hold onto sodium and water to increase the amount of fluid in the blood.

If the reason for the pressure drop sensed by the body were a leak—say, from a stab wound—it is easy to see that all these measures would probably help. In a person who is hemorrhaging, raising pressure, increasing the heart's rate and force, and holding onto as much fluid as possible would help preserve blood flow to vital organs.

Unfortunately, if a failing pump is the reason for a pressure drop, then all these measures are actually harmful. They only worsen matters by placing more stress on the already weakened myocardium, which now has to work against higher resistance and a higher fluid load.

So far, medicine has little to offer that directly repairs the failing myocardium. However, there are many treatments that reduce the strain on the heart and preserve its function for a long time. Most of them are aimed at counteracting the body's misguided response to cardiomyopathy and heart failure.

What are some treatments for heart failure?

Today, doctors have a wide range of treatments to choose from. The precise combination of drug and nondrug therapies will depend on the symptoms, the underlying cause of the symptoms and the stage of heart failure being treated.

In the past, much therapy relied on resting the patient (advising against exercise) and boosting the heart's activity with medication. Today that thinking has nearly reversed. There is less emphasis on resting the whole patient and more on specifically allowing the heart to rest, or at least to work with greater ease.

Mild, regular exercise is usually encouraged, if it is possible (which it may not be in some types of neuromuscular disease). And instead of giving drugs that increase the heart's contractile force, doctors are more likely to prescribe those that reduce the heart's work and allow it to rest.

Common treatments include:

Nondrug Treatments

Low-sodium diet. If fluid overload is a problem, a diet low in sodium may be prescribed. The usual recommendation is a daily intake of 2 to 4 grams of sodium (2,000 to 4,000 milligrams). You will have to read labels on prepared foods and avoid adding salt in cooking or at the table.

Mild exercise. Exercise is not always possible in neuromuscular disease, but if it is, it is often recommended. Walking, swimming, or using a stationary bicycle may be recommended by your doctor. If active exercise is not possible, your doctor may suggest passive exercise in the form of physical therapy. Strenuous exercise is usually best avoided, and swimming should not be done alone.

Assisted ventilation. When blood oxygen levels are low, the heart has to work harder to get the same amount of oxygen to the tissues. (This is why the heart works harder at high altitudes, where atmospheric oxygen is low and leads to low blood oxygen levels.) Low blood oxygen levels also lead to high blood pressure in the pulmonary circulation.

In many types of advanced neuromuscular disease, respiratory muscle weakness leads to low blood oxygen, placing an additional strain on the heart. Assisted ventilation—the use of mechanical devices to help failing respiratory muscles move air in and out of the lungs—can be a crucial intervention that can boost blood oxygen levels, ease breathing, and help the heart work better. Ask your doctor about these devices.

Oxygen therapy. In some cases, the doctor may prescribe supplemental oxygen to ease the heart's workload. This has to be done with extreme care in patients with neuromuscular diseases in whom the respiratory system is impaired, because giving oxygen can complicate matters. Good communication between the pulmonary specialist and the cardiologist is important.

Drug Treatments

Easing the heart's burden. The drugs most often used today are those that reduce blood pressure (and therefore the resistance against which the heart has to pump), reduce the fluid content of the blood (reducing volume and pressure), and counteract those influences of the nervous system that raise blood pressure and increase the heart's rate and force.

Increasing force. Drugs that increase the heart's contractile force are also sometimes used, but with extreme care, as they can have dangerous effects.

Drug interactions and anesthesia pose risks. All these drugs can have their actions interfered with or occasionally increased by other medications, including many over-the-counter remedies for such things as colds and diarrhea, so the cardiologist should be kept aware of any other medications being used or considered. Anesthesia can also be a problem, because of potential chemical interactions, and also because of the underlying heart problem itself.

Be sure your cardiologist and surgeon communicate with each other if any surgery is planned. You may wish to wear a MedicAlert tag or bracelet explaining your condition. These become especially important in case of accident or unplanned hospital admission.

Surgical Treatments

Heart transplants. Heart transplants are by no means routine, but they are becoming increasingly common as a treatment for heart failure when other measures have failed. Transplants have saved the lives of several young men with Becker MD, in whom the skeletal muscle weakness (including respiratory weakness) was minor compared with the heart failure. Donor hearts are usually given to people who have a good overall prognosis.

Reduction surgery. There is a new procedure to reduce the size of floppy, dilated ventricles that is reported to be of some benefit in some types of heart failure. This could provide an alternative to transplant for some people with advanced cardiomyopathy.

Septal myotomy. In some people with severe hypertrophic cardiomyopathy, a surgeon can relieve some of the obstruction caused by the overgrown muscle layer by cutting the septum—the part of the muscle between the two ventricles. This procedure can partially relieve the constriction of the ventricles.

How can heart problems be detected and monitored?

There are many good tests in use today for detecting and following the progress of cardiac problems. The familiar EKG—the electrocardiogram—is perhaps the most often used. In this test, surface electrodes placed on the chest and limbs indirectly measure the current that flows through the heart. But the power of the EKG to reveal cardiomyopathies is not very great. An EKG measures electrical activity of the heart, not its muscle function. Abnormalities in muscle function are sometimes reflected in the EKG and sometimes not.

A somewhat more elaborate but much more accurate test for cardiomyopathy is the echocardiogram, an ultrasound picture of the heart in action that resembles the kind of imaging study often done in pregnant women to check on the fetus. The technician can videotape the echocardiogram so the cardiologist can compare changes between tests.

Table 21.1. Medications Used for Heart Failure

Type of Medication	How It Works	Example(s); Generic (Brand Name)
ACE (angiotensin-converting enzyme) Inhibitor	Blocks actions of ACE, a molecule that normally leads to fluid retention and raised blood pressure through activating the chemical angiotensin	fosinopril (Monopril); lisinopril (Prinivil, Zestril)
Vasodilator	Dilates veins, reducing amount of blood returning to the heart as it relaxes between beats	isosorbide dinitrate (ISDN)
Loop diuretic	Increases urine output by acting on kidneys (in part of kidney known as loop of Henle); reduces fluid overload	furosemide (Lasix)
Potassium-sparing diuretic	Acts on kidneys to increase urine production and reduce fluid overload; decrease excretion of potassium, counteracting excess potassium loss caused by some other diuretics	spironolactone (Aldactone); triamterene (Dyrenium)
Beta blocker	Reduces heart rate, force of heart's contractions and speed of nerve impulses through heart by blocking beta receptors (docking sites) that receive signals from nervous system	propranolol (Inderal); metoprolol (Lopressor, Toprol XL)
Alpha-beta blocker	Same as beta blockers, but also blocks alpha receptors (docking sites), stopping nerve signals that constrict blood vessels and raise blood pressure	carvedilol (Coreg)
Inotrope (Influencer of Muscle Force)	Increases force of muscle contractions of heart; high rate of complications, including abnormal heart rhythms	digoxin (Lanoxin, Lanoxicaps)

More invasive tests, such as cardiac catheterization studies, can be done under specific circumstances, if the situation warrants them. Cardiac catheterization studies involve putting probes into the cardiac blood vessels to directly measure pressures in different parts of the circulation.

Cardiomyopathy can be silent, completely without symptoms, in someone who is not exercising or exercising minimally. Many doctors today recommend frequent EKGs and some recommend frequent (for example, yearly) echocardiograms for patients at risk for cardiomyopathy, even if there are no symptoms.

Early symptoms to watch for in the exercising person are fatigue and shortness of breath. Later, fluid buildup in the lungs (in left heart failure) or feet (right heart failure) comes into the picture, with overall edema and cough following if treatment is not sought.

In the person with neuromuscular disease, fatigue and shortness of breath are just as likely to come from weakened respiratory muscles as they are from weakened cardiac muscles. A doctor should determine the origin of the problem and refer you to the appropriate specialist.

Additional Information

MedicAlert Foundation International
2323 Colorado Avenue
Turlock, CA 95382
Toll-Free: 888-633-4298
Phone: 209-668-3333
Fax: 209-669-2450
Website: http://www.medicalert.org
E-mail: customer_service@medicalert.org

Muscular Dystrophy Association
3300 E. Sunrise Drive
Tucson, AZ 85718-3208
Toll-Free: 800-572-1717
Phone: 520-529-2000
Fax: 520-529-5300
Website: http://www.mdausa.org
E-mail: mda@mdausa.org

Chapter 22

Anesthesia Risks with Muscular Dystrophy

People with neuromuscular disorders (NMDs) must take great care if they are to have a local or general anesthetic. Even someone with very mild, or non-existent symptoms, or someone who has a family history of a disorder, needs to let the anesthetist know well in advance so that tests can be carried out and proper care after the operation can be arranged.

Who Should Read This?

• Everyone who has a neuromuscular disorder, even if their symptoms are very mild.

• Everyone who has, or had, a relative with a neuromuscular disorder.

• Professionals involved with the care of people with NMDs around operations or treatment under local anesthetic.

Which Are the Neuromuscular Disorders?

Neuromuscular disorders include all the muscular dystrophies plus: myotonic disorders; congenital myopathies including mini-core,

"Anaesthetics," is reprinted with permission from the Muscular Dystrophy Campaign, a United Kingdom charity focusing on all muscular dystrophies and allied disorders. © 2003 Muscular Dystrophy Campaign. All rights reserved. Additional information is available at www.muscular-dystrophy.org.uk.

central-core, and multi-core disease plus nemaline and myotubular myopathies; mitochondrial myopathies; lipid storage myopathies; inherited metabolic myopathies including glycogen storage disease; familial periodic paralysis; inflammatory myopathies including infective myositis; autoimmune myositides including polymyositis and dermatomyositis; spinal muscular atrophies; hereditary and idiopathic peripheral neuropathy (HMSN also known as Charcot-Marie-Tooth disease); inflammatory, autoimmune and toxic neuropathies including Guillain-Barre syndrome and CIDP; and disorders of the neuromuscular junction including myasthenia gravis.

Many people are afraid of having an anesthetic, mainly through ignorance, but when we look at the rate of complications and even deaths arising from anesthesia we see that it is in fact very safe. This safety is the result of a thorough understanding of the patient's medical condition with a careful assessment before the operation, marked technical improvements in monitoring facilities during the operation, and the provision of good recovery facilities such as Cardiac Care Units (CCU) and Intensive Care Units (ICU).

Patients with neuromuscular disorders (NMDs) deserve special attention when it comes to anesthesia because many of the agents used (gases and chemicals) have effects on both muscle and nervous tissue. The main areas of concern are how the anesthetic agents will affect the muscle and the heart which is itself a muscle. A skeletal deformity such as scoliosis, or curvature of the spine, can also affect the way the patient responds to anesthesia so it is important to consider that too.

Anesthetics and the Heart

An article printed in the Winter 1995 No. 20 edition of *The Search*, showed how people with NMDs can sometimes have associated heart disease. This can occur as a cardiomyopathy, when the heart muscle does not work effectively, or as a defect in the way the electrical activity of the heart is transmitted, a conduction defect. The anesthetic vapors—the smelly agents such as ether and halothane which are inhaled—can reduce the effectiveness of the heart's muscle contractions and also aggravate any conduction defect. The vapors are all slightly different from each other, some having more effect on the heart than others. So it is important that the anesthetist makes a good assessment of the heart's condition before the operation which would include the level of physical activity that the patient can manage, and an electrocardiogram. Occasionally a more extensive assessment is needed.

Anesthetics and Breathing

Doctors need to measure how weak the patient's muscles are, usually by assessing the amount of physical activity that the patient can perform, and by taking a blood test to measure levels of a muscle enzyme, creatine kinase (CK). Any anesthetic agent which affects the muscles will also affect the muscles we use to breathe. Strong analgesic or sedative agents will affect these muscles indirectly, and muscle relaxants will have a direct effect on them. As breathing (or respiration) may already be difficult for patients with NMDs, these drugs should be used cautiously, and monitoring of breathing after the operation is absolutely essential. As a result, the patient is usually best cared for in a Cardiac Care Unit or Intensive Care Unit immediately after the operation. The muscles used for swallowing can also be affected which is another reason why good post-operative care is important.

Muscle Relaxants

Muscle relaxant drugs should only be used if essential because they tend to have a more profound and prolonged effect in NMD patients compared to other patients. One type of muscle relaxant, called suxamethonium, should usually be avoided. It causes the release of potassium ions (K+) from the muscle tissue into the blood. In normal patients this is usually of little practical significance. In patients with NMD the muscle may normally leak K+ so that a further increase in the levels of K+ in the blood may cause abnormal heart rhythms. Therefore, a pre-operative blood test to check K+ levels is important.

Local Anesthetics

A local anesthetic works by preventing the normal electrical activity in the nerve around which the anesthetic agents are placed. For minor procedures, such as stitches for cuts, they are probably the first choice for patients with NMD because they have few if any side-effects. However, for major local anesthetic techniques, e.g., spinal or epidural, careful assessment of the patient is needed and the type of NMD considered well before the operation.

Changes in Body Temperature and Pre-Operative Fasting

Patients with NMD do not tolerate changes in body temperature or the fasting often associated with anesthesia or surgery as well as normal patients, so steps need to be taken to minimize these problems by keeping the patient warm and well hydrated using intervenous drips.

Malignant Hyperthermia and Central Core Disease

Malignant hyperthermia (MH) is an inherited disorder which causes an unexpected, sometimes fatal, reaction in the patient to certain anesthetic drugs. Because some patients with NMD have experienced similar problems during anesthesia there have been claims that patients with NMD may also have MH. However, it is generally accepted that the only neuromuscular condition truly related to MH is central core disease (CCD), although this is not always the case. Patients with CCD should be considered potentially susceptible to MH unless proved otherwise by a special type of muscle biopsy which screens for MH.

Summary

- Clearly anesthesia in NMD is not to be undertaken lightly. Such patients should expect the anesthetist to make a careful and thorough assessment of their particular condition and their current state of health.

- They are not suitable to be treated as out-patients because doctors should carry out pre-operative investigations, and enough time and recovery facilities should be available after the operation.

- It is absolutely essential that the person affected by NMD should inform the anesthetist even if there are only minor symptoms or no symptoms at all. Occasionally a neuromuscular disorder in a person who had no symptoms has come to light only because of an unexpected problem with anesthesia, particularly in young children. The anesthetist should also be warned if there is an inherited NMD in the family.

- If possible ask for the anesthetist to be forewarned before admission to hospital and consider wearing a Medic Alert bracelet or similar in case of accidents.

Additional Information

Muscular Dystrophy Campaign
7-11 Prescott Place
London, England
SW4 6BS
Phone: 011-44-020-7720-8055
Fax: 011-44-020-7498-0670
Website: http://www.muscular-dystrophy.org
E-mail: info@muscular-dystrophy.org

Chapter 23

Inflammation in Neuromuscular Disease

Usually, inflammation of tissue occurs with an injury or an infection, but it is also an important part of certain neuromuscular diseases.

Ask anyone for a snap definition of inflammation, even a doctor, and he or she will probably say it is redness, swelling, sensations of heat and pain, or all of the above. It is true that those are the hallmark symptoms of inflammation, but they describe a mosquito bite or a sore throat better than they describe an inflammatory neuromuscular disease. To understand the role of inflammation in neuromuscular disease, it is important to look beyond symptoms, and consider the underlying process.

Inflammation in Health

Inflammation is really the immune system's first line of defense in tissue that has been damaged by injury or infection. Essentially, it is an increase in blood flow and a mass invasion of blood-borne immune cells into the damaged tissue.

In inflammatory neuromuscular diseases, macrophages home in on signals from abnormal or dying muscle fibers, and release chemicals that recruit lymphocytes. Both cell types might inadvertently attack the muscle in the same way they would attack an infection.

At the beginning of the inflammatory process, chemicals released by the body's own dying cells or by foreign microbes attract immune cells to the injured or infected area. Among the first cells to respond are macrophages, which eliminate the dying cells and microbes by engulfing them and/or breaking them apart with destructive chemicals. (Derived from Greek, *macro* means big and *phage* means eater.) The macrophages also release proteins called cytokines, and fat-like chemicals called leukotrienes and prostaglandins.

Cytokines and certain leukotrienes are strong attractants for other immune cells, including the lymphocytes, which mount a focused attack against infectious microbes. As the inflammatory response intensifies, lymphocytes continue to invade the area and proliferate. Other leukotrienes and prostaglandins cause widening of nearby blood vessels (vasodilation) and increased permeability of capillaries. Histamine, the target of antihistamine cold and allergy remedies, is produced from yet other immune cells and has similar effects. The resulting increase in blood flow allows a steady influx of immune cells into the damaged area.

The increased blood flow is also largely responsible for the telltale symptoms of inflammation. The rush of warm blood causes redness, heat, and swelling. At the same time, pressure from the swelling and the accumulation of immune cells, along with the destructive chemicals released by the cells, irritate local nerve endings and cause pain.

Inflammation In Disease

In many disease states, the inflammatory process spins out of control and becomes harmful. In some neuromuscular diseases (like certain muscular dystrophies), inflammation is probably a secondary response to muscle degeneration, while in others (like the inflammatory myopathies), it might be a primary cause of degeneration. In either case, the inflammation can contribute to disease progression.

In Duchenne muscular dystrophy, degenerating muscle fibers are often surrounded by inflammatory cells (mostly macrophages). Although the macrophages are probably there to clear away dead tissue, they might hasten muscle decay in the process. Severe cases of myotonic dystrophy and facioscapulohumeral MD sometimes show similar patterns of inflammation. In the inflammatory myopathies—polymyositis

(PM), dermatomyositis (DM) and sporadic inclusion-body myositis (IBM)—macrophages and lymphocytes intensely invade muscle tissue.

In DM, macrophages and lymphocytes appear to attack the capillaries in muscle tissue, ultimately causing muscle fibers to degenerate by cutting off their blood supply. In PM and IBM, the immune cells actually swarm around the muscle fibers themselves, even fibers that otherwise appear healthy. The invading cells appear to directly damage muscle in PM, but it is not clear how they contribute to muscle degeneration in IBM.

Finally, there is some evidence of inflammation in amyotrophic lateral sclerosis, a disease caused by the death of muscle-controlling nerve cells. In some cases of ALS, the brain and spinal cord contain enhanced numbers of macrophage-like cells called microglia and elevated levels of cytokines and prostaglandin. The significance of these observations hasn't been established.

Surprisingly, inflammation is not typical of myasthenia gravis or Lambert-Eaton syndrome, autoimmune diseases in which the immune system attacks the body's own tissues.

Treatments

Several immunosuppressants (drugs that suppress immune system activity) have been used in attempts to reduce the inflammation associated with DMD, the inflammatory myopathies, and ALS.

Steroid-based drugs like prednisone have broad anti-immune and anti-inflammatory effects, including blocking the proliferation of lymphocytes and the production of cytokines, prostaglandins, and histamine. Other immunosuppressants have more focused inhibitory effects on lymphocyte proliferation (methotrexate and azathioprine) or macrophage activity (IVIG).

For DM and PM, the most effective treatment is often a combination of prednisone and other immunosuppressants. Prednisone can help slow the course of DMD, but other immunosuppressants that have been tested are not effective. (Actually, it is unclear whether prednisone works via its anti-inflammatory effects or by some other means.) Immunosuppressant therapies for IBM and ALS have generally been unsuccessful, but are still under investigation.

Chapter 24

Progress in Treatments for Muscular Dystrophy

Around the time the first issue of *Quest* was published, in 1994, neurologists had just established that the steroid prednisone could slow the course of Duchenne muscular dystrophy (DMD). Molecular biologists were beginning to come up with realistic approaches to gene therapy—techniques for replacing or repairing the defective genes that cause DMD and other diseases in MDA's program. And, although MDA-funded investigators had begun a pioneering trial of cell transplantation for DMD in 1990, stem cell therapy was a treatment for blood disorders, seemingly irrelevant to neuromuscular disease. Obviously, times have changed—so much so, in fact, that it is hard to keep pace. This chapter highlights some of the most recent and groundbreaking advances.

Duchenne Muscular Dystrophy

Prednisone

Treatment with prednisone—considered the only effective medication for DMD by many neurologists—could be undergoing a makeover.

Reprinted from "From Steroids to Stem Cells" by Dan Stimson, *QUEST*, Volume 10, Number 1, February 2003. Reprinted with permission from the Muscular Dystrophy Association, www.mdausa.org. © The Muscular Dystrophy Association. For additional information, call the Muscular Dystrophy Association National Headquarters toll-free at (800) 572-1717. To find an MDA office in your area, look in your local telephone book, or click on "Clinics and Services" on the MDA website.

Standard protocols used since the early 1990s call for daily adminis-tration of prednisone, but given this way, the drug can cause weight gain, delayed growth, osteoporosis, and behavioral problems.

Two pilot trials reported late in 2002 show that a different dosing schedule may deliver prednisone's benefits without these unhealthy side effects. An MDA-funded trial in the United States tested high-dose prednisone given only on Friday and Saturday of each week, and a British trial tested the closely related drug prednisolone, given at a standard dose for the first 10 days of the month, or for 10 days on and 10 days off.

Both treatments produced significant strength gains with few side effects, and the weekend protocol is now slated for a larger trial. Mean-while, the American Academy of Neurology is developing a set of guidelines for prednisone use in DMD.

Gentamicin

In mice with DMD, the antibiotic gentamicin stimulates the pro-duction of dystrophin—the protein missing in the disease—but the jury is still out on whether the drug will work in people. These mice fail to produce dystrophin because they have a mutation that inserts a stop signal in the dystrophin gene; 5 percent to 15 percent of boys with DMD have the same type of mutation. Gentamicin allows a cell's gene-reading machinery to bypass the stop signal and produce a full-length dystrophin protein. In two small trials, the drug reduced the levels of creatine kinase, an indicator of muscle breakdown, but failed to increase dystrophin levels in boys with DMD.

Utrophin

MDA-funded researcher Kay Davies continues to search for drugs that will stimulate muscle cells to produce utrophin—a protein that has similar functions to dystrophin, but is restricted to small patches of adult muscle. In the late 1990s, Davies' research at the University of Oxford in England showed that mice with DMD are protected from muscle degeneration when they are genetically engineered to make more utrophin. Since then, she has been using a rapid search method called high-throughput screening to identify chemicals with utrophin-boosting activity.

A screen of over 160,000 chemicals, set up three years ago in collabo-ration with the Long Island, N.Y.-based company OSI Pharmaceuti-cals, was unsuccessful. More recently, Davies has begun collaborating with a fledgling company founded by Oxford chemists and with a large

Swiss company, MyoContract Ltd. Testing a small custom-designed chemical library, both companies found a family of chemicals that increase the levels of utrophin in laboratory-grown cells. Those increases are probably too small to compensate for dystrophin, Davies says, but she is in discussions with MDA about setting up a larger screen to find more effective chemicals.

Other Muscular Dystrophies

For nearly a decade, researchers were stymied by the search for the culprit gene behind facioscapulohumeral muscular dystrophy (FSHD), and thus, they had few clues to treatment. In August 2002, MDA grantee Rossella Tupler at Massachusetts General Hospital in Boston discovered that the mutations underlying FSHD—mapped to chromosome 4 in 1992—are not in a single gene, but in a DNA region that controls genes. Deletions (missing pieces of DNA) in that region cause genes that are normally off to turn on. Finding ways to block these overactive genes could lead to effective treatments.

Myotonic muscular dystrophy (MMD) turns out to arise from a similarly complicated mechanism. In 1992, the disease was linked to repeating units of DNA in the DMPK gene on chromosome 19. Around the same time, John Day and Laura Ranum at the University of Minnesota in Minneapolis saw evidence for a chromosome 3 form of the disease (MMD2), and in August 2001, they reported that MMD2 is caused by repeats in a different gene, ZNF9. This was an important clue that the repeats—not the specific genes containing them—are central to MMD.

Shortly after that discovery, scientists began focusing on how the repeats might interfere with the functions of different cell types in the body, leading to MMD's diverse symptoms. It turns out that the repeats create abnormally long pieces of RNA (the intermediate between DNA and proteins), leading to a traffic jam that keeps cells from turning other RNAs into protein. Targeting the repeats with small inhibitors derived from DNA or RNA might alleviate symptoms of the disease.

Autoimmune Diseases

Better Immunosuppressants

In clinical trials, several new drugs have shown promise against autoimmune diseases, which occur when the immune system attacks other tissues in the body. Prednisone is a mainstay of treatment for these diseases, which include myasthenia gravis (MG) and the inflammatory myopathies, but in some cases it fails to produce improvement, and in others it has intolerable side effects.

In 2001, two trials conducted at MDA clinics—at Johns Hopkins University in Baltimore and Duke University in Durham, N.C.—showed that MG sometimes responds to mycophenolate mofetil (CellCept), a drug originally developed to prevent immune rejection of transplanted organs. In both trials, about 65 percent of MG patients experienced improved strength or a reduced need for prednisone after receiving CellCept for several months.

More recent trials at Hopkins and in Argentina suggest similar benefits from intravenous cyclophosphamide, a drug traditionally used to treat cancers of the immune system.

In a multicenter trial funded by NIH, researchers are testing the multiple sclerosis drug beta-interferon-1a (Avonex) against inclusion-body myositis (IBM). In an MDA-funded pilot trial completed in 2001, the drug was found to be safe, but not effective for IBM patients. The new trial doubles the dose and is expected to yield results later this year.

Vaccines

J. Edwin Blalock, an MDA grantee at the University of Alabama in Birmingham, is making progress in his efforts to develop vaccines for MG. Traditionally, a vaccine is an inactivated virus that stimulates the immune system to boost its defenses against future viral infections. The MG vaccines are designed to resemble proteins on the errant immune cells that cause MG; they are meant to stimulate the immune system to destroy those cells.

Blalock has shown that the vaccines increase strength in mice primed to develop MG. In preparation for a human trial, he has begun treating pet dogs that naturally developed MG, and with help from a Belgian entrepreneur who has MG, he has established a biotech company called CuraVac. Blalock's vaccine strategy also holds promise for treating other autoimmune diseases.

Gene Therapy: Progress and New Challenges

In 1999, MDA clinic director Jerry Mendell of Ohio State University began a trial of gene therapy for limb-girdle muscular dystrophy (LGMD)—one of the first efforts to test this fledgling science against a human disease. That same year, a young man died in an unrelated gene therapy trial, and the government suspended all gene therapy research involving human subjects.

Although Mendell's trial was never completed; he was able to salvage some data from it. Last year, he announced that his experimental protocol—intramuscular injection of the alpha-sarcoglycan gene—was safe, but not beneficial for people with alpha-sarcoglycan deficiency (a form of LGMD). Meanwhile, Mendell and other MDA scientists have redoubled their efforts to bring gene therapy back to the clinic.

Vector Questions

In Mendell's trial, the alpha-sarcoglycan gene was packaged into an adeno-associated virus (AAV), considered among the safest and most effective vectors (gene-delivery vehicles) partly because of its small size. Since then, vector technology has improved remarkably, with new versions of AAV that home to muscle with higher efficiency.

Barry Byrne, director of the Powell Gene Therapy Center at the University of Florida in Gainesville, was recently awarded an MDA grant to fine-tune these viruses in preparation for a new LGMD gene therapy trial.

Meanwhile, other researchers have laid the groundwork for a Duchenne MD gene therapy trial by testing viral delivery of the dystrophin gene in mice with the disease. Two MDA-funded research groups, one led by Jeffrey Chamberlain at the University of Washington in Seattle and the other headed by Xiao Xiao at the University of Pittsburgh, have developed small versions of the very large gene—called mini- or microdystrophins—that are easily accommodated by AAVs. When given to mice with DMD by intramuscular injection, this type of gene transfer slows degeneration and improves contractile force in the injected muscles.

Immune System Obstacles

Still, researchers face several obstacles before gene therapy can live up to its promise, including the body's immune system—which has the potential to destroy gene therapy vectors and the therapeutic genes inside. In fact, immune reactions could lead to harmful side effects—even death. Scientists and FDA officials now believe that the 1999 gene therapy-related death of Jesse Gelsinger, a teenager being treated for a liver disease, was caused by an immune reaction to the vector used in the trial. Mendell, Chamberlain, and Xiao believe AAV provokes almost no response from the immune system. Unfortunately, recent studies suggest that even dystrophin itself might cause an immune response in someone whose body has never made the protein.

And in other ways, the AAV-microdystrophin system is not a perfect solution to DMD. While microdystrophins retain the most essential parts of the full-length protein, Chamberlain predicts that, at best, they may bring DMD closer to Becker MD (a less severe version of dystrophin deficiency). For these reasons, Chamberlain has been testing a larger vector, a gutted adenovirus, for its ability to deliver full-length dystrophin to the muscles of DMD mice. Other researchers have made vectors from retroviruses (like HIV) and from plasmids, or condensed circles of DNA.

Reaching Enough Muscles

But the biggest obstacle to gene therapy for muscle diseases, Chamberlain says, is that so far, no one has come up with a way to deliver a gene to all of the muscles in the body. "There's a lot of talk about scaling up intramuscular injection, for example, just targeting some of the most critical muscles, like those that control posture and hand function, to improve the quality of life for boys [with DMD]," he says. "But clearly, we have to get beyond that and find ways to deliver dystrophin to the heart and the diaphragm [a chest muscle that controls breathing]."

Two MDA-funded researchers, Hansell Stedman at the University of Pennsylvania in Philadelphia and Leaf Huang at the University of Pittsburgh, are at the forefront of efforts to develop systemic gene-delivery methods. In a rodent model, Stedman has shown that he can deliver the delta-sarcoglycan gene to the muscles of an entire limb by using clamps and tourniquets to increase local blood pressure and medications to increase local blood flow. Huang has used a similar procedure to deliver dystrophin to the diaphragm in mice with DMD.

For other neuromuscular diseases, would-be gene therapists have learned much from research on DMD. Gyula Acsadi, who is developing a gene therapy approach to treat ALS, spent his early scientific career studying ways to deliver dystrophin to muscle cells. Byrne and Andrea Amalfitano (at Duke University) are both working on gene therapy for Pompe's disease, a fatal infant disease caused by altered muscle metabolism. Amalfitano spent his early career working with Chamberlain. Chamberlain predicts that DMD gene therapy trials will begin in two years, and probably will involve intramuscular injections of AAV-microdystrophin. In the meantime, he says, researchers need to validate systemic gene delivery methods in large animals with DMD.

Stem Cell Therapy for Muscles and Nerves

Stem cells occupied an obscure corner of science until 1999, when *Science* magazine recognized progress in stem cell biology as the "scientific breakthrough of the year." Before that, scientists knew little about embryonic stem cells—those that give rise to and assemble our tissues and organs—and even less about stem cells in the adult body.

Scientists once thought that adult stem cells could be found only in tissues with a high rate of cell turnover, such as bone marrow and skin. Now, it is clear that they are found in tissues once thought incapable of regeneration, like the brain, and that they have some capacity to cross tissue boundaries.

With new techniques for isolating and growing embryonic stem cells and adult-derived stem cells, scientists could one day have a tool kit for counteracting neuromuscular diseases. Stem cell transplants to repair damaged muscles and nerves could become as commonplace as organ transplants.

But for the present, stem cell therapy poses a set of challenges much like those of gene therapy. In fact, "stem cell therapy basically is gene therapy—you're just using the cell to deliver the gene," says Louis Kunkel of Children's Hospital in Boston, who hopes to use stem cells to treat muscular dystrophy.

Like any gene therapy vector, transplanted stem cells could trigger an immune response. Also, scientists do not entirely understand how stem cells choose their fate; and the signals that control their mobilization to different tissues in the body are poorly understood.

MDA-funded researchers have addressed these problems by experimenting with both embryonic and adult-derived stem cells, each of which has distinct potential advantages. (In accord with federal policy set by President Bush, MDA's support of human embryonic stem cell research is limited to some 75 stem cell lines created before August 2001.) In principle, adult-derived stem cells could be harvested from the person in need of treatment, corrected for any genetic defects, and transplanted where they are needed, circumventing the problem of immune rejection. Embryonic stem cells, on the other hand, are believed capable of generating more cell progeny and a greater variety of cell types.

Making New Muscle

Kunkel and his colleague Emmanuela Gussoni have isolated muscle-forming stem cells from the muscle tissue and bone marrow of healthy adult mice. In a 1999 study funded by MDA, they used a bone marrow transplant procedure to deliver the cells to mice with DMD. Some of the injected cells migrated through the bloodstream to form new muscle fibers, but not in sufficient numbers to improve muscle function.

More recently, nature performed a similar experiment on a boy with DMD. At 1 year of age, the boy received a bone marrow transplant for an immune disorder, and 11 years later, he was discovered to have a slowly progressive form of DMD. When Kunkel and Gussoni were asked to perform a muscle biopsy on the boy, they found that a small number of transplanted marrow cells had made muscle cells—not enough to account for the boy's slow course of DMD.

"The fact that cells from a bone marrow transplant can be found in muscle is a big finding," Kunkel says. "But the levels are not high enough to be therapeutic. In mice, dogs, and humans [with DMD], we've found that after a transplant, less than 1 percent of the fibers in a given muscle produce dystrophin."

Other stem cells, delivered by other methods, have produced better repair. Johnny Huard, an MDA grantee at the University of Pittsburgh, has found stem cells in adult mouse muscle that can form muscle fibers, nerves, and blood vessels. When given to mice with DMD by intramuscular injection, these cells can restore dystrophin in up to 25 percent of the fibers in the injected muscle.

Recently, he has also shown that a chemical in the body called TGF-beta can stimulate the cells to form scar tissue, an important clue as to why muscle-derived stem cells sometimes fail to produce muscle. "During an injection of stem cells, we may have to block [TGF-beta activity] to keep the cells from making scar tissue," he says. Other chemicals, he and Kunkel note, might be used to attract stem cells to muscle and push them toward a muscle cell fate.

Renewing Nerves

Several research groups have shown that embryonic and marrow-derived stem cells can be induced to become motor neurons, the muscle-controlling nerve cells destroyed by ALS and SMA. But given the complex connections neurons must make with each other and with muscle cells, many scientists believe stem cells might be more efficient at rescuing sick neurons than replacing dead ones.

This thinking recently gained support from a study by Jeffrey Rothstein, who co-directs the MDA/ALS Center at Johns Hopkins. Rothstein found that intraspinal injections of human embryonic stem cells significantly improved the motor function of rats with an ALS-like disease. But when he examined the rats' spinal cords, he found that very few of the stem cells had produced motor neurons. Instead, most of them had formed astrocytes—support cells in the nervous system. The cells appear to release neurotrophic factors that nurture dying neurons back to health.

Stanley Appel, director of the MDA/ALS Center at Baylor College of Medicine in Houston, is hopeful that bone marrow stem cells will be similarly beneficial to people with ALS. But he does not expect the cells to form neurons or astrocytes; Appel and others believe that autoimmunity might contribute to ALS. In an MDA-funded clinical trial, he is giving bone marrow transplants to 10 ALS patients, hoping that the procedure will reboot their immune systems. Scientists at the University of Turin in Italy recently announced they are testing direct intraspinal injection of bone marrow stem cells in ALS patients.

Chapter 25

Physical Therapy:
Flexibility, Fitness, and Fun

Say *physical therapy* and most people think of World War II movies with wounded heroes struggling with weights and pulleys, athletes nursing injuries in whirlpool baths, and heart attack survivors sweating on treadmills. Say physical therapy and muscular dystrophy in the same sentence and you may get the same uncertainty from anxious parents that you do from skeptical insurance company representatives. "Does it really help in those diseases?" is a frequent response. "I mean, what can you do in a degenerative, genetic disease?"

That's what Yvonne Nichols of Horseheads, New York, heard from her insurance company when she tried to get physical therapy for her 8-year-old son, Scott, who has Duchenne muscular dystrophy (DMD). "The insurance company termed the therapy 'inactive care,'" Nichols says. "They call it inactive care when it's not going to improve a condition, and they refused to cover it."

Fortunately for Nichols, she and Scott live in an area where the schools are very good about complying with the requirements of the Individuals with Disabilities Education Act (IDEA), which mandates that every child is entitled to a full education, including physical education,

Reprinted from "Physical Therapy—Flexibility, Fitness, and Fun" by Margaret Wahl, *QUEST*, Volume 7, Number 3, June 2000. Reprinted with permission from the Muscular Dystrophy Association, www.mdausa.org. © The Muscular Dystrophy Association. For additional information call the Muscular Dystrophy Association National Headquarters toll-free at (800) 572-1717. To find an MDA office in your area, look in your local telephone book, or click on "Clinics and Services" on the MDA website.

with whatever special services and adaptive equipment may be necessary to make that happen.

Scott's DMD was diagnosed in kindergarten, when his physical education teacher noticed that his motor skills were not developing as expected and encouraged the family to investigate. That summer, after the diagnosis, Nichols swung into action. "We went through the Committee on Special Education," she says. "I contacted the school, because I had a friend who had a son with behavioral problems. They went through the CSE, so I knew a little about it and what to do."

Scott was classified as "orthopedically impaired" and assigned to a physical therapy program involving a half-hour of therapy two days a week during the school day. The therapy mostly involves stretching his heel cords and the muscles at the backs of his thighs, but Scott is also learning to manage his energy level and stay safe. There's some fun involved, too, like walking on 4-inch stilts.

"I've heard about red tape with the CSE," Nichols says, "but we had no trouble whatsoever. We've had nothing but good experiences."

A New Way to Look at Physical Therapy

"In the old way of looking at things, rehabilitation meant you were going to get better," says Sheila Hayes, a physical therapist associated with the MDA/ALS Center at Columbia-Presbyterian Medical Center in New York. That's no longer the case, she says. In fact, the American Physical Therapy Association recently started a special section on degenerative diseases.

Shree Pandya is a physical therapist and educator who has been involved with the MDA clinic at the University of Rochester (NY) for many years. Now, she works mostly with patients—including Scott Nichols—who have been in research studies at the university. Pandya sees physical therapy as "helping people to remain at their highest functional level possible at any given point in time within the constraints of their disorder."

Physical therapy overlaps a great deal with occupational therapy, but there are some differences. For the most part, although both disciplines deal with maximizing function, OT is concerned more with the small muscles, particularly those of the hands, while PT is concerned more with large muscles, such as the legs, and with mobility.

Today, physical therapy is an integral part of the treatment of almost any neuromuscular condition, and is usually included in the medical plan for everyone with these conditions and in the school or preschool program for children.

How Much and What Kind?

Unfortunately, there is a lack of research on exactly what kind of PT and how much is ideal in each of the various neuromuscular disorders.

Most therapists agree that a certain amount of stretching and range-of-motion exercises (these ROMs keep joints supple by putting them through their normal range of motion in space) is almost always a good idea in neuromuscular diseases. Such maneuvers tend to slow down or sometimes even prevent the development of contractures, the freezing of joints that are not moved.

Most therapists also agree that a certain amount of exercise is good for cardiovascular health, and that some weight bearing, where possible, can head off the development of the bone-weakening disorder osteoporosis. Most also agree that strenuous exercise in certain types of metabolic muscle disorders (for example, phosphorylase deficiency, or McArdle's disease) can lead to serious muscle damage and perhaps kidney damage as well. (This is because proteins leaking out of damaged muscle cells reach the kidneys, where they are toxic.)

In periodic paralysis, attacks of paralysis are often brought on by resting after strenuous exercise. Cramping of muscles, paralysis of muscles, or cola-colored urine are warning signs to stop exercising immediately in any muscle disorder.

For some people, just activities of daily living, like walking up and down a few stairs, getting in and out of chairs, and turning from side to side in bed have to suffice for physical therapy. Even those simple things can help preserve both strength and flexibility.

But when it comes to more concerted efforts to increase strength or muscle bulk in the muscular dystrophies, disagreements and uncertainty surface. Several of the dystrophies (Duchenne, Becker, some limb-girdle dystrophies, and at least one congenital dystrophy) are known to result from fragile muscle membranes. These membranes are sheaths that surround each muscle fiber (long cell) inside the muscles. In several muscular dystrophies, the sheath is weakened because it lacks one of several membrane proteins. Extra stress on the membranes, many experts have reasoned, may hasten muscle degeneration.

On the other hand, muscles are designed to be stressed, and leaving them alone can also hasten their deterioration and interfere with overall fitness. Pandya, despite many years of experience in the field, is not sure about the exercise question. "I would rather be cautious," she says, "but sometimes I wonder if we have been too cautious." She says the most serious quandaries are posed by "college-age kids with facioscapulohumeral dystrophy or limb-girdle dystrophy, who do not have as much of a progressive disorder as Duchenne dystrophy and are into exercise with weights and equipment."

Pandya prefers that they do walking or swimming instead of weight lifting, but she says there are not a lot of studies. "Basically, we try to summarize what we know from the literature, that a certain amount of exercise is good for all of us, as well as keeping weight down, eating a healthy diet, all those things." She is not enthusiastic about exercises that may tear membranes and damage muscles cells that have a hard time renewing themselves (which describes muscles in muscular dystrophy).

She recalls a research study on boys with DMD conducted many years ago. Exercising the thigh muscles three times a week temporarily strengthened these muscles, but when the children were tested six months and a year later, they had lost the gains. Because of this study and others, Pandya is not keen on overzealous strengthening exercises in severe muscular dystrophies like DMD. She is more interested in increasing the child's overall flexibility. Of equal concern to Pandya is a youngster's experience of childhood. "The child has to be a child first, and a child with muscular dystrophy next," she says, and she tries to build a PT program around that philosophy.

Don't Overdo It

Jenny Robison, a physical therapist who has long been associated with the MDA clinic at Vanderbilt University in Nashville, Tennessee, has much the same philosophy. "I try not to overload my patients," she says. "But in my years of experience, I can see kids whose parents have done exercises and night splints [to keep feet in proper alignment] and surgeries, and they're in so much better shape than kids who haven't had any intervention. I think it works, but it's a lot to do." Physical therapy "prevents or slows down problems like contractures and keeps people in a better functional position to do things that they want to do, to live life as well as they can. It also helps people by getting them the right equipment," Robison says.

Concerns about exercise also exist in motor neuron disorders like spinal muscular atrophy (SMA) and amyotrophic lateral sclerosis (ALS). In these disorders, motor neurons, the nerve cells that control muscle movement, are lost, leaving muscle fibers orphaned—without a nerve supply. Some investigation of exercise in motor neuron disorders has been done, Hayes says, and the consensus is this: When motor neurons die or do not function, their neighboring motor neurons can take over, at least for a while, supplying more than their share of muscle fibers with nerve signals. But these new connections are fragile and under stress. Over-exercising the muscles can stress the new connections still further, perhaps hastening damage (Hayes does not think this is likely), but almost certainly making it harder for a person to function by the next day. Hayes' recent experience is with ALS patients, but she says conclusions about exercise in ALS should apply equally to people with SMA.

In her view and that of other experts in motor neuron disease physical therapy, she says: "It's okay to do moderate strengthening for muscles that are uninvolved, that show no overt weakness. But once a person is starting to exhibit weakness, it's best to stay away from weight machines, free weights, or any type of resistance exercises. If the goal is to improve function, then exercising to the point where muscle fatigue impairs function is counterproductive."

A Child First

Children especially need to have a PT program that works for them in the context of their other activities. No one understands Pandya's message about children needing to be children first better than Sherrie Shannon of Fairview, Pennsylvania. Her son, Christopher, an 11-year-old with DMD, has had the wrong kind of physical therapy, and too much of it, she says.

Shannon says she was directed to a physical therapist in her area who was approved by Medicaid, but knew next to nothing about MD. "Christopher was only the second kid with muscular dystrophy that she had ever seen," Shannon says, adding that the therapist told her she had had only about four hours of education on neuromuscular disorders in her five years of PT training.

"She started him on wall squats—where you lean against the wall and squat down and have to get back up—and on sit-ups," Shannon recalls. Christopher has recently begun a pool therapy program, a welcome change, but Shannon says of the therapist, "She's not listening for Christopher's cues saying, 'I'm tired.'"

Shannon describes her son's schedule: "From 7:30 to 8 in the morning, he does leg exercises and manual stretches at home; then at a quarter to 9 he gets more stretches at school, at 12:30 more stretches, more when he gets off the bus, and then again before bed. On the days when he has PT after school, he goes from school to therapy."

Shannon is all for the stretches—in moderation—and for flexibility exercises in general, but she says, "I don't see that strengthening has helped him in any way, because he's still declining at an average rate." Fortunately, Shannon has recently been able to bring in a consulting therapist with years of experience in DMD who has been helping their primary therapist. Christopher's program is undergoing modifications and shifting more toward water therapy.

But Shannon is also concerned with the quality of Christopher's life. She describes how the physical therapist had him doing an exercise called "side-lying subluxation—where he lies on his side and has to lift his leg and kick behind him. That's supposed to help strengthen the muscles that bend the hip." Shannon says, "You can do that standing, doing kickball. I'd rather let him kick the ball."

Christopher also likes sled hockey, a game his mother describes this way: "He sits down in a sled, someone pushes him, and he hits the puck." Winners on Wheels, a program she found through her MDA office, sponsors sled hockey in her area. Nowadays, when Christopher asks if he can play instead of doing exercises, Shannon tells him, "We'll wait a half-hour for the exercises. Go play."

Tapping Into Technology

PT is not just about exercises. It is also about technology and modifying the environment. Canes, walkers, wheelchairs, scooters, neck supports, and ankle-foot and knee-ankle-foot orthoses (AFOs and KAFOs) are among the more common devices used in neuromuscular conditions. But sometimes modifying an armchair so that it has more support, or constructing a way to hold a book at eye level can make an enormous difference to someone's physical well-being.

"A therapist can try various devices and see what works the best," Hayes says. "ALS patients are a challenge, because some of the assistive devices have to be modified if they have hand weakness. You may have to put forearm platforms on a walker, for example. There's a lot of equipment available; you just have to know what to try with each patient." And, says Hayes, you have to be alert to changes in the patient's condition, a common factor in neuromuscular disorders.

A popular intervention in many conditions is the AFO. AFOs are typically constructed out of molded plastic, with a support that goes up the calf and continues under the sole of the foot. The AFO holds the foot in a functional position, preventing foot drop—the foot flopping down because of weakness in lifting it—and slowing the development of contractures at the ankle joint.

Pandya says she calls AFOs night splints when she's thinking about DMD, because in this disease they are more often used to prevent contractures than to aid walking and are worn overnight for this purpose.

Pandya says she thinks they probably are not needed if the boys are still standing several hours a day, and if the parents and child are willing to do regular stretching exercises. In other conditions, such as myotonic muscular dystrophy (MMD), they are used to aid walking by preventing foot drop, Pandya says.

Pandya and Robison are both involved in the prescription of wheelchairs and other mobility devices, and in the particulars of their modifications and seating. Robison has a special certification in wheelchair seating from the Rehabilitation Engineering Society of North America, but even without special credentials, wheelchair seating and modification is an area that falls squarely in the physical therapist's domain.

A scooter may be fun to zip around in for the person with ALS who is not too far along in his disease, Hayes says, but therapist and patient have to be realistic: The person is likely to need the more complete support of a wheelchair in time, and his insurance is not going to be thrilled about paying for two expensive devices within a few years of each other.

In DMD, Pandya says, she likes to see a child start with a lightweight, flexible wheelchair that is relatively inexpensive and easy for everyone to maneuver. In fact, she says, some children can push it themselves with their remaining arm strength, which is good exercise. Then, in high school, when the child has reached his full size, she recommends getting a power wheelchair for maximum mobility. By then, weakness usually mandates its full-time use. Pandya is also conscious of insurance restrictions and says the companies are not going to pay for too many vehicles in too short a time.

Specialized Knowledge

Finding a physical therapist is fairly easy. But finding one with the specialized knowledge it takes to treat the problems in neuromuscular disorders, and one that an insurance company or government health plan (such as Medicare or Medicaid) will cover is another story. The MDA clinic is a good place to get a referral to a therapist who knows about neuromuscular disorders and to set up a free yearly consultation with one. But insurance or personal resources are required to finance an ongoing therapy program that is not connected to a school or early childhood program, and that is where the going can get tough. MDA clinic physicians can help you appeal to insurers regarding the need for a therapist who specializes in neuromuscular conditions.

Financial concerns aside, finding the ideal person is doubly difficult if you do not live near a big city, Robison says. The American

Physical Therapy Association may be able to help you find a specialist in your area. Where children are concerned and you cannot find someone with neuromuscular disease expertise, Robison advises parents to search for a pediatric physical therapist.

Yvonne Nichols advises parents who are searching for a physical therapist: "It's important that it's a physical therapist that the child likes. They talk and joke together, and they need to do that. Scott is not demonstrative in any way, but he runs through the clinic and hugs Shree." (Scott sees Shree Pandya for evaluations as part of a drug study.) She says he also loved the private pediatric therapist the family was temporarily able to see.

Schools can be a good source of help and advice, Robison says, but you have to be on your guard. "Some schools are great and some will do as little as they have to do. Some of these schools will run you over if you don't learn to fight for yourself."

Robison strongly endorses parent advocacy groups that interpret disability law for families and help them make school systems comply with regulations. Social workers associated with medical centers or school systems can also be a help. "The more informed parents are the better they can advocate for the child," Robison says.

Robison and Pandya see the role of the physical therapist as more of a consultant to the parents and the school staff than as someone who necessarily does hands-on therapy during the school day (although sometimes they do conduct therapy sessions this way). "Therapists in the schools can act as a bridge between us [at university medical centers] and the school and parents, and help the school staff understand the changes in function and how to handle the child," Robison says.

"Occupational and physical therapists in the school system are important," she says, but they are usually "more in a consulting role in the school system, usually not in a direct therapy role." "They can be an advocate for the child in the school system, because they understand the disease and the equipment. They can go to the principal and say why he really needs to have a computer. They're a medical bridge to the school."

For children under 3 who are not yet in regular school programs, state-administered, federally mandated programs, generally called early intervention for children under 3, and preschool education programs for children 3 to 5, are part of IDEA. Therapies can be conducted in the home, preschool, daycare center, or other settings. Such programs "help with equipment, with therapy, with getting the right things for children," Robison says.

Taking to the Water

"Swimming is probably the most important thing responsible for the condition I'm in," says Chad O'Connell, who's 26 and has Duchenne muscular dystrophy. Unlike many people of his age with DMD, says O'Connell, he doesn't need a ventilator, has fairly good cardiac function, and has kept his weight down despite using prednisone, a drug that almost always causes significant weight gain. He attributes all this to his time in the water. "I'm probably one of the strongest people with DMD that I know. I'm stronger than people that are 18 years old," he says.

O'Connell remembers taking a bus to a pool near his elementary school in Fairport, New York, as part of the school day. Then, starting in ninth grade, he attended schools that had pools. The swimming was considered adapted physical education, something that is required by the Individuals with Disabilities in Education Act. O'Connell also had some physical therapy through his school system.

The buoyancy of the water can aid in exercise. "I still think swimming is the best," he says of the various physical education and physical therapy activities he has done. "I pace myself. I don't try to overdo it."

Shree Pandya, a physical therapist at the University of Rochester (NY) Medical Center who has evaluated O'Connell as part of a drug study, could not agree more with O'Connell's assessment of his swimming program. "What we have always recommended here as one of the best exercises is swimming," Pandya says. "That's because it's fun for the kids and they can exercise all the muscles in the body at the same time. They can even throw in some pulmonary work, like holding the breath and blowing bubbles in the water. "Water is a medium in which they can function even in the late stages of a neuromuscular disease. I've had kids who can't walk who still can go in the water and swim or walk in the pool. While they're losing other activities, this is an activity they can stay with. "Even a child who doesn't have the strength to function on land will be able to function in the water, because the buoyancy of the water can be used to minimize weight and the effect of gravity," she says. "You can use water as a medium of assistance or resistance, depending on what movement you're doing and how you do it."

Family Fun

Cheri Gunvalson and her family live in Gonvick, Minnesota, where it is too cold to swim outside most of the year. Her son Jacob, 8, has

Becker muscular dystrophy. Devices like a spa lift can help with getting in and out of the pool safely.

"I think swimming is one of the best activities for Jacob," Gunvalson says. "We swim at a local pool at a motel. It has a warm whirlpool, too, and he's thin and gets cold fast, so then he can go in the whirlpool. The cost is usually $2 to $3 per time. I bring all three of my kids and they play together. Our local pool is an outdoor one that's only available three months a year, so the motel pool works well."

Pandya, located in upstate New York, says they, too, are "talking indoor pools." She says, "We really push for swimming in community pools. We have two or three pools that are available, with nominal charges."

Safety First

Of course, take sensible precautions. Make sure an able-bodied person is at the pool at all times in case something goes wrong, and make sure there are no heart problems that would rule out swimming.

Special problems occur in cold temperatures (including cold water) in some disorders. In periodic paralysis, cold can bring on an attack of paralysis, while in myotonic dystrophy (MMD) and paramyotonia congenita (PC), cold water can cause muscles to stiffen and interfere with swimming. People with these conditions should swim in warm water.

Getting Started with Physical Therapy and More

Getting started with a physical therapist can take some work on your part, but it is worth the time and effort to improve your or your child's quality of life. One way to find a therapist in your area is through the American Physical Therapy Association which maintains a state-by-state listing of certified therapists with specialties.

American Physical Therapy Association
1111 North Fairfax Street
Alexandria, VA 22314-1488
Toll-Free: 800-999-2781
Phone: 703-684-2782
Fax: 703-684-7343
Website: http://www.apta.org

Your MDA clinic is always a good place to start with physical therapy. MDA covers one visit with a therapist a year, designed to help you set up a home physical therapy program or work with a community or school-based therapist. These therapists are knowledgeable about neuromuscular disorders and can serve as consultants for local therapists, teachers, and families.

MDA also covers some of the expenses associated with leg braces (orthoses) and wheelchairs. Call your local MDA office, the national office, or visit MDA's website for details about MDA's programs.

Muscular Dystrophy Association–USA

3300 E. Sunrise Drive
Tucson, AZ 85718-3208
Toll-Free: 800-572-1717
Phone: 520-529-2000
Fax: 520-529-5300
Website: http://www.mdausa.org
E-mail: mda@mdausa.org

Government, schools, and other agencies can help you. The National Information Center for Children and Youth with Disabilities is a clearinghouse for information and referrals on disability-related issues for children and youth from birth to age 22.

National Dissemination Center for Children with Disabilities (also known as NICHCY)

P.O. Box 1492
Washington, DC 20013
Toll-Free: 800-695-0285 (Voice and TTY)
Fax: 202-884-8441
Website: http://www.nichcy.org
E-mail: nichcy@aed.org

Prior to the implementation of the Individuals with Disabilities Education Act (IDEA) in 1975, most children with serious disabilities were shut out of public education. The IDEA of 1975 was significantly amended in 1997, and today it is a comprehensive federal program, administered separately by each state, designed to provide a "free, appropriate public education" to every student regardless of disability.

The law now covers infants and preschool children as well, on the theory that what happens before school starts has a major influence on educational success.

Services judged necessary for a student to take full advantage of the educational system, even if they are primarily medical in nature, such as physical therapy, can be included in a child's IEP, the individualized education program that each school system sets up for a child with a disability.

To set up an IEP, you can contact your local school district, usually working through a Committee on Special Education. Call your local school and speak to the principal or the person in charge of special education. If you do not have success (or even if you do), you may want to involve yourself in a parent advocacy group.

A program for an infant with a disability is known as an individualized family service plan (IFSP). To set up an IFSP, contact the agency in your state that is in charge of early intervention services for infants and toddlers with special needs. Therapists, social workers, pediatricians, and support groups can help direct you to the right agency.

For more information on IDEA and government resources, contact the Office of Special Education and Rehabilitative Services of the U.S. Department of Education.

U.S. Department of Education

Office of Special Education and Rehabilitative Services
400 Maryland Ave., S.W.
Washington, DC 20202
Toll-Free: 800-872-5327
Phone: 202-205-5465
Website: http://www.ed.gov/about/offices/list/osers/index.html

Chapter 26

Managing
Breathing Difficulties

Chapter Contents

Section 26.1—Making Breathing Easier 246
Section 26.2—Noninvasive Ventilation 254

Section 26.1

Making Breathing Easier

"Making Breathing Easier," reprinted with permission from the Muscular Dystrophy Campaign, a United Kingdom charity focusing on all muscular dystrophies and allied disorders. © 2003 Muscular Dystrophy Campaign. All rights reserved. Additional information is available at www.muscular-dystrophy.org.uk. And, "Treatment for DMD: Respiratory News" reprinted with permission from Parent Project Muscular Dystrophy. © 2003. All rights reserved. For additional information about Duchenne and Becker Muscular Dystrophy, visit the Parent Project website at www.parentprojectmd.org.

Breathing Difficulties and Neuromuscular Disorders

Breathing difficulties can affect some individuals with neuromuscular disorders. Simple measures can be taken to reduce these problems, and in many situations it is possible to provide excellent control of symptoms.

Breathing problems include an increased susceptibility to chest infections, difficulty coughing and clearing phlegm, breathlessness, and under-breathing (known as hypoventilation) particularly during sleep. This section provides background information on how families can help in the management of respiratory problems and identify symptoms which require investigation.

Who develops breathing problems, and at what age?

Respiratory muscle weakness is relatively common in most neuromuscular conditions, and is inevitable in the late stages of Duchenne muscular dystrophy. The age at which respiratory problems develop varies enormously. The youngest children we have treated for nocturnal hypoventilation have intermediate spinal muscular atrophy (Type II) and required breathing support at the age of 1–2 years. Young men with Duchenne MD tend to develop symptoms of nocturnal hypoventilation aged 15–20 years, and respiratory muscle involvement in conditions such as spinal muscular atrophy Type III, limb-girdle muscular dystrophy, and acid maltase deficiency may not occur until adulthood.

Respiratory muscle strength can be very variable within and between neuromuscular disorders; therefore, investigations and treatment must be tailored to the individual. Long-term management of breathing problems should always be medically supervised.

Recent research (*Neuromuscular Disorders* November 2002) shows that non-invasive nocturnal ventilation can have a significant effect on extending the life span of children with Duchenne muscular dystrophy (DMD). Overall, better coordinated care has probably improved the chances of survival to 25 years from 0% in the 60s to 4% in the 70s and 12% in the 80s. Nocturnal ventilation has increased this possibility to 53% in the 1990s, and these figures are continuing to improve all the time.

How do breathing problems arise?

When we breathe, certain muscles act as bellows to expand our lungs; these are called inspiratory muscles. They cause oxygen to be drawn into the lungs. The most important inspiratory muscle is the diaphragm. Weak inspiratory muscles reduce lung volume.

Breathing out the waste gas (carbon dioxide) from the lungs is known as expiration. This is usually passive and does not require particularly strong muscles, but coughing does require effective contraction of these muscles and normal functioning of the upper airway (bulbar) muscles. Scoliosis (a curved spine) reduces lung volume even more, and causes the respiratory muscles to contract inefficiently due to the asymmetrical shape of the chest.

After a period of breathing at low lung volumes, the chest wall tends to become stiff and less compliant making it more difficult for the respiratory muscles to expand and draw enough oxygen into the lungs. Children and adults with low lung capacity are prone to chest infections and these are slow to clear because coughing is ineffective. If the bulbar muscles are weak, food may be drawn down the wrong way into the lungs leading to recurrent infections.

During sleep, inspiratory and upper airway muscles normally relax and the intake of oxygen goes down. If these muscles are already very weak, then the oxygen intake becomes even lower, this is known as under ventilation or hypoventilation. In mild cases hypoventilation does not cause any symptoms and is only noticeable in rapid eye movement (REM) sleep when we often dream. However, if hypoventilation at night progresses it can lead to low oxygen and high carbon dioxide levels during the day.

If upper airway muscles are particularly weak, short episodes of upper airway obstruction may occur during sleep; this is known as obstructive sleep apnea. Often hypoventilation and obstructive sleep apnea coexist.

Spotting the Symptoms and Acting on Them

Symptoms of nocturnal hypoventilation include morning headaches, lethargy, breathlessness, disturbed sleep, and poor appetite. Erratic noisy breathing during sleep may be observed. In young children, failure to thrive or gain weight is not uncommon. These symptoms should be reported to your doctor.

Breathing problems can also be picked up during routine clinic visits. Vital capacity and overall respiratory muscle strength can be measured by simple blowing tests. Once vital lung capacity is less than 50% predicted and respiratory muscle strength falls below 30% of normal, hypoventilation becomes a possibility and regular checks should be made. Hypoventilation is unlikely if vital lung capacity is over 50% of normal, other than at the time of a severe chest infection.

If problems with breathing during sleep are suspected, a sleep study will usually be carried out. Here oxygen and carbon dioxide levels (and sometimes the pattern of breathing) are monitored overnight using small probes attached painlessly to the surface of the body. Arterial oxygen and carbon dioxide levels during the day can be measured on a small blood sample taken from the finger or earlobe. The sleep study may show a variety of findings. The most common of these is a fall in oxygen level and rise in carbon dioxide particularly during REM sleep due to under ventilation. In others, short episodes of stopping breathing (apneas) due to either obstruction of a floppy upper airway (obstructive sleep apnea) or lack of breathing effort (central sleep apnea) are seen.

Measures to Help Avoid Breathing Problems

Healthy eating. It is important to eat a sensible, balanced diet. Obesity should be avoided as it impedes breathing and increases the work of the respiratory muscles. It may also increase a tendency to obstructive sleep apnea. Remember that it is always easier to prevent obesity than to lose weight. Constipation leading to abdominal distension is not only uncomfortable but reduces diaphragm movement. It is best dealt with by a good fiber intake, although sometimes mild laxatives are needed.

Influenza and pneumococcal vaccine. The influenza (flu) and pneumococcal vaccines are recommended for individuals with breathing problems. These vaccines are not 100% effective, but will significantly reduce the risk of infection. The influenza vaccine is given once a year, usually in October. The pneumococcus bacterium is one of the most common causes of bacterial pneumonia. The pneumococcal vaccine lasts about five years. Both vaccines can be given by your family doctor and are very safe; however, individuals who are allergic to eggs should not receive them.

Breathing exercises and physiotherapy. Deep breathing helps to fully inflate the lungs and puts the lungs, respiratory muscles, and chest wall through a good range of movement. Cycles of 10 deep breaths aiming to expand the lower rib cage are recommended, with a short rest every few breaths. Assisted coughing or huffing is especially beneficial in clearing secretions at the time of a chest infection. Huffing is achieved by taking a few deep breaths and then forcing the air out as rapidly as possible with the mouth open. Phlegm is shifted from deep within the lungs to the main airways and then can be expectorated more easily. A family member or friend can help expand the chest in this region by placing their hands over the lower rib cage. Your physiotherapist will advise on breathing exercises and other forms of treatment if appropriate, such as postural drainage and chest clapping if secretions are excessive. Cough assist devices may be of value in some individuals with a weak cough.

Confidence about breathing can be boosted by breathing control advice and activities such as singing and playing musical instruments like the recorder.

Posture and curvature of the spine. Good posture is essential to allow the rib cage to expand optimally. It requires attention in the sitting, lying, and standing positions. For wheelchair users appropriate special seating not only improves posture and comfort, but may prevent the development of skeletal deformity. Around half of boys with Duchenne muscular dystrophy develop a significant curvature of the spine (scoliosis) and a scoliosis is relatively common in other neuromuscular disorders which arise before adolescence. Surgical correction of the scoliosis is used in some individuals to stabilize the spine and prevent further loss of lung volume. However, spinal surgery does not prevent further loss of lung capacity when it is caused by progressive muscle weakness.

Treatments

Chest infections. Prompt use of an antibiotic is recommended if phlegm is discolored or copious and the individual feels unwell and/ or feverish. Colds and flu are often followed by a bacterial infection so that an antibiotic may be required if symptoms do not clear up. Huffing and chest physiotherapy should be started as soon as possible.

If these measures are not beneficial, then further medical help should be sought. Children and adults with a tendency to wheeze may be prescribed a bronchodilator drug such as salbutamol (Ventolin) which can be delivered by inhaler, spacer device, or nebulizer.

Ventilation. There is no evidence to support the use of breathing assistance at night in individuals without symptoms or clinical features of nocturnal hypoventilation. Mild hypoventilation in obese individuals may be helped by weight loss. For moderate or severe hypoventilation, associated with symptoms, non-invasive nasal ventilation can be used.

Nasal ventilation. This system consists of a closely fitting nasal mask joined to a ventilator which augments the patient's breathing, thereby increasing oxygen and reducing carbon dioxide levels. A range of ventilators can be used such as the BiPAP (Respironics), Nippy (Thomas Respiratory Systems), DP90 (Taema), and BromptonPac (PneuPac). Many of these are portable and all are easy to operate. In most individuals, ventilation is initially needed only at night. If respiratory muscle weakness progresses, then use during the day may be required. Most patients are able to quickly acclimatize to nasal ventilation and find that their sleep quality improves.

Nasal ventilation can produce excellent control of symptoms in adults and children, sometimes over long periods of time. Evidence suggests that nasal ventilation may also reduce the frequency of chest infections and decrease hospital admissions. However, if the bulbar muscles are very weak, nasal ventilation cannot prevent aspiration, and in this situation another form of ventilation that will protect the airway can be considered. Ventilatory options should always be discussed on an individual basis, taking into full account the wishes of the patient and family, and the clinical circumstances.

Other forms of ventilatory support. Continuous positive airway pressure (CPAP) is a mask and compressor system which resembles nasal ventilation, but delivers a constant pressure rather than breathing support. This treatment is helpful in obstructive sleep apnea as the pressure acts to hold the upper airway open. Negative pressure devices such as the tank ventilator, cuirass ventilator, and other devices such as the rocking bed were used in the past to treat breathing problems caused by neuromuscular disorders, but have now been mainly superseded by nasal ventilation. However, negative pressure ventilation is still available for patients who do not adapt to mask ventilation, and newer negative pressure models such as the Hayek Oscillator may have a role in very young children and some adults. Ventilation via a mouth-piece is a variant of nasal ventilation that can be used at night or as a breathing aid during the day.

There is much that can be done now to control respiratory problems in neuromuscular disorders. Although a decline in respiratory capacity is inevitable in some conditions, symptom control produced by treatment such as nasal ventilation has been shown to improve quality of life. Children and adolescents using nocturnal nasal ventilation are able to return to school or higher education and adults are able to return to their usual daily activities.

Parent Project Respiratory News: Airway Clearing Devices

It has become clear, over the last 10+ years, the critical importance of good airway clearance of secretions as respiratory muscles become weaker, particularly for people with neuromuscular diseases (but also for people with intrinsic lung disease as they become weaker). The importance of both the expiratory muscles as well as the inspiratory muscles needs attention. Effective assisted cough techniques should be taught early, certainly when peak cough flow (PCF) falls below 300 lpm. Both breath stacking, to increase inspiratory capacity, and assisted cough flow are needed. When manual methods are not sufficient, then the CoughAssist made by J.H. Emerson (previously called the In-Exsufflator), may be considered to ensure a good PCF. In the past reimbursement has been a barrier. Now CMS (Centers for Medicare and Medicaid Services) has created a new HCPCS code E0482 for Medicare to reimburse for the CoughAssist device when it is clinically appropriate. Most health plans and health insurance companies follow Medicare policies for those covered for medical equipment. The following information summarizes the details. Ventilator users and their caregivers should become familiar with this information.

CoughAssist: Cough Stimulating Device

- Cough stimulating device, alternating positive and negative pressure.

- Effective date: January 1, 2002.

- Medical necessity documentation is required.

- 15 months capped rental is covered Medicare fee schedule: reimbursement range: $427.89 (ceiling) to $363.71 (floor).

- Maintenance and servicing fees may be billed once every 6 months after the 15 months rental cap has been reached.

The CoughAssist: This is a device that helps patients who cannot cough for themselves. It enhances or replaces a patient's natural removal of bronchial secretions. The noninvasive device simulates a natural coughing process and reduces the risk of airway damage and respiratory complications associated with more invasive procedures.

The CoughAssist assists patients in clearing secretions by gradually applying positive pressure to the airway to achieve a good inspiratory lung volume, and then cycling rapidly to negative pressure to achieve effective expiratory cough flow. This rapid shift in pressure, usually via a mask or mouthpiece, produces a high expiratory flow rate from the lungs, which simulates a cough.

- Model 1006916 cycles manually from positive to negative pressure.

- Model 1006915 cycles automatically.

The J. H. Emerson Company CoughAssist is a revised model of the Emerson In-Exsufflator, based on the Cofflator (O.E.M Corporation). The CoughAssist (or In-Exsufflator) is a portable electric device which utilizes a blower and a valve to alternately apply a positive and then a negative pressure to a patient's airway in order to assist the patient in clearing retained bronchopulmonary secretions. Air is delivered to and from the patient via a breathing circuit incorporating a flexible tube, a bacterial filter, and either a face mask, a mouthpiece, or an adapter to a tracheostomy or endotracheal tube.

The CoughAssist is indicated for use by patients who are not only unable to cough, but also unable to clear secretions effectively using available manual cough assistive techniques. This patient population experiences reduced peak cough expiratory flow (PCF) resulting from high spinal cord injuries, neuromuscular deficits, or severe fatigue associated with intrinsic lung disease.

Contraindications for the CoughAssist: History of bullous emphysema, susceptibility to pneumothorax or pneumomediastinum (lung barotrauma injury). People with cardiovascular instability should be cautious, and if the CoughAssist is used it should probably initially be used with professional observation at a medical center with at least oximetry monitoring of heart rate and oxygen saturation, before use in the home. Published studies are available.

Other Airway Clearance Devices

- **Yankauer suction tube with a suction device:** Effective for removing oral secretions and phlegm that is coughed up to the oral pharynx. Various medical supply companies. Inexpensive.

- **Resuscitator bag:** Effective to assist with breath stacking, to increase maximum inspiratory capacity prior to a cough. Various manufacturers (such as Ambu bag). Alternatives to achieve breath stacking are: glossopharyngeal breathing (GPB), or the use of a volume ventilator. Inexpensive.

- **Mechanical Percussors:** Made by various manufacturers. Often used together with postural drainage in 6–12 different PD positions. An effective cough is required to bring up the phlegm once it is loosened. They are of uncertain value for people with neuromuscular disease and respiratory muscle weakness. Inexpensive.

- **The Vest Airway Clearance System:** Produces high frequency chest wall oscillation to loosen mucous secretion. An effective cough is required to bring up the phlegm once it is loosened. This can help loosen secretions, which then have to be cleared from the airways (using an additional effective method) of people with neuromuscular disease and respiratory muscle weakness. Very expensive approx. $14,000.

Additional Information

J.H. Emerson Co.
22 Cottage Park Ave.
Cambridge, MA 02140-1691
Toll-Free: 800-252-1414
Phone: 617-864-1414
Fax: 617-868-0841
Website: http://www.jhemerson.com
CoughAssist

Advanced Respiratory
1020 West County Road F
St. Paul, MN 55126
Toll-Free: 800-426-4224
Fax: 877-368-5081
Website: http://www.abivest.com
   Vest Airway Clearance System

Section 26.2

Noninvasive Ventilation

Mike Neufeldt likes his job at motorcycle manufacturer Harley-
Davidson's Milwaukee headquarters, where he keeps an eye on deal-
ership web sites to make sure they meet company standards. After
work, he sometimes shares a beer with co-workers, and he's been
thinking about how someday he would like to move out of his parents'
house and into a place of his own.

   Not exactly unusual for the average 25-year-old, but Neufeldt is
not average. He has Emery-Dreifuss muscular dystrophy with severe
muscle weakness requiring a power wheelchair and 24-hour assisted
ventilation. Had a few key events taken a different turn, his life would
likely be far more limited than it is today.

Adamant about Another Way

   Mike's muscle disorder progressed relatively slowly for many years.
But in his early teens, he began to have trouble sleeping at night, was
falling asleep in school, and was getting headaches. He did not realize it

then, but those are classic signs of impaired breathing muscles and insufficient air exchange, or underventilation.

Then, one summer day in 1993, he was so tired he decided to take a nap. "When I woke up, I was blue," he remembers. "I had blue lips and blue fingertips."

His parents rushed him to a local hospital, where doctors tried unsuccessfully to stabilize his condition. "I started getting worse, not better, and they felt that I was showing signs of needing a tracheostomy," Neufeldt says. (A tracheostomy [or trach] is a surgical procedure that makes a hole in the windpipe, or trachea, through which a tube is passed that can be attached to a ventilator.)

"My mom was adamant that there had to be another way, something else we could do," Neufeldt recalls. So was the 15-year-old. The doctor was reluctant to allow Mike a voice in the decision, but Carol Neufeldt was adamant about that, too. "I had been making medical decisions all my life," Neufeldt says. His parents respected that.

The doctor acquiesced and suggested that Mike try a newly developed device, a bilevel positive airway pressure machine, with a noninvasive—nontracheostomy—interface. Pulmonary specialists knew these new arrivals were not as powerful as the ventilators used in hospitals or the ones that went home with tracheostomized patients. But the machines were easy to use, were fairly portable, and seemed sufficient for many people with moderate respiratory muscle weakness.

Life with a Bilevel Positive Airway Pressure Device (BiPAP)

The new devices were dubbed "BiPAPs" by one manufacturer, Lifecare, which has since been purchased by Respironics. (The term is a Respironics brand name, but has become a generic term for bilevel positive airway pressure devices.) Neufeldt uses a Respironics PLV-100 volume ventilator, which fits on the back of his power chair.

By the time Neufeldt left the Milwaukee area hospital, he was using a Lifecare BiPAP at night only. He was given an interface (the part where the device meets the user) called nasal pillows, perforated cushions that fit into the nostrils.

"I was able to breathe a lot better," he says. But after about a year, he felt he was "slowly going downhill." His energy was waning and his activities became more limited. His pulmonologist told him to extend his BiPAP into some daytime hours, but Mike did not find that practical. The device, though portable, seemed cumbersome to tote around, especially for a teenager. Once again, the Neufeldts began to search for alternatives.

A Visit to Newark

With help from MDA National Headquarters, Neufeldt and his parents located John Bach, co-director of the MDA clinic in Newark, New Jersey. Bach is known across the United States and in Europe for his expertise in noninvasive ventilation (NIV) to treat respiratory problems in neuromuscular diseases. He has been a physician specializing in physical medicine and rehabilitation since 1980, but he has never forgotten his undergraduate studies in engineering.

Bach brings to his patients a strong grasp of physics and engineering principles, as well as medical knowledge. He has a keen interest and a broad background in ventilation history, from the days of iron lungs—cylinders that surrounded the patient and applied negative pressure that caused the lungs to inflate—to today's highly portable systems that push pressurized air into the respiratory tract and weigh no more than a laptop computer. Neufeldt, who served as MDA National Goodwill Ambassador in 1987 and 1988 and is now a member of MDA's National Task Force on Public Awareness, stayed in Newark only a day. But he saw enough to equip him to continue discussions with his physician in Wisconsin.

A Stronger Vent

Bach did not recommend that Neufeldt spend more time on the BiPAP or get a tracheostomy interface. Instead, he recommended switching to a different type of ventilator—a volume-cycled device, as opposed to the BiPAP, which is pressure-cycled. Volume vents deliver a set volume with a variable air pressure, whereas pressure vents deliver a set pressure with a variable volume of air. Because of tradition and their historical uses in medicine, volume vents are capable of delivering far greater pressures and volumes than are pressure vents, such as BiPAPs. Traditionally, though, they have only been used with tracheostomy or endotracheal (down the throat) tubes. Bach's idea was to use these powerful ventilators with noninvasive interfaces.

A New Solution

Armed with the information from Bach's clinic, Neufeldt returned to Milwaukee, where he was fortunate to find his physician a willing partner in the switch to the volume vent. The doctor admitted Neufeldt to the hospital and helped him begin using a PLV-100 volume ventilator without a trach. (The PLV-100 is also a Respironics device, originally made by Lifecare.)

Neufeldt began using a sip-type mouthpiece (the user draws on it like a straw to trigger a full breath from the device) during the day and continued with his nasal pillows at night. The system worked. Neufeldt went on to graduate from high school and then from Marquette University with a degree in broadcast and electronic communications, and then to begin his work with Harley-Davidson—all while on a vent.

The Trouble with Trachs

Bach and a growing number of other physicians are skeptical of tracheostomy tubes, at least for many (not all) people with respiratory muscle weakness as their primary breathing problem. For Bach, there is only one indication for a trach: the kind of weakness of the mouth and throat (bulbar) muscles seen in amyotrophic lateral sclerosis. For most people, a system at the back of the throat routes food and liquid down the esophagus and into the stomach, and air down the trachea and into the lungs.

But when the muscles or nerves that control such a system are not working, food and liquids are easily inhaled into the lungs (aspirated), causing infection or obstruction, and air taken in through the nose or mouth may end up in the stomach instead of the lungs.

"Once the bulbar muscles are so bad you can't speak or swallow or keep saliva out of your airway, you need to be trached, or you'll be in respiratory failure," Bach says. ALS, he says, is the only neuromuscular disease in which that routinely occurs, noting that he has not found it necessary to use a trach tube in anyone with Duchenne muscular dystrophy in more than 20 years.

Trachs, Bach notes, lead to dangerous accumulations of mucus in the lungs and interfere with the ability to enjoy eating, tasting, and sometimes talking. They also place an enormous burden on caregivers and on the family's finances if they hire assistants.

The main problem with trachs, Bach says, is their interference with the body's normal mechanisms for constantly clearing the respiratory tract of mucus through the action of tiny beating hairs (cilia) whose job is to move these secretions up and out. To make matters worse, the presence of the tube itself—an unwelcome foreign body in the trachea—causes more than the usual amount of mucus to be produced.

Most trach users are taught that they need suctioning—passing a catheter attached to a suction device through the trach tube and down into the airways—to remove mucus many times a day, Bach says. But, he adds, suctioning itself can push bacteria from the upper airway down into the deeper and normally sterile lung passages, adding to the risk of respiratory infections, including serious pneumonias. Of course, the need for constant suctioning also requires constant attention—an extremely awkward requirement for trach users going to work or school. Fortunately, there are ways to avoid excessive suctioning, Bach says.

If trachs must be used, Bach recommends a device called a CoughAssist (made by the J.H. Emerson Company and distributed by Respironics), which can do what suctioning does with less damage to the airways and less discomfort for the patient. CoughAssists are usually used without a trach, but adapters can be purchased that allow the device to fit onto the trach tube. Use of the CoughAssist can reduce, if not eliminate, the need for suctioning. CoughAssists deliver a large volume of air into the lungs and then quickly reverse the air flow to pull out secretions, just as a cough would.

Skill Gap a Hazard Zone?

Joshua Benditt, director of Respiratory Care Services at the University of Washington Medical Center in Seattle, agrees with Bach that the person who needs a trach is the one whose bulbar muscles are severely weakened. "If you can't handle your secretions well, and you don't have any strength in your mouth, almost all of the noninvasive interventions, even the nasal or face masks, become quite difficult," Benditt says.

Like Bach, Benditt tries to avoid using trachs whenever possible. "When the patient is well motivated, noninvasive methods can do incredible things," he says. "I have about 25 Duchenne dystrophy patients, and that's all they use. I haven't trached a Duchenne patient in five years. "Noninvasive ventilation allows for a much better quality of life. You live longer and you're more independent, and we work really hard on that. In fact, one of the most satisfying things to me is to avoid a trach." In ALS, he says, he can often ventilate patients with a mouthpiece for a year or two, until bulbar involvement becomes severe.

Edward Oppenheimer, a pulmonary consultant and an associate clinical professor of medicine at the University of California at Los Angeles, sounds a cautionary note. Oppenheimer, who was in clinical practice for more than 30 years and has treated many patients with ALS and muscular dystrophy requiring ventilation, says, "If you need continuous ventilation, tracheostomy may be a more dependable method." He says the connections in a trach system are generally more secure than they are with noninvasive systems, and the access to the airway to remove secretions is more direct through the trach tube than with NIV interfaces. He adds that there is a "huge education and skill gap" for doctors and therapists with respect to NIV. More education for professionals is desperately needed in this area, he says. In the meantime, he is concerned that if patients ask doctors to "do something they're not prepared to do, they're going into a hazard zone."

Making a Change

Like Mike Neufeldt, Tedde Scharf, now 61, has never let her disability get in her way. As assistant dean of student life at Arizona State University in Tempe, a position she has held for 21 years, she works more than full time despite having almost no voluntary muscle movement and relying on 24-hour assisted ventilation.

Scharf's muscle disease—thought to be a form of limb-girdle muscular dystrophy—progressed gradually throughout her childhood and young adulthood, but by the time she reached her mid-40s, she began having some new problems. She was falling asleep at her desk and at meetings, was dead tired all the time, and had terrible headaches. Thinking she was just getting older, Scharf tried to press on. Then, in 1988, she had two bouts of pneumonia five months apart. Scharf's doctors recommended tracheostomy-delivered ventilation, to which, with great reluctance, she agreed.

Cold Air and Constant Care

From the beginning, Scharf intensely disliked the trach. For one thing, it directed cold air into her lungs. Heaters were available, but they had to be plugged in—not a good option for the active user. "During the day, I couldn't be tied down that much," she says. The constant need for suctioning was even less practical for the busy professional. "If I needed to be suctioned, I had to arrange for attendants to come to the office during the day," she says. "It was a royal pain." Worst of all, for the first six months, Scharf was unable to speak, something doctors told her she would just have to accept. Remarkably, she continued working, with constant note writing.

Finally, she met David Muir, who had muscular dystrophy and was able to talk despite the presence of a trach tube. As Scharf later learned, Muir was the inventor of the now widely used Passy-Muir speaking valve, a device she obtained, after much persistence, in 1989.

A Fortunate Encounter

Then, in 1993, another chance meeting would eventually lead to momentous changes for Scharf. That year, while attending a meeting in connection with her service on the MDA Board of Directors, she discovered that rehabilitation specialist John Bach was speaking at a medical conference in the same location. "I just slipped in the door in the back and listened to him speaking," she says. Bach was presenting his unorthodox ideas on noninvasive ventilation, and he soon had Scharf's full attention.

After the lecture, the doctor approached Scharf directly and asked her why she had a trach. Surprised, she stammered, "I had respiratory failure." Bach told her, "You don't need that thing" and followed up with a stack of articles supporting his position.

For the next two years, Scharf tried to convince her insurance company to allow her to see Bach in Newark and to switch to an NIV system. They refused. At long last, in 1995, Scharf's university changed insurance plans. While the new plan did not allow her to go to Newark, it did permit her to travel to Texas to see a trusted colleague of Bach's, pulmonologist Joseph Viroslav, at what was then the Dallas Rehabilitation Institute. (Viroslav is now director of pulmonary medicine at St. Paul University Hospital in Dallas.)

So Ready to Do It

By 1995, Scharf had been on invasive ventilation for seven years. The day she arrived in Dallas, she was ready to have the trach removed. "I was so ready to do it," she says. But the staff declined, cautioning her that a more gradual conversion to a noninvasive system was necessary. With the trach tube still in but plugged, Viroslav taught Scharf how to use a pneumobelt (also called an exsufflation belt), an unusual type of noninvasive ventilation that places a corset containing an inflatable bladder around the user's midriff. The positive pressure ventilator pumps air into the corset's bladder, which pushes the wearer's diaphragm upward, allowing exhalation. When the ventilator cycles to a lower pressure, the diaphragm descends by gravity, causing inhalation. "I knew that I wanted the pneumobelt," Scharf says. Its lack of visibility (it can be worn under clothes) had appealed to her, and she had gone to Texas hoping to obtain one.

As an additional alternative, Scharf learned to use a mouthpiece, and she obtained a nasal mask for nighttime use. Scharf also learned how to take in a volume of air sufficient to generate a cough (breath stacking) and how to cough. "Nobody had ever showed me how to cough until then," she marvels.

Scharf's NIV was delivered by a Lifecare PLV-100, although she later switched to the smaller LTV950 from Pulmonetic Systems. (It is the size of a laptop computer, while the PLV-100 is about the size of a desktop monitor.) Scharf adapted to her new systems almost immediately. "I think I was so psychologically ready that I just changed," she says, although she was told that many longtime trach users had a hard time making the switch. "I was ready to go home, but I had plane tickets for leaving in 10 days—so I went to malls and had a good time in Dallas."

Beyond BiPAP

Although Bach welcomes any trend that moves physicians away from relying solely on tracheostomy to treat ventilatory failure, he says total dependence on bilevel pressure devices is not the answer either. "Some people are using nighttime BiPAP and calling it non-invasive ventilation," he says. "When you do that, you can't get a deep breath. You may do okay until you get a cold. Then respiratory failure occurs." Bach only uses BiPAPs for babies and for specific types of adult patients, but he says the devices generally are not strong enough. "They're enough to ventilate most people and rest the inspiratory [inhalation] muscles, but they're not strong enough for getting a deep breath to cough with or to maintain lung compliance [suppleness]."

BiPAPs are appealing, he says, because they are small, easy to use, highly portable, and as ventilators go, relatively inexpensive. But they are derived from devices meant for people with abnormal breathing patterns during sleep, not severe respiratory muscle weakness, and in his view, they are rarely up to the job they need to do as a neuromuscular disease progresses.

Physicians who are not familiar with vent options, he says, often recommend either using the BiPAP for more hours of the day or going to trach ventilation once nighttime BiPAP is not sufficient. Instead, Bach puts his patients on a volume ventilator and ensures they have a method for clearing secretions.

Benditt has a slight preference for BiPAPs and other pressure-cycled ventilators for nighttime use, because they automatically compensate for air that leaks around the person's nighttime mask or other interface. "For the individual patient," he says, "a pressure-regulated ventilator might work better at night, with a mask, while you might want to use a volume ventilator during the day."

Bach, however, considers the leak compensation feature of BiPAPs a drawback. He says the increases in air pressure can wake the person several times a night if the device senses a small leak. He prefers to use a volume vent, but to minimize air leaks with good seals.

Cough Power

If there is anything virtually all respiratory care experts agree on, it is the crucial need to clear secretions. "Most of the time, people with neuromuscular disease do not develop respiratory failure because of an inability to breathe, but because of an inability to cough," Bach says. "In Duchenne dystrophy, 90 percent of respiratory failures occur during chest colds, because people can't cough, and they get pneumonia."

There are a variety of methods to ensure a good cough, no matter how weakened the expiratory muscles—the main ones responsible for coughing—and the bulbar muscles may be.

Breath stacking—closing the throat after each breath taken in through a mouthpiece and then coughing—is a good method for those who can manage it, and caregivers can be taught how to increase coughing efficiency by pressing on the abdomen.

For others, the **CoughAssist,** which delivers a high-volume breath and then quickly reverses to negative pressure through a mask, requires no strength and no ability to close the throat. "It simulates, rather than stimulates, a secretion-clearing cough," Oppenheimer says. For those using trachs, catheter suctioning or a CoughAssist with a trach adapter can be employed.

People who have the ability to cough well sometimes benefit from devices that shake up mucus in the chest and move it up toward the mouth and throat, such as the Vest, an airway clearance system made by Advanced Respiratory. The vest is attached to an air-pulse generator that rapidly inflates and deflates the device up to 20 times per second to create air flow in the lungs. Oppenheimer is cautious, however. "It shakes stuff around, so it's good for cystic fibrosis [a lung disease] patients, who have a good cough," says Oppenheimer. "But if you shake stuff around and then can't get it out, you drown in it, so it has limited application in respiratory care." The oscillation vest is now being studied for its possible application to neuromuscular disease, and the company is considering adding a cough-assistance feature.

Biofeedback

So, how do you know you're not getting enough air before you develop headaches, daytime sleep attacks, or pneumonia? Bach's answer: the oximeter.

Oximeters are electronic devices about the size of a small cell phone that measure the amount of oxygen in the blood through a completely painless sensor that can be clipped to a finger or earlobe. Bach advises his patients to get one and use it as a biofeedback monitor if they feel tired or have a cold.

If the oxygen level is normal (at least 95 percent saturation is the medical terminology) without any supplemental oxygen, there is a very good chance that air exchange is adequate. If saturation levels dip below normal, patient and doctor have to decide whether the problem is chronic underventilation because air exchange is not adequate or whether there is mucus plugging the airways. Either way, steps have to be taken.

Supplemental oxygen (that is, taking in oxygen concentrations of more than the 21 percent that is usual for room air) is a very bad idea in neuromuscular disease for a variety of complex biochemical reasons, Bach says. But there is also a simple reason not to use it, he cautions: It destroys the value of oximeter readings, offering dangerously false reassurance about the adequacy of air exchange.

Self-Management

Self-management skills are important in any chronic condition, and some people have more ability in this area than others. Tedde Scharf may have elevated it to an art form. Rising at dawn to begin a full day of meetings, projects, and grants administration to help some 1,500 students with disabilities, she says not being afraid and "adapting as you go along" have helped sustain her.

"I think that unless people are consistent with their doctors, they're not likely to get what they want," she says. "Managing your own care takes a certain amount of motivational ability. You have to take responsibility for yourself, but you also have to be willing to ask for help and then manage it." For vent users, knowing the options and finding doctors willing to explore them can make the difference between just living and really enjoying life.

Making Noninvasive Ventilation (NIV) Work

To make noninvasive ventilation work in neuromuscular disease, you have to become your own best troubleshooter. Here are some common problems. The solutions, based on the principles endorsed by John Bach and others, require the participation of a health care professional well versed in the use of NIV in neuromuscular disease.

Problem: Constant sleepiness, morning headaches, foggy feeling, shortness of breath, low oximeter readings.

Solution: Ensure that an adequate volume and pressure of air are being delivered. This may require switching from a pressure-cycled to a volume-cycled ventilator. Ensure that you are spending enough time on the ventilator. Nighttime ventilation alone may not be enough.

Problem: Signs of chest infection, such as shortness of breath, fever, malaise, low oximeter readings.

Solution: Get treatment for acute infection. Then find a regular method of clearing secretions, such as caregiver-assisted coughing, breath stacking with coughing, oscillation vest with coughing, or CoughAssist use.

Problem: Skin or eye irritation from mask or other interface.

Solution: Ensure that the interface fits comfortably but firmly, ordering a custom-made one or a gel-padded one as necessary. Eye irritation can mean there is air blowing into the eyes from a leak in the interface.

Problem: Emergency medical personnel want to administer oxygen in response to signs of respiratory distress.

Solution: Be familiar with your respiratory program and its principles. Keep a written explanation of it and your specialist's contact information with you or a caregiver, and offer it to emergency personnel as necessary.

Ventilation Resources

International Ventilator Users Network (IVUN) Division
Post-Polio Health International (PHI)
4207 Lindell Blvd., #110
Saint Louis, MO 63108-2915
Phone: 314-534-0475
Fax: 314-534-5070
Website: http://www.post-polio.org/ivun
E-mail: info@post-polio.org

Dr. John R. Bach
Website: http://www.doctorbach.com

Pulmonetic Systems, Inc.
17400 Medina Road, Suite 100
Minneapolis, MN 55447-1341
Toll-Free: 866-752-1438
Fax: 763-398-8400
Website: http://www.mbbnet.umn.edu/company_folder/
pulmonetic.html
E-mail: info@pulmoetic.com

Chapter 27

Pain Control and Neuromuscular Disease

Pain, Pain, Go Away

While pain is, thankfully, not a major symptom of most neuromuscular diseases, it can be a problem for many people who have these disorders.

Pain is a central aspect of several neuromuscular diseases, and a secondary consequence of muscular changes in others. In all these situations, pain can make it more difficult to cope with the challenges of living with a disorder. Pain that prevents normal motion or disturbs sleep interferes with the body's ability to maintain health.

Inflammation

For those with polymyositis or dermatomyositis, muscle pain often accompanies the inflammation at the heart of these diseases. In the myositis diseases, the immune system mistakes certain parts of

Reprinted from "Pain, Pain, Go Away" by Richard Robinson, *QUEST*, Volume 3, Number 3, Summer 1996. Reviewed in February 2004 by Dr. David A. Cooke, MD, Diplomate, American Board of Internal Medicine. And reprinted from "Marvelous Massage" by Carol Sowell, *QUEST*, Volume 7, Number 6, December 2000. Both articles are reprinted with permission from the Muscular Dystrophy Association, www.mdausa.org. © The Muscular Dystrophy Association. For additional information, call the Muscular Dystrophy Association National Headquarters toll-free at (800) 572-1717. To find an MDA office in your area, look in your local telephone book, or click on "Clinics and Services" on the MDA website.

the muscles for foreign tissue, and responds by attacking them with chemicals that kill the muscle cells. The result of this attack is called inflammation, and is marked by tissue swelling, tenderness, and pain in the affected areas.

Prednisone, a synthetic steroid drug, suppresses the inflammatory response and is often prescribed to combat the effects of myositis. Reduction of inflammation also reduces the associated pain.

Pain is also a central symptom of the metabolic diseases of muscle, such as phosphorylase deficiency, debrancher enzyme deficiency, and mitochondrial myopathy. In these diseases, the normal energy-producing reactions in muscle cells are interrupted, preventing quick resupply of the fuels needed for strenuous activity. As a result, even moderate exercise quickly exhausts the muscles; pain and cramping often ensue and can last several hours. Little can be done to ease the pain except to wait; it fades on its own over the course of an hour or more as the muscle returns to its normal resting state. People with these diseases learn to monitor their activity levels to avoid the kinds of exercise that bring on pain.

Cramping

Cramping is also a painful symptom in other neuromuscular diseases, including ALS. These cramps result not from fuel exhaustion, but disorders in nerve cell control of the affected muscle. Cramps often occur at night, when muscle is at rest. Some people find that 1–2 tablespoons of brewer's yeast before bedtime helps prevent night cramps.

Infrequent cramping is most easily treated by passive stretching of the affected muscle; application of ice may help. More frequent cramping can be treated with phenytoin (trade name Dilantin) or carbamazepine (trade name Tegretol).

Each of these drugs reduces nerve excitability. Unfortunately, they cannot be used by people with heart abnormalities, a common problem in some neuromuscular diseases. Those with myasthenia gravis also should avoid these drugs, as their effect can make myasthenic symptoms worse (though cramping is rare in MG). People with other neuromuscular disorders should consult their doctors before using these medications.

The same cautions apply for quinine, an over-the-counter medication used for years to treat leg cramps. It has now been removed from the market by the Food and Drug Administration because of questions concerning its effectiveness. Those with frequent cramping may wish to try cutting back on stimulants such as caffeine, which can overexcite muscle.

Prolonged Contractions

Myotonic dystrophy (MMD) involves a different sort of cramping—muscles relax very slowly after contraction. While this is rarely painful for voluntary muscles, it can lead to painful conditions if involuntary, or smooth, muscles are involved. These include the muscles of the digestive system. Prolonged contraction can lead to painful abdominal cramps and constipation. Gallstones can form if the smooth muscle of the gall bladder is involved.

The available anti-cramping medications can help, although it is especially important for those with myotonia to consult a physician before using these drugs, since heart conduction and rhythm problems are a common and serious problem in this disease.

A healthy diet may help avoid some of these problems. High-fiber foods help to minimize constipation, and low-fat, low-cholesterol foods cut down on gall bladder activity. Surgery may be indicated in some cases.

Finally, cramping can sometimes be a good sign in myasthenia gravis. In MG, the normal nerve cell signaling molecule is broken down before enough of it builds up to cause muscle contraction. The drug Mestinon is often prescribed to delay the breakdown; cramping is a sign that the drug has begun to work.

Skeletal Problems

While the muscle wasting of the muscular dystrophies does not itself cause pain, the resulting muscle weakness often leads to changes in posture which, if uncorrected, can be quite painful.

When skeletal elements shift out of their normal positions, they may stimulate pain receptors in the joints. For instance, facioscapulohumeral muscular dystrophy often leads to shifting of the shoulder joint, as the weight of the arm becomes too great to be resisted by the weakened shoulder muscles. A partial dislocation results, and irritation of the ball-and-socket joint there can lead to chronic inflammation.

Treatment for this type of pain may involve non-steroidal anti-inflammatory drugs (NSAIDs) such as ibuprofen, or a prescription steroid. A sling may help relieve the stress on the shoulder muscle. In many cases, surgery can increase support of the shoulder joint when other methods fail to provide relief from pain.

In Duchenne muscular dystrophy and spinal muscular atrophy, muscle weakness progresses to include those muscles that support the spine and chest. The resulting changes in posture often lead to scoliosis, or curvature of the spine, a painful and potentially life-threatening condition. Changes in posture put weight on structures unsuited to the stress, and full expansion of the chest cavity becomes difficult, which impairs breathing already made difficult by weakened respiratory muscles.

In the past scoliosis was treated with bracing in the wheelchair, however, current recommendations are almost unanimously in favor of early surgery to prevent the curvature before it becomes severe enough to impair breathing.

Surgery, of course, can bring its own painful complications. The person with neuromuscular disease facing surgery, whether for treatment of disease-related problems or not, will need careful evaluation for the planning of anesthesia and control of post-operative pain. For instance, certain anesthetics increase the risk of malignant hyperthermia, a rare but potentially serious complication during surgery. Opiate pain relievers such as codeine and morphine suppress normal respiratory function, decreasing breathing rate and depth. This can be life-threatening if the respiratory system is already weakened by neuromuscular disease. Many anesthetic agents normally used in surgery are unacceptable for the same reason. It is important that the medical team plan for pain control with full knowledge of the patient's medical history.

Headaches

Of course, people with neuromuscular disease have the normal range of other medical problems not related to their disorder. Pain can arise from headaches, fever, menstrual cramps, arthritis, etc. Treatment with non-prescription medication is usually as effective and as uncomplicated as for those without neuromuscular diseases.

However, there are some caveats. Aspirin and NSAIDs can cause gastrointestinal bleeding. These drugs should therefore be avoided by those on prednisone, which can have the same side effect; acetaminophen (for example, Tylenol) can be substituted. Aspirin also should not be given to children with fever, as a rare condition called Reye's syndrome may result.

Atropine and scopolamine are present in some over-the-counter drugs for constipation and allergy. Because they affect transmission of nerve signals to muscle, they should be used only after consultation with a physician.

Anxiety

Finally, the psychological pain of anxiety or depression can be a major consequence of a neuromuscular disease, and its treatment is every bit as important as is the treatment of physical pain. For the person finding it difficult to accept his diagnosis, or who is anxious or depressed about the future, proper counseling and family support are critical. MDA support groups are an important resource for those learning to cope constructively with the challenges of life with a neuromuscular disease.

Pain Relief, Relaxation, and Comfort Can Result When You Get Rubbed the Right Way

What is not to like about a massage? What could be more inviting than a dimly lit, quiet room offering calm peace and privacy, your eyes closed, your body lying relaxed and comfortable under fresh cool sheets, your skin being touched by soothing oils and warm, caring hands?

For people with neuromuscular disease there is much to like—everything from improved blood flow to relaxation of knotted muscles to nurturing touch. Massage has many immediate benefits, say practitioners, physicians, and people who have discovered its pleasures. The downside is almost nonexistent.

Massage is the manipulation of soft tissue by stroking, kneading, and pressure. It has been around for thousands of years, and it is good for babies, kids, adults of all ages, people with almost any medical condition or with none, and even for pets. Its general result is better blood circulation, overall relaxation, stress reduction, and relief from muscle pain. Those effects in turn can—depending on the individual—yield better sleep, more flexibility of joints, improved bowel function, relief of mood symptoms such as depression and anxiety, and in some cases even prolonged muscle function. Though it cannot stop or reverse the progress of a neuromuscular disease, massage can temporarily ease some symptoms and make a person feel more comfortable.

Most people who enjoy frequent massage wholeheartedly agree that it feels great, even if they are not quite sure why. Doctors and physical therapists suggest it can ease neuromuscular pain, with no side effects to be concerned about. There is also a growing field of research aimed at scientifically measuring and explaining why and how massage produces its many benefits.

Bill Altaffer of Tucson, Arizona, has been getting massages twice a month for about 15 years. An attorney who has spinal muscular atrophy, Altaffer says massage has benefits "for circulation, relaxation, contractures, chest loosening up so you can breathe. I can't explain this to you scientifically, but when she works on me, my ribs all crack because things get loosened up, the cartilage sort of gets moved around."

If massage is so great, why is it not used every day? One reason may be the cost. Fees can range from $25 to $75 for an hour's treatment. This may be within even a modest budget if you only go once a month. If you are a regular customer, you can probably get a cut rate or have shorter sessions.

Williams also suggests negotiating with a therapist for regular sessions. The therapist may offer a sliding scale, or be willing to give a discount if you bring in other referrals or place announcements in a newsletter or bulletin board. Paying for several sessions up front could get you a deal. It is unusual for health insurance to cover massage therapy, but it may be covered if it is prescribed by your doctor or physical therapist. An alternative is for family members to learn massage. Schools often give short courses on the basics, and there are instructional books and web sites.

Massage by a family member can be a bonding or loving experience. Hernandez-Reif points out, "In most of our child studies, we train parents to massage their children because it is cost-effective. There are benefits for the person receiving massage and for the person giving it." Some people can do self-massage of pressure points on the head, face, torso, and feet. You can also use products that apply pressure on trigger points, usually involving hardwood or rubber knobs.

Altaffer points to another significant benefit of massage. "People with disabilities who are skinny and shy about their bodies live in their heads more than they live in their bodies. So it is nice to celebrate your body, give your body a treat every once in a while."

Steve Pinczewski of Erie, Pennsylvania, worked as a massage therapist for several years and describes massage as passive exercise. Pinczewski takes Mestinon for his myasthenia gravis, and finds massage relieves the cramps that sometimes occur with the drug. Pinczewski cannot say enough good about massage. "There's nothing better. It gets rid of all the toxins built up in the muscles. Anybody who can't get rid of their anxiety with a good massage, they've got a serious problem."

Pat Moeschen of Salem, New Hampshire, teaches music in a middle school. He has been getting regular massages for over a year. "It helps relieve stress with the muscles, especially in my legs and my lower back. It has just been fabulous. I feel great every time I have one," he says. "The next few mornings when I get up after having one I certainly feel better. By better I just mean more refreshed, my muscles are a little bit looser. It makes things easier to stretch."

Moeschen, who has Becker muscular dystrophy, also does regular physical and aquatic therapy. He finds massage a good addition to those treatments. "I push myself to the limits and when I have this treatment I feel that it will make me less prone to injury because things are just looser and easier to be used." He asks his massage therapist to place particular emphasis on "my calves. It's probably the tightest muscle on my body at all times." Moeschen, who plays the drums, finds massage also helps alleviate fatigue and tightness in his lower back, shoulders, arms, and hands.

Gregory L. Pittman, MDA clinic director at Baptist Hospital East in Louisville, Kentucky, considers massage "an untapped resource," especially for dealing with the pain that often accompanies weakening muscles. "Typically, we are always trying to find the least pharmacological means to deal with pain because we know that pain medicines don't generally work very well, at least in the long-term. Any time you can come up with something that has nothing to do with medications is always a bonus," he says.

Pittman says massage can provide people with neuromuscular disease with needed physical activity. Family members can stretch the person's limbs and perform basic massage.

Another benefit is simple physical contact. "I wouldn't underestimate the fact that many of the patients have a serious problem with isolation," says Pittman. "People seem to be afraid to touch the disabled and that may even apply to their own family members. Yet I think that everyone has a certain need to feel physical contact from people."

Robert Lee Archer, MDA clinic director at the University of Arkansas for Medical Sciences in Little Rock, also likes the symptomatic, palliative treatment massage can provide. "I think that in many people, if they're having a lot of problems with muscle spasms, or increased tone [tension] in their muscles, they may well feel better after a massage. Certainly it's not curative. I don't think there is any real good hard scientific data to support using it in any certain neuromuscular conditions," Archer adds. "At the same time almost all of us have a subjective impression that massage, when our muscles are tight, tense, it seems to help them relax. I will talk to people who chronically have stiffness in their shoulders about having people in their family do massage, or rub their necks on a daily basis."

Wendy M. King, a physical therapist who works with MDA's clinic at Ohio State University Medical Center in Columbus, says, "Massage is one aspect of physical therapy. Personally, it's always been one of my favorites because, aside from all of the anatomical and physiological benefits you might get from massage, it's hands-on. I don't think you can deny the psychological aspect of just having a professional place their hands on you and attempt to help you." King explains that in neuromuscular diseases, various muscles degenerate at different rates, leading to an imbalance between muscle groups. This can lead to development of nodules or trigger points, places in the muscles where tension builds up. Massage can relieve those trigger points.

Marla Kaplan, a licensed massage therapist in Commack, New York, works with many clients who have chronic diseases or disabilities. For those with neuromuscular disorders, she says, "We can increase circulation to the area, which has to improve the health of the tissue. We can keep the tissue to a certain degree from the natural atrophy that is going to happen, and that is going to aid in movement." In addition, Kaplan says, "A massage will bring about an awareness to a muscular dystrophy patient on just how tight they are, just exactly what is happening from their body. So that when they are getting sore, when their legs are getting tired, they can do something about it whether it's moving, or calling an aide."

Maria Hernandez-Reif, director of research at the Touch Research Institute at the University of Miami School of Medicine, finds that massage before a physical or occupational therapy session can warm up and relax the muscles, thereby making the therapy session more comfortable and effective.

What Science Says

The popular idea that massage releases toxins is fact-based. According to an article by two physicians in *Physical Medicine and Rehabilitation Clinics of North America*, tense or contracted muscles can release substances, such as potassium, that cause pain, leading to more tension, more toxins, and more pain, and so on. Relaxation of these muscles can "flush out the algesic [painful] substance as new circulation is brought to the area." Massage may also prompt production of endorphins, substances that can reduce pain perception.

The relaxation of tense, tight, or contracted muscles is what leads to that looser all over feeling, along with increased flow of blood. The better flow of blood and lymph (a fluid collected from tissues and carried by the bloodstream) into tissues and organs throughout the body makes these areas healthier and better functioning.

The Touch Research Institute is studying the effects of touch therapies on people with a variety of health conditions. They are attempting to measure and understand scientifically what happens when people are touched therapeutically. Hernandez-Reif, a research psychologist, says there are two theories about how massage reduces pain. The gate theory suggests that pressure and cold nerve fibers are larger and more myelinated (insulated) than other nerves. "If you apply pressure and cold to a painful area, typically those signals reach the brain quicker than the pain signal because the connection is larger and more myelinated, which means it slides quicker," she says. The signal then "shuts the gate, so that the pain signals are blocked."

The second theory is that the neurotransmitter serotonin is involved in pain (as well as depression). "Individuals who experience a lot of pain have depleted serotonin. We find that massage naturally increases or replenishes serotonin levels. By replenishing these levels, it helps the body perceive less pain as well." This idea is backed by studies measuring serotonin levels in painful conditions, Hernandez-Reif says.

The institute's research is based on a view that applying pressure to the skin through massage stimulates the touch receptors, which in turn stimulate the vagus nerve, a primary nerve that branches to organs of digestion, the heart, lungs, and larynx, Hernandez-Reif explains. This stimulation "tends to generate a parasympathetic state, which is sort of a calming relaxing state."

The institute's research has found beneficial effects of massage for everyone from premature babies to people with cerebral palsy, multiple sclerosis, juvenile rheumatoid arthritis, depression, Down's syndrome, social isolation, history of sexual abuse, migraine, fibromyalgia, and more. Measured results include decreases in spasticity and hypotonia, improved range of motion, and increased self-esteem and optimism. The group has not yet studied muscular dystrophy but plans to do so.

Types of Massage

There are dozens of types of massage, many developed with a spiritual component. Most well-trained therapists apply a combination of techniques suited to the individual client. Following are some of the most commonly used and most applicable types of massage for people with neuromuscular disease.

Swedish massage: This is perhaps the most familiar type. Through basic stroking on superficial layers of muscle with pressure to relax muscles and stimulate blood flow, it can help restore temporary length and comfort, if not function, to muscles that have atrophied. The strokes in Swedish massage include moderate rolling, shaking, squeezing, and tapping.

Shiatsu: This form of massage is based on stimulating the so-called energy meridians or channels of the body. A gentle touch is involved, and the client can be dressed in loose clothing (many other forms require near nudity).

Trigger point: This deeper type of massage focuses on knots or nodules of muscle fibers, cramps, and spasms. These tight spots build up in people with neuromuscular disease because muscles are too weak to flush out toxins and may remain contracted. King says massage can help break down these knots. "We are talking microscopic here, but it doesn't matter because you as a person can tell the results. Now it's true that it may not always be a permanent effect but if it could be done on a somewhat regular basis the results can carry over." Trigger points are sensitive and feel painful when the therapist presses on them with fingers or elbow. But the brief pressure soon leads to relief.

Myofascial release: This form of massage focuses on muscles (myo) and connective tissue (fascia). The fascia are believed to retain tension from physical and emotional trauma, and to become shortened in dysfunction. Myofascial release helps restore correct shape and equilibrium.

Finding the Right Massage Therapist

If you decide you would like to try massage, first ask your neuromuscular doctor if there is any reason you should not have a massage. Usually there is not.

Physician Greg Pittman says, "I don't think there would be much likelihood of actually damaging anybody with massages. I can't imagine you could do anything by massaging a muscle that would make a difference in that person's neuromuscular disease."

When not to massage. However, massage is not advisable for anyone with a skin condition, blood clots or circulatory problems, active infections or inflammation, malignancies, congestive heart disease, or dermatomyositis. It should also be avoided in the abdomen in the early months of pregnancy and in areas with unhealed wounds such as pressure sores.

Once you have your doctor's go-ahead it is time to find a massage therapist. You can start with recommendations from friends, your doctor, physical therapist, or independent living center. You can also check with the American Massage Therapy Association for names of practitioners near you.

The right practitioner. Most massage therapists probably are not familiar with disability or neuromuscular disease, but you may be able to find one who is. Ask about experience and do not hesitate to ask for references.

Tracy Williams, a rehabilitation counselor who founded Touch/Ability in Tucson, Arizona, trains massage therapists and other practitioners in disability awareness. "The effective practitioner is one that is hard to determine. You have to go to them, you have to talk to them, you have to ask them questions, and then you have to feel if your personality melds with theirs," she says. "If the therapist kind of has a hesitancy to take you on as a client then you probably want to find another referral," Williams advises.

About half the states regulate massage therapists and require a license, which is earned by completion of at least 500 hours of classroom instruction. The Commission on Massage Therapy Accreditation/Approval accredits training programs according to federal guidelines. Be sure to find out whether your state or city requires a license, certificate, or registration, and whether the therapist you are considering qualifies.

Accessibility. Accessibility of the therapist's facility—the building, the massage rooms, the restroom—is another consideration. (Some massage therapists are willing to come to your home.)

It is possible to do some upper body massage on a person sitting in a wheelchair, but best benefits result when the recipient is lying on a massage table. Is there a lift or an adjustable table that lowers so you can transfer onto it? Will the personnel help you transfer, and do you want them to, or will you need to bring someone with you?

Be sure the therapist will work with your preferences and restrictions on body positions. For example, if you have breathing limitations, you probably don't want to lie on your stomach. Massage facilities usually have a variety of pillows and wedges to give you support and make you comfortable.

Communication. It is important that your therapist be willing to learn everything that will help her treat you. Urge her to phone your doctor with any questions and to read MDA literature. Be sure she is open to feedback about comfort and areas where you would like special attention. She should be asking whether various movements are comfortable, painful, or too intrusive, and heeding your answers.

Marla Kaplan asks clients to rate pain and sensation of various touches, especially when they have limits on sensation. "You have to be very careful to make sure that they completely understand that when it comes to massage therapy, unless it is trigger point, that it should feel comfortable at all times and that feedback is extremely important. No therapist is going to know better than them what they are feeling," she says.

Outrageous claims. Massage enthusiasts will cite many cases of remarkable results in which some symptoms were noticeably changed. However, any massage program that claims to cure or reverse the effects of a neuromuscular disease should be avoided. Though a legitimate therapist may have seen people achieve great symptom relief, anyone claiming to do more than that is a charlatan.

Additional Information

American Massage Therapy Association (AMTA)
820 Davis Street, Suite 100
Evanston, IL 60201-4444
Phone: 847-864-0123
Fax: 847-864-1178
Website: http://www.amtamassage.org
E-mail: info@amtamassage.org

Touch Research Institutes
University of Miami School of Medicine
7th Floor, Suite 7037
1601 N.W. 12th Ave.
P.O. Box 016820
Miami, FL 33101
Phone: 305-243-6781
Fax: 305-243-6488
Website: http://www.miami.edu/touch-research
E-mail: tfield@med.miami.edu

Chapter 28

Treating Scoliosis in Muscular Dystrophy

Muscular dystrophy can cause a curvature of your spine called scoliosis. Scoliosis and other back problems are treated by a bone and joint specialist called an orthopaedic surgeon. The purpose of this chapter is to give you some information concerning scoliosis and possible treatments. Knowing a little bit about scoliosis treatment will help you and your parents be better prepared for your visit with the orthopaedic doctor.

What Is Muscular Dystrophy?

Muscular dystrophy is an inherited disorder that produces a progressive weakening of muscles, making it difficult to control how you move and hold yourself upright.

What Is Scoliosis?

Scoliosis is a problem with your backbone, or spine, causing it to bend sideways and twist. Scoliosis can happen for many different reasons. Neuromuscular diseases, like MD, can cause scoliosis because the muscles that support the spine start to weaken and can no longer hold it straight up and down. Scoliosis can occur in either the upper back (thoracic), lower back (lumbar) or, very rarely, in the neck (cervical region). Scoliosis can develop slowly or quickly depending on its cause. Patients with Duchenne muscular dystrophy (DMD) usually have faster progressing curves than people with other kinds of neuromuscular problems.

Why Worry about Scoliosis?

Up to 90% of people with DMD will develop a severe scoliosis. The curve generally begins shortly after a person can no longer easily walk and needs to use a wheelchair. This usually happens at about 10 years of age. Due to muscle weakness in the back and chest, a person with DMD may no longer keep the spine in an upright, straight position. As the curve gets bigger, it changes the way you sit in your chair and where the pressure points are underneath you. If you use a wheelchair, these changes require frequent modifications of your chair to keep you well supported, prevent skin problems, and to keep you as independent as possible. While your chair can help support your spine, it cannot stop the progression of the curve. Scoliosis is a concern because if the curve becomes too large it can crowd your heart and lungs, making it hard for you to breathe properly. This may cause lung problems like pneumonia.

Treatment

Bracing is not a treatment option for DMD. The treatment of choice for DMD is surgical correction of the curvature. Surgery is done to straighten your spine and to prevent the curve from getting any worse. The doctors decide it is time for surgery when the curve gets to a certain size, which is usually around 25 degrees in patients with DMD. Surgery is done earlier in children with DMD than in other conditions, because research and experience show that if a curve reaches 25 degrees in a person with DMD, it will almost certainly continue to get bigger. Deciding to have surgery is a big decision and can be very frightening for you and your family. This chapter was prepared to answer your questions about surgery if you and your doctor decide it is necessary. If you have any further questions, please write them down so you will remember to ask your doctor.

Advantages of Early Surgery

People with scoliosis and muscular dystrophy can develop problems with their lungs, problems with sitting, balance, and with back pain.

Having your spine straightened before these conditions develop may save you lots of problems later on. If you are already having lung problems, having surgery can improve your breathing and help prevent problems like pneumonia. Also, straightening your spine will help you keep your balance better, help prevent back pain, and pain while sitting, allowing you to sit comfortably for longer periods of time. All of this can improve your quality of life.

Changes and Risks Related to Surgery

As a result of your surgery, you might be taller because your spine will be straighter. Being taller may make it harder for you to fit into your car or van. Being taller may also interfere with eating because your arms must move a longer way to get to your mouth. There are always risks involved with the surgery itself and with being put to sleep for surgery. Some of these risks include the possibility of infection or a problem with the metal rod the doctor will attach to your spine. The chance that these complications will occur is very low, and your doctor will do everything he or she can to prevent them. The doctors and nurses will make sure you know what the risks are and will answer all your questions before your surgery.

How the Surgery Works

The goal of surgery is to straighten your spine to prevent breathing and sitting problems. To do this, the surgeon will use a long curved stainless steel rod, called a Luque (loo-key) rod. The doctors attach the rod to your spine. In most patients, the rod is attached to the back of the pelvis. This is done if the hips are slanted or tipped. X-rays taken before your surgery are used to determine where your curve starts and where it ends, and also what shape the rod should be. That way the doctor knows where on your spine to attach the rods. Bone from the bone bank is placed along the side of the rod. This bone will grow into the spaces between your backbones (vertebrae) and will hold them straight. This is called a spinal fusion. Until these bones heal together, they need to be supported and kept from curving again. This is the purpose of the Luque rod. The rod is attached to your backbone and holds everything straight until the bones are fused together.

Before Surgery

All patients lose some blood during surgery, and sometimes you need to get some back afterward. You will get blood either from our blood bank, or if you are medically able, you may donate your own blood ahead of time. This is called autologous donation. The doctors and nurses will talk to you about donating and receiving blood when you set up your surgery date.

What Happens on My Workup Day?

One to three days before surgery you will go to the orthopaedic clinic for your pre-op workup. You can plan on being at the hospital approximately five hours on this day. The doctor will listen to your heart and lungs, and in general make sure you are in good shape for surgery. If you are sick on this day, or a few days before, notify the doctor, as he may decide to postpone your surgery until a later day.

The nurses and doctors will ask you and your parents some questions and answer any questions that you may have. This will enable them to give you the best care while you are hospitalized.

Urine and blood samples will be obtained. After the blood sample is taken, a bracelet will be applied to your wrist or sent home with you. It is very important to keep the band clean and dry so that your name and hospital number are legible. Remember to bring the band with you on your surgery day, or another blood sample will need to be taken.

You will have several x-rays taken. A medical photographer will take some pictures of you and your back, so the doctor can compare how you look before and after surgery. You may need to go to a special laboratory for an EEG (electroencephalogram) so they can check the nerve messages going through your spine before and during your surgery. They do this by attaching special wires to your head and your legs. This does not hurt. They will be removed after this first test, and then put back on the day of your operation.

You will also spend some time talking to the surgeon who will do your operation, as well as to the doctor who will be putting you to sleep. This doctor, the anesthesiologist, will explain to you how they put you to sleep, and will answer any questions you might have. They will ask you about any medications that you take on a daily basis. The anesthesiologist may instruct you to take these medications with a small sip of water the morning of your operation. You should tell the doctors or nurses about any allergies you may have to medications, foods, tape, or latex (rubber products).

The nurses will describe what will happen the day of your surgery and give you general information about being in the hospital. You should make plans to be in the hospital for 7 days.

You will be taught how to use a small breathing device called an incentive spirometer. This device will assist you with breathing deeply and coughing to clear your lungs after surgery, which decreases the chance of pneumonia. Also after surgery, you will roll side to side without bending or twisting your back. This is called logrolling (turning as a unit). The nurses will help you, but it is a good idea to practice this before surgery. The nurse will discuss methods of pain control to be used after your surgery, including the use of a machine called a patient-controlled analgesia pump (PCA). You will be shown scales for rating your pain and you will be asked to choose one that you would like to use while you are in the hospital.

The operating room staff will call you the day before your surgery to tell you what time you need to be at the hospital. You do not need to spend the night before your operation in the hospital.

The nurses will also give you a special scrub brush to scrub your back and right hip the night before surgery. This will help remove any germs on your skin and cut down the risk of infection during your surgery. If you are allergic to iodine, let your healthcare team know. You can do the scrubs in the shower or tub, but will need help from another person to get all your back clean. You will also need to wash your hair and remove any finger or toenail polish.

Your stomach needs to be empty when you go to sleep; therefore, you may not eat or drink anything after midnight the night before surgery. This will help keep your stomach from getting upset afterwards. You may want to avoid salty foods the night before surgery to prevent waking up really thirsty. You cannot have a sunburn, bad rash, or sores on your back at the time of surgery, as they could lead to an infection.

Make sure all your questions are answered before you leave the hospital on your workup day.

The Day of Surgery

Before you go to the hospital, you will need to wash your back again with another scrub brush for five minutes. Brushing your teeth and rinsing out your mouth are okay, but do not swallow the water. Do not chew gum.

When you get to the hospital, you will need to check in at the presurgical area. The nurse will record your vital signs (temperature, pulse, and blood pressure), talk briefly with you, and put on your identification and blood bands. You will get into a hospital gown and the nurses will help you onto a special bed. From here you will go back to the EEG lab, where they will put the special monitoring wires on your head. Sometimes they will put these wires on in the operating room. The operating room transport person will take you to the surgery area when it is time for your surgery.

Surgery

While you are in surgery, your family can wait for you in a lounge. The doctors will talk to them periodically during and after your operation and let them know how you are doing.

A nurse will greet you as you arrive in the operating room. The room is sometimes cool and noisy. Please let the nurses know if you are not comfortable. Warm blankets are available. In the operating room, you will be connected to many monitors. If this was not done earlier, a needle will be put into a vein in your arm. This is called an IV. The anesthesiologist will give you medications to put you to sleep. Once you are asleep, the doctor will begin the operation. A mask may be placed over your nose and mouth to help you breathe. After you are asleep, a tube is placed in the back of your mouth and throat to provide air to your lungs. This tube will be removed before you wake up. You will lie on your stomach on the operating bed with your arms and legs supported with pads. Your back will be scrubbed before starting the operation. The operation generally takes 4 hours, but you will be in the operating room a total of 4–5 hours.

A tube, called a Foley catheter, is placed in your bladder while you are asleep. The Foley drains urine out of your bladder so the nurses can measure it, and keep track of how well your body is getting rid of fluid. This tube is usually removed on post-op day 3.

A drain is placed in the incision during surgery. This is called a Hemovac. It is a small tube that drains extra fluid from your back into a little collection container. The doctors will remove it on post-op day 2. There is a mild burning feeling when the drain is removed.

Post Anesthesia Care Unit (PACU or Recovery Room)

When you wake up from surgery you will be lying on your back in the recovery room area. You will already be in your bed. You may feel stiff from being in one position for longer than normal. A nurse will check you frequently and make you comfortable with warm blankets. You will receive oxygen and be encouraged to take deep breaths to help your lungs expand.

The nurse may ask you to rate your pain on a scale of 1 to 10. If you feel sick to your stomach let the nurse know. You can have medicine to make you more comfortable if you have pain or are feeling sick to your stomach.

You will have some more x-rays while you are in the recovery room. You will be in the recovery room for 2–4 hours, or until the anesthesiologist says you are awake enough and doing fine. If you are 16 or younger, your parents or 2 adults may see you in the recovery room.

If the doctor thinks you need to be hooked up to monitors overnight (in case of breathing or heart problems) you will go to the Pediatric Intensive Care Unit (PICU). Your parents may see you in the PICU. Your doctor will decide when you are ready to come to your room on the Orthopaedic Unit from either the PACU or PICU. You will be taken to the Orthopaedic Unit in your bed.

Orthopaedic Unit Surgery After Surgery

After surgery the nurses will frequently take your vital signs (blood pressure, temperature, respiration rate, and pulse). This is so important that they even wake you up during the night to do this. The doctors and nurses will be touching your hands and feet, and asking if you have any numbness or sleepy sensations in your arms or legs. Let the nurse or doctor know if your arms and legs tingle or feel numb or just plain funny.

The IV will give you fluids during and after surgery. The IV will remain in until you are able to eat and drink which is usually around 4 to 5 days after surgery. The anesthesia medicine slows the motion of your intestines and may cause you to be nauseated or even vomit after surgery. The nurses will listen to your stomach every few hours to hear if your bowels are working. You may not drink anything until it is determined that your bowels are returning to normal. This may take up to 4–5 days. You may rinse your mouth out with water and brush your teeth. If you drink or eat before your bowels are ready, you may become nauseated and bloated.

You will have pain medicine to keep you comfortable. Your IV will be hooked up to a PCA (patient controlled analgesia) pump that has a tube of pain medicine inside. This syringe is attached to your IV line and continuously gives you a small amount of pain medicine. If you still are uncomfortable, there is a button to push to give you a little extra pain medicine. If you are unable to push this button, a family member or the nurse may push it for you. You may need an occasional shot in the muscle for pain along with the PCA. This depends on how severe your pain is. Your PCA will continue until your stomach wakes up and you are able to drink and take pain medicine by mouth.

You will also get antibiotics through your IV line to decrease the chance of infection. The antibiotics will continue until one dose after your Hemovac drain and Foley catheter are removed. A blood sample will be taken from you each morning after surgery for 3 days to check your blood count. If you are short on red blood cells, it might be necessary to give you a blood transfusion.

In the operating room a big bandage is put on your back. This will be changed on post-op day 2 and removed on post-op day 3. The stitches used to close your wound are under your skin. Your body will just absorb them, so they do not have to be removed. Pieces of tape called steri-strips are placed over your incision after surgery, and will gradually fall off on their own after you go home.

The day of surgery you will be flat in bed. The nursing staff will help you move from side to side by logrolling every 2 to 4 hours. When turning, your shoulders and hips must go all at the same time, like your back is one big log. You will be helped into a position either on your back or your side and propped up with pillows to keep you comfortable.

You will be sitting up in bed the first day after surgery. You will sit up 3 times that day to get your body used to sitting up again. The second day after surgery you will be carefully lifted out of bed into a wheelchair.

A child life specialist may come to your room and offer you activities to do while you are in bed. When you can be up and out of your room, you will be invited to attend group activities in the playroom. Your parents and/or caregiver will be taught how to take care of you. The nursing staff will encourage them—and you—to do as much as you are comfortable with. Please ask the nurses about anything that you may have a question about.

Going Home

Before you go home, x-rays will be taken while you are sitting, which is usually in 5–7 days after surgery if no problems arise. No cast or brace is usually necessary following surgery.

After surgery you can sit at only a 60 degree angle for 6 weeks. You can use your own wheelchair if the back reclines 60 degrees and the arms can be removed. If not, you can rent one. The rental chair will be a standard wheelchair without any pads or supports to help you sit, and so you will have to use pillows for support.

While you are in the hospital, you will be lifted into the chair by 3–6 people, depending on how much you weigh. Your parents or caregiver will be taught how to lift you by the fireman method when you get home, or you could use a mechanical lift. You may not be lifted under your arms for 6 months or until your spine heals completely.

In the days right after your surgery, the nurses or a parent will give you a bed bath. Keep your incision clean and dry. The steri-strips will gradually fall off. You may shower two weeks after surgery if your back incision is well healed and has no drainage. Direct the water stream on your front and shoulders, letting it trickle down your back. Do not direct the water stream on your back incision. You may not get into a tub or swimming pool for 6 months after surgery. Your back incision may be numb for 4 to 6 months.

You will be sent home with a prescription for pain medicine. You should also continue taking your iron as you were before surgery.

You may return to school in 2–4 weeks depending on how you feel. The people at school may need instructions on how to lift you. They may also need to know if there are changes in your height so adjustments can be made (for example, your desk may need to be higher).

Your first return appointment will be about 6 weeks after you go home, then 4 months, 6 months, and one year after surgery, and then every year after that. It is really important that you return for your scheduled appointments.

If any of the following problems occur before your appointment, notify your doctor right away:

- fever, chills, redness, warmth, or foul-smelling drainage at the surgical site

- increased in pain

- numbness, tingling, or increased

- weakness in your arms or legs

- change in bowel or bladder control

Chapter 29

Achilles Tendon Release

Two important goals of physiotherapy for adults and children with neuromuscular conditions are to keep the joints as flexible as possible, and where feasible, to keep the person standing or walking. These goals are largely achieved using passive stretching and exercises, orthoses (e.g. splints or long-leg braces), standing frames, and swivel walkers. Sometimes, if the Achilles tendon is becoming too tight and preventing a person from benefitting from these techniques, the tendon may be surgically released. This allows the foot to rest at a right angle. Other times when the tendon may be released are if a person who is dependent on a wheelchair is in pain from the feet, which could be alleviated by the operation. In rare cases, the operation is performed so that the child's feet look more normal and s/he can wear ordinary fashionable footwear.

The Importance of Flexible Joints

When joints are allowed to tighten and contractures set in, limbs can start to become deformed and even painful. This usually happens in neuromuscular conditions because there is an imbalance in muscle strength, so the stronger muscle pulls the weaker one in a particular direction. In delaying or preventing these contractures there are, of course, psychological benefits for a child to look like his or her peers, but keeping the body straight and flexible and the limbs loose can also help the body to function better. Keeping contractures under control by ensuring that the joints are as supple as possible can help to prolong standing and walking.

The Benefits of Being Able to Stand or Walk

Standing or walking can help prevent calcium loss from bones, keep weight down, and promote better circulation than if a person was sitting in a wheelchair. Importantly, standing can also help keep the chest and lungs less constricted and therefore assist breathing. Caregivers find it easier to manage a child who is able to stand; there is usually less lifting and some day-to-day activities can be performed independently by the person with the neuromuscular condition, for instance, standing over a washbasin to brush his or her teeth. In some conditions, standing can help delay curvature of the spine which may happen more quickly once someone starts to use a wheelchair full-time.

Children with Non-Progressive Conditions

Where a condition is static (or non-progressive), but the muscles are very weak, splints or braces may help a child to start walking. If the Achilles tendon has not responded to stretching techniques or splints and is preventing the child from fitting into splints or braces, the tendon can be surgically released. In these non-progressive conditions, the child may subsequently stop walking because as s/he grows, weight and height can sometimes outstrip muscle strength.

Boys with Duchenne Muscular Dystrophy

With Duchenne MD, which is progressive, a child finds it increasingly difficult to walk as his muscles weaken. The child prevents his legs from buckling by locking the knees and walking on his toes with his stomach pushed forward and shoulders pushed back to keep his center of gravity. This can cause the joints to tighten, especially at the ankle.

As the child finds it more difficult to walk, physiotherapists familiar with the condition will start to see the child more often, looking for the time that useful walking is almost finished. It is usually at this stage that the operation on the Achilles tendon is performed. It allows the child to carry on walking with the help of appropriate orthoses, and/or to use a standing frame or swivel walker. It is important that the operation is performed within three months of the child starting to become dependent on a wheelchair. This is because once in a wheelchair, the muscles waste more rapidly and contractures can set in which will make walking much more difficult to achieve after the operation.

Studies indicate that children with Duchenne MD have been able to walk or stand an average of two years and as long as four years after the operation. However, there are a few cases where the operation is not helpful in enabling the child to walk.

The Operations

There are two variations on the tendon-Achilles operation; they vary in the length of the cut and the amount of discomfort. By far the most common operation is the percutaneous tenotomy. The literal meaning of this title is: cutting the tendon through the skin. The actual operation to nick the tendon lasts no longer than five minutes and is done under general anesthetic. After the tendon has been cut, leg plasters are fitted; long or short plaster may be used. Where long plasters are fitted, the upper end of the plasters will probably have ischial supporting hips which allow the child to sit back on them and support his weight (the ischial bone lies beneath the buttocks).

The small nick on the tendon leaves very little or no scarring. Within 24 hours of the operation, the child is able to stand and walk with help from a physiotherapist. Sometimes it may be a little longer before the child is able to stand, but the sooner a child is walking or standing after the operation the better, because if a child is relatively immobile, his muscles waste more quickly.

An orthotist measures the legs either before, during, or after the operation in order to make long-leg braces for walking or ankle-foot orthoses. It is important that the orthotist is skilled, that the orthoses are ready soon after measuring (this is usually from a few days up to two weeks), and that they fit well. If they fit badly the child's motivation to walk will be affected. Long-leg braces should be reviewed at regular intervals (usually about every four months) and altered or changed as frequently as possible, which may mean one or more changes a year.

Ideally, this kind of treatment requires an orthopaedic surgeon and an orthotist experienced in neuromuscular disorders, a system which allows the child to be booked in when the timing is right, and a physiotherapist who understands the requirements of children with neuromuscular conditions. In summary, it needs timing and teamwork.

The second type of operation is called a formal lengthening of the Achilles tendon. This involves a two-inch cut along the tendon and is usually performed where the contracture is more severe. Stitches are involved and the procedure results in greater soreness than the Percutaneous Tenotomy where the child probably experiences only slight discomfort, but in both cases, the discomfort can be easily kept under control with mild pain-killers for a couple of days.

These operations involve a stay in hospital; in the case of children being fitted with long-leg braces in order to walk in them, this may last about two to three weeks because the child has to be taught to walk. These children have to cope with intensive physiotherapy, but are usually well motivated and rise to the challenge without problems. Where the operation is to enable the child to continue standing in frames, they can be discharged from hospital very soon after the operation.

Various Methods

It is important to remember that there is no single best method of management. The decisions about the most appropriate care for an adult or a child and whether to use night and/or day splints, standing frames only, a swivel-walker, or long-leg braces, and whether to have the Achilles tendon operation, will depend on individual circumstances. It will depend too on the outcome of the family's, parents', or adult's discussions with medical advisors including the physiotherapist and the family physician, and on the motivation of the person who is affected by the condition.

Chapter 30

Treatment for Duchenne Muscular Dystrophy

Chapter Contents

Section 30.1—Therapy and Bracing 294
Section 30.2—Nutritional Issues, Supplements,
          Steroids, and Antibiotics 299
Section 30.3—Stretching, Exercises, and Postural
          Correction in Duchenne Muscular
          Dystrophy 308

Section 30.1

Therapy and Bracing

This section includes "Treatment for Duchenne MD: Physical Therapy," and "Treatment for Duchenne MD: Splints & Braces." This information is reprinted with permission from Parent Project Muscular Dystrophy. © 2003. All rights reserved. For additional information about Duchenne and Becker Muscular Dystrophy, visit the Parent Project website at www .parentprojectmd.org.

Physical Therapy

A combination of different therapies plays an important role in keeping the body as flexible, upright, and mobile as possible. This is accomplished through a mixture of physical therapy, a regimen of exercise, bracing, and the use of a wheelchair.

There are three main areas where contractures (loss of elasticity in the joints) are most prevalent: the Achilles tendons (in the ankles), knee flexors (hamstrings), and the iliotibial bands (hip flexors).

Exercise can help postpone or even prevent contractures in boys with Duchenne MD. Physical therapists may teach methods to gently take each joint and move it through its range of normal positions on a regular basis and help keep tendons from shortening prematurely. Please consult a physical therapist before conducting these motion exercises as doing it incorrectly may do more harm than good.

If exercise does not help, surgery may be a viable option to treat ankles and other contractions while the child is still mobile. This involves cutting the Achilles tendon at the back of the heel in order to allow the foot to resume a normal position. After the surgery, the child will have to wear a cast and then leg braces to keep the contracture from reforming.

Occupational Therapy

While physical therapy focuses on allowing greater motion in the joints and prevention of other ailments, occupational therapy focuses on helping with specific tasks or activities. Through this type of therapy, boys with Duchenne MD can learn and re-learn how to dress themselves, use a computer, use the bathroom, and other tasks of daily life.

Frequently Asked Questions about the Use of Splints and Bracing

Orthotists, the people who are specially trained in making splints, have devised a system of naming splints depending on which joints they control. AFOs are ankle-foot orthoses and come from the toes or mid-foot to below the knee. These may be called ankle splints. KAFOs are knee-ankle-foot orthoses and extend from the foot up to the thigh. These are the ones that are usually called long leg braces or calipers. One pair may look different from another, they can be of several different types of materials, and they may have varying functions, but the way of naming them is standard.

Why should my child wear night splints for the ankles and when should they start?

Studies have shown that the regular use of night splints for the ankles, in conjunction with stretches, helps to maintain the range of movement at the ankle and reduces the tightness of the tendo Achilles (TA). In DMD, most boys will develop some tightness of the ankle quite early. The foot that just comes to the neutral position (90°) has already lost 20° of range. It is therefore important to start wearing AFOs at night as soon as the ankle starts to get tight.

How long should they be worn?

Some therapists advise that the boys start with one hour and gradually build up the time. As long as the night splints are comfortable and well fitting from the beginning, they are generally tolerated for longer than this, and therefore, parents should try to get the child to wear them for as long as possible, all night ideally.

What are the features of a good splint?

A good splint holds the foot at 90° to the leg, no more, no less. It should be unlined to prevent excess sweating. It should be of lightweight molded plastic, made individually for each child with a strap at the top and a strap over the ankle joint.

It should not cause any rubbing over bony parts or the back of the heel, and it should not be so high that when the knee is bent it digs into the back of the thigh. It should extend a little way past the toes to allow for growth. Occasionally, with a very thin child, thin padding may be put over bony parts and a thin sheepskin pad put in the heel. It is suggested that the children wear a lightweight cotton sock inside them to prevent the feet sticking to the plastic.

Would it not give a better stretch if the knee were included as well?

It is important to note that these splints are resting splints not stretching splints. The idea is that they hold the foot at 90° for as much of the night as possible rather than having the feet plantarflexed, i.e., with the toes pointing down. If the knees are included, the boys find them very restrictive and uncomfortable. Sometimes they are unable to move in bed and wake frequently.

What if my child will not wear the splints or will only wear them for part of the night?

Children vary considerably in how they tolerate the splints. Some will let you put them on when they go to bed, some parents do not put the splints on until after the child is sleeping. There are children who wear them all night, others who wear them for a few hours only. A few hours are always better than nothing.

Some children find they cannot turn in bed, in this case try to wear one on one foot for one night, then on the other foot the next night.

If your child really does not tolerate the splints at all, try to have the splints worn for as long as possible when the child returns home from school while they are doing activities such as watching television or doing their homework. Wearing splints at night is something that the children will be asked to do for many years so try not to resort to bribery—it could become expensive.

Should my child wear splints during the day to try and stop them walking on their toes?

At Hammersmith Hospital it is not felt that the boys should wear splints for walking. Most boys (apart from those with noticeably flat feet) need to walk up on their toes, as it helps assist the quadriceps muscle in stabilizing their knees. Concern is not about the boys who walk on their toes, but those whose heels remain off the floor when they are standing still.

There are other centers however, that do use splints during the day, and it is important to accept that there are different approaches to management. That does not necessarily make one approach right or wrong, just different.

What advantages are there in using braces when the boys are having difficulty walking?

Wearing KAFOs when walking becomes difficult has been used for many years in DMD. The benefits, apart from prolonging the ability to walk, include maintaining a more mobile and straighter spine for a longer time, controlling contractures of the hips, knees, and ankles, to make management and transfers easier, and also for the boy's own self esteem.

Can all the boys who are fitted with KAFOs manage to walk in them and for how long do they walk?

As long as the boys are fitted with the KAFOs at the correct time, they will manage to achieve independent ambulation. On average they will walk in them for two years, but some will only do it for six months, others have kept walking for several years.

When is the best time to start bracing?

For the best possible outcome, it is very important that the boys have not completely lost the ability to walk. Ideally the boys will be fitted with KAFOs just before they lose useful ambulation, but the only way to ensure this is with regular careful monitoring. A guide to when they are ready for them is when a child is struggling to walk 30 feet without assistance.

Are all children suitable for bracing?

Most children, at the time they are losing functional walking, have tightness of the TAs that prevents the foot from achieving the 90° position. It is necessary to correct this and surgery is therefore needed. At Hammersmith Hospital a very small percutaneous tenotomy is performed. This requires a general anesthetic, but the incision is very small. Rarely are there any stitches and casts are not applied. The child will stand in the KAFOs the day after surgery.

Most children are suitable for bracing, but not all our children and families want it. Although about 90% of our boys with DMD do have rehabilitation of walking in KAFOs, it is an informed decision taken by the families. There are children who may have challenging behavior or severe learning difficulties that make walking in KAFOs inappropriate. There are also those families who decide not to proceed as they do not want the surgery, but the numbers are small. Around one in ten children do not have tight TAs and so do not require surgery.

In a few cases, the boys have marked tightness of one or both iliotibial bands and again this may require minor surgical release. This can be performed at the same time as the TA release.

What are the disadvantages of KAFOs?

Apart from the need for surgery, the most important part of rehabilitation in KAFOs is getting the correct ischial (sciatic) weight bearing KAFOs that fit well from the first day. For this it is necessary to find an orthotist who has experience of DMD and the specific type of KAFOs used.

The parents are warned that following surgery to the TAs the boys are rarely able to take their own weight and so when they are not wearing the KAFOs can no longer stand for transfers or for dressing/toileting. (It must be remembered that the boys may lose this ability anyway shortly after loss of walking.)

The other requirement for rehabilitation in KAFOs is having facilities for the walking training. It takes up to two weeks from surgery for the boys to achieve full independent walking. There are twice daily physical therapy sessions during this period and it may be done as an in-patient or out-patient depending on how far the child lives from the hospital. For children not requiring surgery, the training period is usually 2–3 days.

How often do the KAFOs need replacing?

This will depend on how quickly the child grows, but generally they are replaced yearly. The KAFOs are designed to have some room for growth in them, but this is only for increased thigh length.

Do the children in KAFOs still use night splints?

Yes. They should wear the night splints whenever the KAFOs are not being worn. It is often recommended that the KAFOs are worn all day as they are (or should be) comfortable to sit in. This means that when the boys want to, or have the opportunity to walk, they can do it straight away. When they are not wearing the KAFOs, it is recommended to wear the night splints to try and prevent the TAs getting tight again, but they should definitely be worn at night.

Are splints necessary if I choose not to have KAFOs or when walking in KAFOs is stopped?

To maintain a good foot posture, it is preferable that ankle splints are worn during the day and at night. The day splints are then cut to the mid-foot to allow shoes to worn over the top of them. Again, if it is not possible to wear both types of splint, then either day or night splints should be worn.

Section 30.2

Nutritional Issues, Supplements, Steroids, and Antibiotics

This section includes "Nutritional Issues for Duchenne Muscular Dystrophy," and "Treatment for Duchenne MD: Steroids/Nutritional Supplements/Antibiotics." This information is reprinted with permission from Parent Project Muscular Dystrophy. © 2003. All rights reserved. For additional information about Duchenne and Becker Muscular Dystrophy, visit the Parent Project website at www.parentprojectmd.org.

Nutritional Issues

Duchenne Muscular Dystrophy (DMD) is a genetic, progressive neuromuscular disorder affecting approximately one in 3,500 male infants across all populations. It is a recessive, single gene defect on the X chromosome of the mother.[1] There are also cases of spontaneous mutation with no carrier identification identified in the mother. In 1987, the protein associated with this gene was identified and labeled dystrophin.[1]

In voluntary muscles, dystrophin is located under the cell membrane and attaches to a small group of other muscle proteins that, in turn, attach to the extracellular matrix outside the muscle fiber. Without dystrophin, muscle contractions can cause cracks in the cell membrane, muscle-degrading enzymes are activated to destroy the damaged cells. The destroyed muscle fibers are then replaced with fat and connective tissue.[1, 2]

With identification of the gene and concurrent research and therapy, boys with DMD are surviving longer, into their late 20s and older. Medical management of DMD spans multiple sub-specialties and clinics including: rehabilitation medicine, neurology, orthopedics, pulmonology, and cardiology. Nutrition care and management of DMD is an integral component of care. The following are some of the multiple issues associated with nutrition management in DMD:

- Accuracy and consistency of anthropometrics including weight and length

- Determination of ideal body weight

- Nutritional implication of corticosteroid therapy

- Osteoporosis and low-impact fractures

- Escalation of nutrition support with progression of muscle weakness

- Obesity with decreased activity

- Nutrition and emotional issues

Obtaining Accurate Weight and Length Measurements

A child who is able to stand and walk can be weighed and measured by the same means with the same tools as any pediatric patient. Infant scales and recumbent length boards can be used for infants. Regular scales and wall-mounted stadiometers are recommended for older children. However, when a boy with DMD is unable to stand, accurate weights and lengths are a challenge. Ideally, a wheelchair scale should be used. The child (in the wheelchair) is weighed, and then a Hoyer lift is used to lift the child. The wheelchair is weighed alone, and its weight is subtracted from the first weight. Growth assessment for older children can be challenging. Armspan has been used as an estimator for height.[3] However; many patients with DMD have scoliosis, spinal fusion, and reduced tibial growth making this measurement inaccurate. One method is to use segmental lengths. There are also recumbent length measure tools, which can be limited in accuracy secondary to contractures. What is important, however, is that no matter how cumbersome, weights and lengths need to be measured consistently by the same method at each clinic visit.[2, 4]

Estimation of Ideal Body Weight

Determination of ideal body weight using standard calculations becomes less relevant in children with DMD. Boys with DMD may lose up to 4% of their muscle mass per year. Specific guidelines for the actual calculation of ideal body weight, hydration needs, and energy requirements are not currently published. One method of determining ideal body weight is to:

1. Determine the height-age (age at which the actual height is at the 50th percentile).

2. Determine IBW for the height-age. This is the 50th percentile weight that matches the height-age.

3. Calculate the percent IBW by dividing the actual weight by the IBW. Depending on the degree of progression of disease and deterioration of muscle mass, up to 20% less of the normal IBW can be factored into the equation.[2, 4]

Nutritional Implications in Corticosteroid Therapy

Of all the therapeutic drugs studied in the management of DMD, only prednisone seems to have the potential for providing interim, palliative, functional improvement for boys with DMD.[3, 5] Several studies describe prolonged function and ambulation in DMD with the use of corticosteroids, although there is no consensus recommending steroids as a standard therapy. However, the nutritional implications of steroid therapy include increased appetite, weight gain, linear growth suppression, decreased absorption of dietary calcium, and fluid retention. The side effects may necessitate some form of caloric restriction, weight monitoring, supplements of calcium and vitamin D, and possibly some sodium restriction.

Osteoporosis

Studies conducted to determine the prevalence, circumstances, and outcome of fractures in boys with DMD indicate that up to 20%

have experienced fractures.[4, 6] Many of these (41%) have occurred in patients who were still walking. Bone densitometry studies in the DMD population show bone density in the proximal femur was profoundly diminished even when gait was not affected and then progressed to four standard deviations below age-matched controls.[7]

Sixty-six percent of the fractures occurred in the lower extremities. Studies in osteoporosis in DMD (independent of steroid use) indicate that the occurrence of a fracture had a significant impact and possible loss of ambulation.[5, 7]

Escalation of Nutrition Support

Many boys with DMD require nutrition support at some point. The primary challenges in nutrition support are hydration (often affecting constipation and urinary tract infections), adequate fiber, adequate energy intake, and adequate protein intake for prevention of skin breakdown. As the disease progresses, many require the use of oral nutrition supplements or gastrostomy tubes. Two calorie per cc tube feedings, if tolerated, provide the greatest number of calories in the fewest hours. The choice of tube feeding products is dependent on gastric motility, choice of feeding style (continuous drip vs. bolus), the need for fiber to prevent constipation, fluid needs, and the need for increased protein.

Obesity

For boys who are still ambulating, significant energy expenditure can occur as walking, climbing, playing, and other childhood activities become more challenging. However, when a boy with DMD becomes wheelchair dependent and is no longer walking, energy requirements can decrease substantially. Unfortunately, by that time, most families have become accustomed to increasing energy intake to meet the needs of the previously ambulating child. Often, eating continues to be one of life's pleasures as the child's world becomes smaller. Creative ways to reward without the use of food, provide calorie-free or low calorie snacks, and adequate after-school supervision are all integral to any successful management of rapid weight gain in a child who uses a wheelchair.

Nutrition and Emotions

In some cases, adolescents with DMD who require assistance with meals at school often stop eating at school. Many are reluctant to ask or rely on friends to help with the mechanics of feeding or are uncomfortable with the length of time a meal can take. Some teenagers may just adjust their mealtimes to a different time of day, however others are at risk for dehydration or inadequate intake. Some will take a high calorie beverage to school (commercial or homemade) so the child only has to have lunch through a straw. Unfortunately, some teenagers, without thoughtful and creative planning, decide to no longer attend school, thereby isolating themselves from critically needed socialization.

While there are many review and research articles related to DMD, there does not appear to be a standard set of guidelines, care map, or clinical pathway specifically for nutrition across the greater than 200 centers taking care of boys with DMD in the United States. To improve care, quality of life, and survival a collaborative process among dietitians to produce a set of nutrition standards for DMD for the use and benefit of all clinics is overdue.

References

1. Muscular Dystrophy Association. *Journal of Love*. Muscular Dystrophy Association: 1998.

2. Washington State Department of Health. *Nutrition Interventions for Children with Special Health Care Needs*. DOH, 2001.

3. Metules, T. Duchenne Muscular Dystrophy. *RN,* Volume 65, No 10, Oct. 2002.

4. Casey, S. Nutrition Issues for Children with Neuromuscular Disorders–A Dietitian's Perspective from Clinical Experience, *Nutrition Focus*. Volume 16, No. 5, Sept./Oct. 2001.

5. Muntoni, F. Fisher, I, Morgan, J, Abraham, D. Steroids in Duchenne Muscular Dystrophy: from *Clinical Trials to Genomic Research. Neuromuscular Disorders*, 12 Suppl 1:S1 62-5, 2002, Oct.

6. Larsen, C, Hendersen, R. Bone Mineral Density and Fractures in Boys with Duchenne Muscular Dystrophy. *Journal of Pediatric Orthopedics*, 20 (1): 71-4, 2000, Jan-Feb.

7. McDonald, D, Kinali, M. Gallagher, A, Mercuri, E, Montoni, F, Roper, P, Jones, D, Pike, M. Fracture Prevalence in Duchenne Muscular Dystrophy. *Developmental Medicine and Child Neurology,* 44 (10):695, 2002, Oct. Parent Project Muscular Dystrophy DMD Regional Roundtable.

Steroids, Nutritional Supplements, and Antibiotics

There are multiple steroid/supplemental treatments for Duchenne MD although there is little agreement (even among researchers and clinicians) about many of them. Options include:

- Prednisone
- Deflazacort
- Albuterol
- Creatine
- Anabolic Steroids
- Calcium blockers
- Gentamycin

Prednisone: A catabolic steroid that slows the loss of muscle degeneration. It is the drug most widely used to treat Duchenne MD. In some cases, walking may be prolonged for up to two years or more. Not only is muscle loss halted, but its strength and function also improve dramatically. Unlike anabolic steroids taken by athletes and body builders, catabolic steroids do not build up tissue, but instead break it down.

Why use these rather than anabolic steroids? Catabolic steroids, like the natural hydrocortisone, help the body break down tissues to release glucose (sugar) and mobilize energy in response to stress or danger. The exact way in which prednisone helps Duchenne MD patients is still not known, but it is likely due to its anti-inflammatory and immunosuppressant effects. Like hydrocortisone, prednisone fights inflammation (swelling) in injured or damaged tissues by suppressing the immune system. The cytotoxic T lymphocytes that rush in to clear away damaged cells may be slowed. Some researchers have speculated that prednisone may also somehow stimulate muscle protein production.

Because of this sugar effect, catabolic steroids are also known as glucocorticoids. They are made and released from the outer portion (or cortex) of the adrenal gland, so they are also known as corticosteroids. Prednisone is a synthetic form of the natural corticosteroid hydrocortisone. Prednisone has many pharmaceutical brand names.

Controlled tests with placebos clearly confirm that prednisone alleviates dystrophinopathic (characteristic produced by the absence of dystrophin) effects. Muscle mass and strength increases, though CK levels remain unaffected (as the muscle does not heal). Likewise, when boys who have been on prednisone stop taking it, they seem to lose its beneficial effects rather rapidly, no matter how long they have been on it. Prednisone works and works well, even though no one knows why.

However, for all its clear benefits, prednisone is known to have several strong side effects, including fluid retention (hence bloating and weight gain) which can lead to high blood pressure and the development of cataracts in the lens of the eye. In some cases prednisone benefits in strengthening muscle are canceled out by obesity and inactivity. Linear growth (in height) may be arrested. There are also severe psychological side effects, such as difficulty concentrating, sleeping, and controlling emotions. Impairment in thinking, reading, and coping skills can lead to depression or aggression. Finally, long term use of immunosuppressants like prednisone can also impair the body's ability to fight infections and heal wounds.

Prednisone use must be monitored carefully to ensure that any gains in muscle function are not outweighed by negative side effects. Prednisone may have to be administered along with other oral supplements, such as calcium (to prevent osteoporosis). For many parents and physicians the hardest decision is when to begin steroid use. Another major dispute involves the dosage regimen. A schedule in which the patient alternates periods of times on and off prednisone may help to provide the desired gains while blunting the harmful side effects. Currently there is no agreement from clinicians whether a ten days on, ten days off schedule, or an alternating one day on, one day off schedule, or even two high doses of prednisone a week (10 mg/kg/week) is best. In most cases prednisone is administered in daily doses of 0.75 mg/kg body mass/day. Still, different parents, physicians, and researchers will all give different answers. It may be that the proper dosage depends largely on the age and severity of the dystrophinopathic (characteristic produced by the absence of dystrophin) phenotype.

Deflazacort: Like prednisone, is a catabolic steroid. It is not marketed in the U.S., though it is available in Canada, Mexico, and other countries. As with prednisone, there is evidence that deflazacort significantly improves muscle strength and function. In addition, it appears to have less severe side effects than prednisone. However, although deflazacort may have fewer side effects (and it still has some), it is not otherwise more effective and is difficult for U.S. residents to obtain.

Albuterol: An immunosuppressant drug that is widely used in inhalant form for asthmatics. Preliminary evidence suggests that it may aid Duchenne MD boys by suppressing the immune cells that rush in to clean up and remove leaky muscle cells and debris. As with prednisone, albuterol interferes with the body's normal inflammation response. Though early data indicates few major side effects, all immunosuppressants are potentially harmful in that they may leave the patient unable to fight routine infections. Albuterol also appears to have some anabolic effects in that it promotes the growth of muscle tissue.

Creatine: A nutritional supplement that has recently gained much notice. Creatine helps the body to build up muscle's energy supply. The creatine kinase or CK enzyme (which is released from damaged muscle cells in Duchenne MD) adds chemical groups called phosphates to creatine. Creatine stores these phosphate groups and donates them to contractile muscle filaments, which need them to contract. Creatine occurs naturally in muscle. Although it is found in meat and fish, it can also be added to the diet as a powdered nutritional supplement. The idea is that the more creatine muscle has, the more energy it has, and thus the stronger its contraction. This is why professional athletes have experimented with extremely high doses.

Recent trials with DMD patients show a slight increase in muscle strength with administration of low levels (5 g/day) of creatine monohydrate. These low levels may prevent the potential kidney damage that can occur with high doses of creatine, but it is still difficult to give young DMD boys sufficient water along with creatine (and other dietary supplements). Behavioral changes may be another side effect of creatine use. As with prednisone (and the other drugs listed), preparing a plan in which the drugs are given for a short time followed by a break of one or several weeks may provide the same benefits as constant use. Medical studies of creatine and DMD continue.

Anabolic steroids: Act to build tissues in the body (unlike prednisone and other catabolic steroids that break them down) and may help to fight DMD by compensating for muscle loss. A pilot study of oxandrolone, a synthetic anabolic steroid, showed some promise in preserving muscle strength. Anabolic steroids have attracted much attention from body builders and athletes who wish to bulk up their muscle mass, and the numerous harmful side effects of their use (including liver and kidney damage, sterility, stunting of growth, severe mood swings, and possible incidence of certain cancers) are well known and widely publicized. However, while research is still ongoing, the levels used by DMD boys—unlike those used by bodybuilders—would be rather low. Still, the levels of improvement (both in athletes as well as in DMD boys) appear minimal. It may be that a combination of anabolic steroids and other drugs can slow muscle degeneration until a better treatment (or cure) is found.

Calcium blockers: Have also been tried to stem the debilitating effects of Duchenne MD. Calcium—a mineral that is found in all tissues of the body—is known to harm cells when it leaks in through membrane channels. But the extent to which such drugs can prevent dystrophinopathy (given that the entire membrane is extremely leaky and not just normal membrane channels) is questionable. Another factor that complicates the use of channel blockers for DMD is the fact that prednisone can lead to osteoporosis, which usually requires oral calcium supplements. However, the amount of calcium in tissues is regulated separately from the amount absorbed from the gut, and precious calcium will be removed from bone when insufficient amounts are ingested in the diet.

Gentamycin: An antibiotic that has figured prominently in recent news items about cases of DMD due to premature stop codons. In these cases the complete gene for dystrophin is never decoded or translated so that this critical muscle protein is not made, or at least not made in full form. Research on mdx mice that simulate human DMD has shown that when Gentamycin is administered, the premature stop codon is somehow ignored so that the entire gene transcript can be read and dystrophin can be produced. A preliminary trial on DMD boys is underway, and hopes are high that this will work in humans as well as it did in the model mice. Unfortunately, this treatment would only work for those instances (about 10% of all DMD cases) in which the gene defect is a premature stop codon.

Section 30.3

Stretching, Exercises, and Postural Correction in Duchenne Muscular Dystrophy

From "Use of Physiotherapy in Duchenne MD." Text and figures reprinted with permission from the Muscular Dystrophy Campaign, a United Kingdom charity focusing on all muscular dystrophies and allied disorders © 2003 Muscular Dystrophy Campaign. All rights reserved. Additional information is available at www.muscular-dystrophy.org. Figures redrawn for Omnigraphics by Alison DeKleine, January 2004, with permission from the Muscular Dystrophy Campaign.

This section is intended to provide guidelines for you to help a child who has Duchenne muscular dystrophy. Long-term management and any specific treatment should always be under the direction of his doctor who will organize and coordinate the professional team looking after your son. It will be much easier if you understand the problems and the thinking behind the treatment, so this introduction is written to help supplement and reinforce the advice and information given to you at the hospital.

How Muscles Work and the Effects of Duchenne Muscular Dystrophy

Skeletal muscles allow us to move, to stand, and by coordinated work, to perform the variety of movements necessary for all the challenges of daily living. Each muscle in the body is composed of a number of muscle fibers. There are different types of muscle fibers and the number and proportion of each type in any muscle depends on what sort of work that muscle normally does. For example, the big muscles (hip extensors) used in standing have a different type of muscle fiber from those muscles that allow us to make quick finger movements. Muscles are attached to bones through specially adapted parts of the muscle, called tendons. Usually a muscle spans at least one joint so when that muscle contracts or shortens it causes a movement to occur. Muscles and their tendons are normally very extensible, being able to lengthen and shorten to allow movement; for example, the muscles of the back lengthen as the abdominal muscles tighten when reaching forwards. Muscles acting over joints are usually evenly balanced.

In Duchenne muscular dystrophy the muscle fibers are gradually replaced by fatty tissue and the normal function of the muscle (produce force) is impaired. The rate at which this happens, and therefore the rate at which weakness occurs, varies somewhat between children with the same condition.

It is important to realize that some muscles are affected earlier than others, and this upsets the normal balance of strength between the muscle groups.

Contractures

Muscles are connected to bones by tendons, while the ligaments (the tissue around the joints which connect bones) control the extent or range of movement. When muscles become weak or are not used, they lose their extensibility and so do all the associated ligaments and tendons. This means that the joint becomes stiff and tight, usually more in one direction than the other, resulting in a contracture or fixed position of the joint, which in turn leads to a deformity. If the joint can no longer move normally, the muscle cannot work normally and becomes weaker from disuse.

In children with early Duchenne muscular dystrophy the most frequently seen contractures occur at the ankles, knees, and hips. These are caused partly by the child walking on his toes, with the knees a little bent and the feet apart, a position he adopts in order to balance in standing and walking as weakness of the hip, knee, and trunk muscles make it more difficult to keep his balance. The contractures are aggravated by the fact that children with latter stages of the condition spend more time sitting.

It is important to seek advice about physiotherapy and to start treatment aimed at preventing contractures as soon as possible after diagnosis, before there is any tightness. Do not wait until there is any obvious deformity.

What Can Be Done?

Increasing weakness makes tasks like walking and dressing more difficult, but there are ways in which your child can be helped to make the most of his abilities and retain as much independence as possible without causing distress or disrupting education or recreation. It is important to remember that the worldwide search for a cure is going on all the time, but when such a treatment is found it will not make stiff or twisted joints move again. This is another reason for trying to prevent deformities and keeping muscles supple and strong for as long as possible.

Use of Physiotherapy in Duchenne Muscular Dystrophy

Physiotherapy means the physical treatment or management of a condition, and this has an important role in helping to maintain our child's maximum potential function. Its main aims are:

1. To provide a physical assessment; information from this can be used in making decisions about care in the future.

2. To minimize development of contractures; by passive stretching.

3. To maintain muscle strength; by exercise.

4. To prolong mobility and function; by means of splints, braces, spinal jackets, etc. as recommended by the specialist at the center attended.

Expert help and advice is necessary for correct physiotherapy treatment, but many simple measures can be undertaken at home. They need to be carried out regularly as part of the child's normal lifestyle to obtain the most successful outcome.

Passive Stretching

This is a simple technique used to stretch tight and/or shortened muscle tissues by slowly, but firmly moving the joint as far as possible and maintaining the position for about 30 seconds. The child must relax completely and should be encouraged not to make any active movement or resist the stretch. If the movement is carried out too quickly, the child is more likely to resist or become frightened.

Passive stretching done properly and effectively is not painful, but there will be a sensation of pulling and of gentle, sustained pressure being applied. The joint or muscle cannot be harmed, provided the instructions are followed carefully and the approach is firm but not aggressive. Some children will be quick to realize that grumbling will make the helper stop the passive stretching; however, irreversible contractures can develop quickly, in the end causing far more discomfort than the exercise or stretching ever did.

310

It is therefore in the child's best interest to continue, but firmness and kindness are essential. Though it does not matter when you do the passive stretching, many people find it easier to establish a routine so that it does not get forgotten. Passive stretching should be done every day and a good idea is to do it after a warm bath when the child is feeling relaxed. Though some children put up a mild protest, once a routine is established and confidence gained, this is usually overcome. It helps enormously if the exercises can be done in an atmosphere of fun; they can be combined with singing, storytelling, and a general sense of enjoyment.

Ankles

The child should lie flat on his back and be encouraged to relax and go floppy. The helper should stand on one side, place one hand on the sole of the foot with the fingers pointing towards the heel, which should be grasped firmly but gently between the fingers and thumb. With the other hand the knee should be held straight, but do not push down on it.

Now gently but firmly pull down on the heel, as if trying to make the leg longer, before pushing the foot up to a right angle (90°) or as near as possible—but do not let the knee bend. You may find it easier to lean towards the child's head rather than trying to use just your arm strength. When you encounter some tightness or resistance to the movement just maintain the pressure for a little while. Then gradually increase the pressure to move the foot a few more degrees and hold this position for about 20 seconds.

The movement should be repeated at least 20 times on each foot. Make sure that when you do this stretching it is the whole foot that is moved and not just the toes and forefoot (see Figure 30.1).

The Knees

Usually only minor contractures develop at the knees before the child becomes dependent on a wheelchair, but it is essential to prevent these because it is difficult to walk with bent knees. To stretch the knees, the child is left in the same position as for the ankles and the grip on the heel is the same, but with the other hand counter pressure is given on the thigh just above the knee-cap, and the foot moved as before, lifting up on the heel to straighten the knee.

This movement should be repeated 20 times on each knee. Alternatively the child may turn so that he is lying face down and a small

311

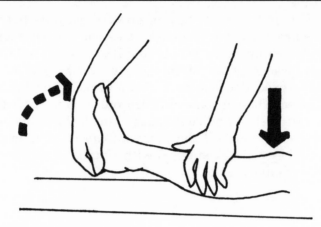

Figure 30.1. *Ankle Stretching*

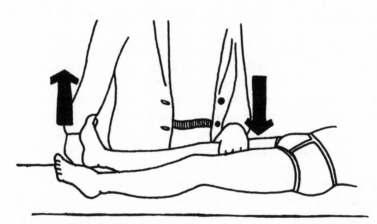

Figure 30.2. *Active Knee Stretching*

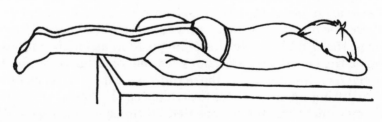

Figure 30.3. *Knee Stretch at Rest*

pillow placed under the thigh, not the knee. This will allow the weight of the lower leg and the foot to straighten the knee joint and is much easier to do if the child is lying on a couch or a bed with their feet hanging over the edge. This can be done when he is watching television (see Figures 30.2 and 30.3).

The Hips

The hip joint is controlled by some of the largest muscles in the body. The two groups that are most likely to become contracted are those that control the bending or forward lifting of the leg (the hip flexors) and those that move the leg out to the side (hip abductors). There are three ways in which the hip flexors can be stretched. All hip exercises should be repeated about 10 times on each side.

1. The child lies on one side with the leg straight and the helper stands behind. Place one hand on the child's hip bone to steady and slide the other hand under the top of the thigh of the same leg. The leg is then drawn backwards towards you to stretch the hip flexors which lie across the front of the hip joint. If you choose this method, you must be sure that the pelvis is steady and you can put your knee against the child's lower back so that your thigh acts as a cushion. Repeat the stretch on the other side (see Figure 30.4).

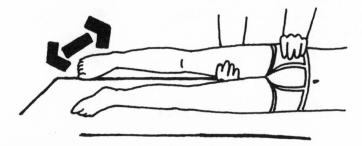

Figure 30.4. Hip Flexor Stretch from Side Position

2. The child lies face down, one hand is placed firmly on the buttocks and the other hand is slipped under one thigh. The

thigh is then lifted and thus extended, so placing stretch on the front muscles of the hip and thigh. Repeat with the other leg (see Figure 30.5).

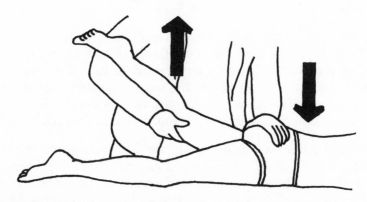

Figure 30.5. *Hip Flexor Stretch from the Prone Position*

3.   The child lies on his back and the opposite leg (the one not being stretched) is bent up towards the chest and held in that position by you or the child, if he can manage it. Your hand is then placed just above the knee of the leg to be stretched and a downward pressure is exerted. Repeat with other leg.

Other hip muscles (linking the lower back with the leg), help to control the angle of the pelvis and can affect the curvature of the spine. The tightening of these muscles may be noticed when the leg is turned inwards as the child walks; also more weight may be put on one leg than the other when standing.

To stretch these hip muscles and the tissues down the outer side of the leg (the iliotibial band) the child should lie face down. The helper stands on the opposite side to the leg that is to be stretched. They then place the hand nearest the child's head firmly on the child's bottom and push downwards. The other hand grasps the thigh from underneath and lifts the leg up as far as possible and then pulls it towards them.

Elbows and Wrists

In the early and intermediate stages of Duchenne muscular dystrophy, it is most unlikely that these joints will present any problems. However, once the child begins to spend more time in a wheelchair, it is essential to start stretching these joints to prevent tightness occurring. All exercises to the elbow and wrist should be repeated 10 times on each side.

1. Standing at the side, the upper arm is held firmly by one hand while the child's palm is kept uppermost. Then, with your other hand holding the wrist, the elbow is straightened downwards very gently (see Figure 30.6).

2. The turning or rotating movement of the forearm although not a big movement is important because it allows the child to bring the hand to the mouth or to grasp objects. In order to preserve this movement, continue to hold the upper arm, but move your other hand down to hold the child's hand. The grip should be as in shaking the hand, but with the fingers extended over the wrist. Keep the shoulders still, and with his elbow bent, simply turn the forearm so that the child's palm is first uppermost and then the back of the hand is uppermost.

3. The wrist is stretched by supporting the forearm near the wrist joint and then with the other hand placed palm to palm moving the child's wrist backwards. Try to keep the fingers straight at the same time because if you allow them to curl over and bend this will take the stretch off the tight tendons in the wrist.

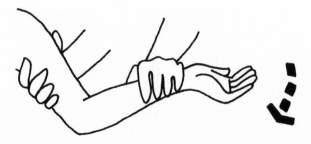

Figure 30.6. Elbow and Wrist Stretch

Shoulders

When dressing it is helpful to maintain full shoulder movement by lifting each arm in turn up above the head making sure that the arm lies parallel to the head.

Night Splints

These, as the name suggests, are designed to wear at night to help prevent contractures. It is usually only necessary for the ankles, so the splint starts at the toes and reaches to just below the knee. It is essential that they fit properly, are comfortable and lightweight.

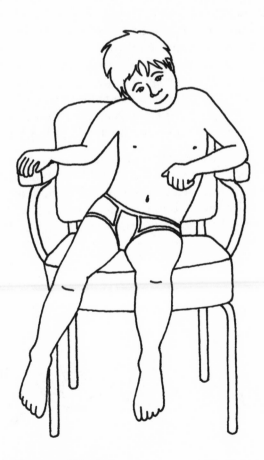

Figure 30.7. Abnormal Posture

Research has shown that night splints used in conjunction with passive stretching are the most effective way of retarding the development of contractures. But they are not a substitute for passive stretching, and are only used in combination with stretching once an obvious contracture is seen.

Postural Correction

The child with muscular dystrophy has the disadvantage of being forced by his muscle weakness to assume unusual postures (see Figure 30.7). It is extremely important that when he is seated every effort is made to correct the abnormal posture (see Figure 30.8).

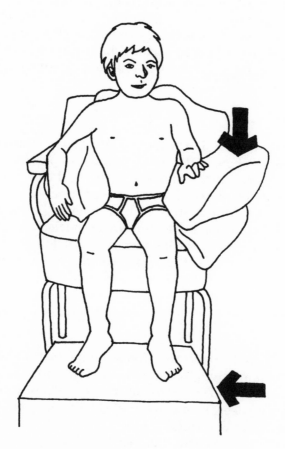

Figure 30.8. Corrected Posture

Sitting

When sitting, the feet should be at an angle of 90°. The seat of the chair should be firm and ideally not too wide. The back of the chair should be firm and either upright or just slightly slanting backwards. The depth of the seat should be the same length as the thigh, so that he is encouraged to use the back of the chair and not slump. The arm rests should be at a height so that the child can support his elbow without hunching his shoulders up or leaning sideways. Wedges of foam are often useful in converting furniture to fit the child, when a correctly sized chair is not available, but this is only a temporary measure.

When sitting, the weight should be equally distributed on each buttock. Sometimes it is necessary to place a small wedge between the knees to help maintain this position. The selection of the correct wheelchair is absolutely essential for the welfare of the child and the specifications for the chair will change at different stages of the condition and as he grows. It is important that expert advice is obtained. Early attention to these factors will help to prevent contractures and scoliosis (curvature of the spine).

Prone Lying

Encouraging your child to adopt the prone lying position (lying face downwards) for an hour a day will do much to prevent the development of contractures at the hips and knees and also help to prevent the development of scoliosis. This need not become a major chore, but can be combined with activities such as reading or watching television. The child should be lying face down on the floor, or a similar hard surface. A small pillow or wedge placed just below the hips will encourage extension at the hips. The weight of the lower leg will straighten out the knees, but it is important to ensure that the feet are free.

Exercises

Exercising against resistance (pushing against a static object) is helpful to maintain strength and mobility. The muscles that are particularly vulnerable in Duchenne muscular dystrophy are those that control the hips, knees, shoulders, and the trunk so some simple exercises for these are described.

It is not necessary to do all the exercises that are given at the same session and some may be too difficult for the boys as they get older.

Common sense must prevail in deciding which exercises to use, but generally it is better to set your aims high. Two or three of the exercises should be done each day. Children with DMD can and usually do enjoy exercise as much as other children. Parents know best the right approach to the child and are naturally good at adapting the general principles outlined here.

Sitting

Sitting either on a firm chair or on the edge of a bed with the hand holding the front edge, an effort is made to pull the toes and foot up at the same time straightening the knee just as in kicking.

It is very important to get the knee as straight as possible, making quite sure at the same time that the child is not leaning backwards (see Figure 30.9).

This exercise can be made harder by the child holding his leg straight for a count of 10. Repeat 20 times with a rest of 30 seconds between each attempt.

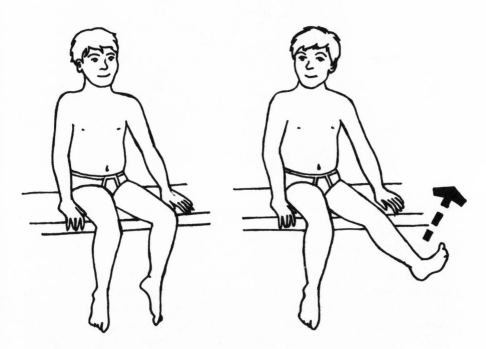

Figure 30.9. *Lower Leg Exercise*

Once this has been achieved, then resistance can be added to the movement. This is done either manually or with a bag hooked over the foot and weighted with a 2 pound weight. However, it is important to note that weights or resistance should not be used if the knee cannot be straightened and should never be left hanging unsupported on the foot (see Figure 30.10).

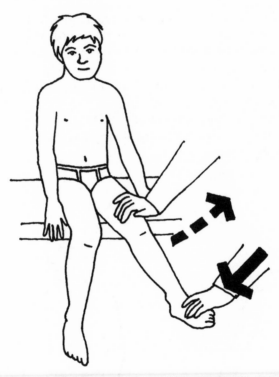

Figure 30.10. Lower Leg Exercise with Resistance

Lying on the Side

The boy lies on his side (a firm pillow placed behind the back may help) and then lifts his leg upwards and slightly backwards; that is away from the other leg. Repeat 10 times (see Figure 30.11).

Again the exercise may be made more difficult by holding the leg in position to a count of five. The child then turns over and repeats the exercise 10 times using the other leg.

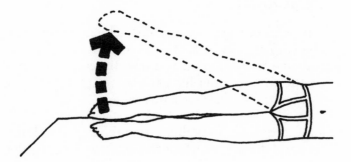

Figure 30.11. Leg Lift Exercise

Lying Face Down

1. First one leg and then the other is lifted up from the hip, while keeping the knee straight. There is a temptation to roll so a hand firmly on the child's bottom will prevent this and ensure the right muscles are working. Repeat 10 times with each leg.

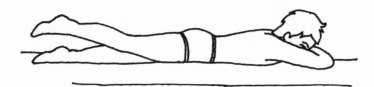

Figure 30.12. Prone Leg Lift

2. With the arms starting at the side of the body, ask him to lift both arms (or one at a time) up behind him. Repeat 10 times with each arm.

3. With the arms at the side, lift the head or head and shoulders off the surface.

Lying Face Upwards

Try to sit up without using the arms (which should be folded on the chest). The chin should be tucked in so that the child appears to roll up. Repeat five times. This is a fairly difficult exercise designed to strengthen the tummy muscles used in standing up or coughing. Two ways of doing the exercise are described.

1. The feet and hands can be held to make it easier, but make sure the child does as much of the work as he can; do not just pull him up (see Figure 38.1.

2. The exercise can be started from a sloping position by placing one or two cushions behind the head and shoulders.

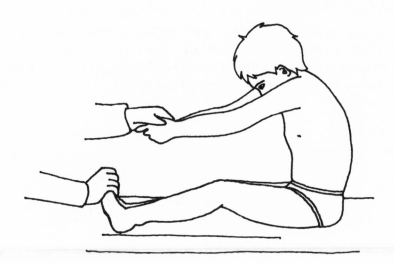

Figure 30.13. *Sit Up*

Upper Body Exercise.

While sitting on the floor or on a firm surface, push down on the hands with the elbows straight and try to lift his bottom off the floor. It may be necessary to place a small (2") block under the hands. Books can often be used for this. Repeat five times.

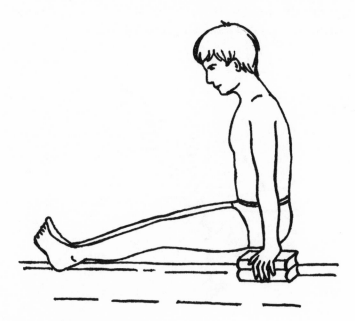

Figure 30.14. Upper Body Exercise.

General Strengthening Exercises

The exercises described in previous sections are designed to strengthen muscles, particularly those which control the hips and knees. However, in normal movement we use combinations of muscle; working together, for instance in walking or in pushing out of a chair. These often involve a twisting or rotating movement and the next two exercises are therefore particularly useful for the leg and arm muscles. The amount of manual resistance given by the parent should be such that the child just manages to do the complete movement (see Figures 30.15 and 30.16).

These exercises should be done daily, but the child should not be stressed. Making the exercises into a game or having a chart of achievement might help towards a cooperative attitude. It is important to keep a happy balance between encouragement and demand.

In addition to specific exercises, physical activities and adaptive sport can be beneficial in helping to maintain as much strength as possible and to give self-confidence. Swimming is an ideal sport, and depending on the muscle strength, horseback riding (probably with a therapeutic riding organization), and bicycling.

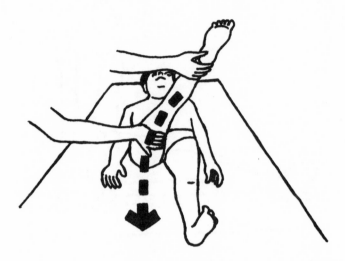

Figure 30.15. *Leg Rotation Exercise. In this exercise the leg is lifted up and across the body towards the opposite shoulder. The child is then asked to point his toes downwards and push his leg downwards and out to the side. Repeat 10 times with each leg.*

How much should we do? Can we do too much?

These are natural anxieties. Exercise, like all training, should never be done to the point of fatigue, but it is most unlikely that you could persuade your child to do too much. The suggested exercises are considered suitable and are easy to do, but there are other ways of achieving the same aim. It is important to remember that as the condition progresses the exercises must be made lighter, but you will know best because you are with the child every day. The approach to passive stretching and exercise is very important. Earlier, it was suggested that it was helpful to set up some routine and that routine must fit with your child's and your family lifestyle so that "doing your exercises" does not become a slogan for boredom or a reprimand. Also, like all routines, it is there to be changed. Most of all, let exercise be fun.

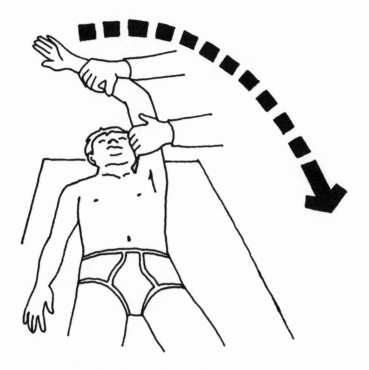

Figure 30.16. Arm Rotation Exercise. The parent takes the child's arm across his body towards the opposite ear. The child is then asked to push the arm downwards and outwards to come to lie by his side. Repeat 10 times with each arm.

Part Six

Care and Management of Muscular Dystrophy at Home

Chapter 31

Handling Disability

From Where I Sit: Alone with Your Disability

Sandy Shipley, a freelance writer and avid traveler who lives in Hermiston, Oregon, shares her experience living with a disability along with tips that have helped her.

I can experience a feeling of aloneness any time, anywhere. Often, I know this feeling occurs because of my disability. I would describe it as a feeling of being left out, not included in life around me.

Living with a disability brings changes to your life, not only in what you can do, but in the way you feel about yourself. You may see yourself differently from the way you used to. The physical changes may make you feel embarrassed, unattractive, or inferior to others. But I have found ways to overcome these feelings of aloneness.

During more than 20 years of living with limb-girdle muscular dystrophy, I have arrived often at the crossroads of choice. Will I be happy or sad? Will I go forward, or give up? Shall I remain active, or sit by the wayside? Some of my greatest successes in dealing with the physical and emotional effects of my disability can be summed up in the following six determinations:

Reprinted from "From Where I Sit" by Sandy Shipley, *QUEST*, Volume 9, Number 6, December 2002. Reprinted with permission from the Muscular Dystrophy Association, www.mdausa.org. © The Muscular Dystrophy Association. For additional information, call the Muscular Dystrophy Association toll-free at (800) 572-1717. To find an MDA office in your area, look in your local telephone book, or click on "Clinics and Services" on the MDA website.

Choose to Use All Aids

Cherish your freedom of mobility. Do not let the embarrassment of being seen with a cane, crutches, braces, or a wheelchair stop you from enjoying every opportunity that comes your way. Accepting medical aides as your friends will open a world of activity that you may never experience without them.

Allow Others to Help You

Recently at a buffet restaurant, my three-wheeled scooter presented a challenge. Inside the door, I could not negotiate the tight turns of the zigzagging maze to the cashier. Seeing my predicament, other patrons began removing obstacles and clearing the way for me. Everyone became involved, and soon an opening appeared. I thanked them, followed their instructions for turning around, and skipped right past the line. It is true, you might become a spectacle. But enjoy it. I felt like a VIP.

Move on Quickly

The feelings of aloneness are never stronger than when I am left behind during a group activity. For instance, when we have had guests in our home, upon leaving, everyone moves outdoors to the car for final good-byes. Due to the stairs, I must stay behind. It may be a small thing, but my momentary feelings of abandonment are acute. Then I remember, "Move on quickly. Don't linger." I offer a final wave, walk away from the door, and immediately begin the task of cleanup. The blues will vanish!

Entertain Yourself

Life from a wheelchair is often full of roadblocks. Many can be overcome, others cannot. But, emotionally overcoming disappointments is often just a matter of planning ahead and looking for new opportunities.

I recall fondly a sightseeing trip with my husband, Walt, and some friends, while visiting the U.S.S. Lexington, a World War II vintage aircraft carrier, now a floating museum at Corpus Christi, Texas. Since accessibility was limited to the hangar deck, and the others would be joining the onboard tours, I knew I would soon be alone. I immediately began planning my own entertainment.

After touring the hangar deck, my group departed on the first of several guided tours. Instantly, the familiar feelings of aloneness enveloped me. But my plan was in place; I would read in detail each exhibit we had briefly scanned.

Turning my scooter around, I poked my nose into the old ship's galley, read personal stories of men who had served on the carrier, and chatted with a knowledgeable U.S.S. Lexington volunteer. He expounded the ship's history with accounts of several attacks that had damaged it, explained the functioning of the immense elevators that lifted the airplanes from one deck to the other, and showed me the massive equipment used to catapult the planes into the air.

Finally, I enjoyed a movie. When my group returned, I was amazed to learn that I had gleaned more information about the ship's history than any of the others, and I had had a great time doing it. I realized I never had been alone, just with different people. What a great experience!

Leave Your Pride at Home

I can accept myself for who I am. In fact, I like to think of myself as unique. But there is still the issue of pride. We all have it. For example, though I usually use a scooter at restaurants, occasionally I cannot. At those times, my husband will assist me slowly inside (since I still have limited walking ability), and seat me. Upon leaving, he will wrap his arms around me and physically lift me to a standing position, until my feet are stable.

Always, I imagine the stares around us, and know that we have become that dreaded spectacle once again. As I regain my balance and readjust my clothing, I try to regain my dignity. But, often as not, the teasing starts from a neighboring table pointing out, "That's one way to get a hug!" And I am again reminded of how accepting people are.

Plan Ahead for Your Own Enjoyment

Accompanying my husband to town is always my pleasure, but often, the shorter stops are accomplished faster and easier if I remain in the car. To combat feelings of aloneness, I go prepared with an electronic solitaire game, a book, or a knitting project. I am never bored during an unscheduled stop. At home, my wheelchair is surrounded with pleasurable activities, as well as the computer, TV remote, and telephone.

Thankfully, my experience has been that, between limited house-work, fun sit-down activities, time with friends and family, a zest for living, and my active imagination there is little time to feel alone or left out. And I am convinced that, even living with a disability, a positive outlook and an enjoyable life are well within my reach. And they are within yours, too.

Chapter 32

Home Adaptations for Living with Muscular Dystrophy

It is important when planning adaptations for a boy with Duchenne muscular dystrophy or an adult or child with other allied neuromuscular conditions to understand the disability and to appreciate the long-term physical limitations. This is because they influence the decisions made and the need for both space and special features in the home.

The main point to consider is that he will use a wheelchair (usually powered which is less maneuverable than a self-propelled wheelchair and therefore requires additional space), and although he will retain functional use of his hands, his grip and strength will be considerably reduced. In addition, he will not be able to reach or raise his arms and is likely to lack balance when sitting. A bedroom/bathroom suite will be helpful.

Access

Pavement

A dropped curb will be required for wheelchair use.

This chapter includes information excerpted from "Adaptations for Boys with Duchenne Muscular Dystrophy and Adults and Children with Muscular Dystrophy and Allied Neuromuscular Conditions," and "Kitchen Adaptations." Reprinted with permission from the Muscular Dystrophy Campaign, a United Kingdom charity focusing on all muscular dystrophies and allied disorders. © 2003 Muscular Dystrophy Campaign. All rights reserved. Additional information is available at www.muscular-dystrophy.org.uk.

Garden

If there is a path around the house this should be at least 35½ inches wide, and a paved area in the garden suitable for an electric wheelchair is essential. For transfers in and out of a car, the driveway needs to have space for the car or van and an additional 8 feet to accommodate a wheelchair at the side. Ideally this should be under cover.

Ramps

A gradient of 1 in 12 is satisfactory as most people with a neuromuscular condition will not be able to propel a wheelchair independently up any slope and are likely to be using a powered chair. The platform at the top of the ramp must extend 48 inches from the door. A handrail will be needed for people able to walk, but for wheelchair users a side safety flange is essential. A double wall with an earth-filled cavity planted with trailing plants makes an attractive camouflage for a high ramp. The surface of the ramp should be nonslip.

Threshold

Raised threshold sills (including steel weather bars) should be avoided, but a flexible threshold will be satisfactory and will not impede access for a wheelchair. It is usually easier to provide level access to an outward-opening patio door (with adjacent window) than with sliding doors.

Doors

Width. Narrow hallways and difficult access problems will influence the need for wide doors, but in most houses a clear opening (i.e., from the face of the door to the door jamb on the other side) of between 33½ inches–35½ inches will be satisfactory. If new building is involved, 36½ inch doors are recommended.

Type. Eventually the only way people with a neuromuscular condition will be able to open doors independently is with the weight of their powered wheelchair—pushing with the footrests. Single-leaf double-swing doors are recommended. A window is no longer felt to be necessary as the disabled boy's movements can be anticipated by the sound of the chair motor.

Disabled adults may choose to have all their doors altered, but parents may decide it is adequate to install swing doors on a child's bedroom and bathroom only. If adaptations are carried out while the disabled child or adult is still able to walk, and are likely to be unsteady on their feet (or there are younger children in the home) swing doors will be dangerous and at this stage the door can be propped open.

Hinges. Double action 4 inch hinges. It is important that this size is not increased as the tension will make it impossible for the door to be opened with a wheelchair.

Kicking plates. These should be fitted at the bottom on both sides of the door. The height from the bottom of the door to the top of the plate should be either:

- 16 inches to avoid damage from wheelchair side curb climbers, or

- 29 inches to cover also the mark left by the wheelchair armrests and/or tray.

Sheets of melamine to match the color of the door—or clear acrylic panels—may be more acceptable than metal plates which often have sharp edges and tend to look institutionalized.

Room Size

It is difficult to be precise about the minimum size of rooms because this is governed by the shape of the room, access, and the number and size of windows/installation of French windows, which affect the available wall space for fittings. The rooms must be large enough to allow the use of an electric wheelchair; the maximum width of an average chair is 27 inches and the length 43 inches.

Bedroom

It is important that the bedroom has an attached bathroom to allow the option of being undressed on the bed and transferred with the ceiling hoist installed over the bed to either:

- a shower chair or Mermaid Ranger and wheeled into the bathroom in privacy and within the warmth of the two rooms, or

- direct on an extended track to the toilet and bath.

Other Size Considerations

In addition to adequate space for movement in a wheelchair, the room must be large enough to accommodate the following:

Door. To bathroom.

Bed. An electric bed is likely to be needed when a disabled person can no longer sit up independently. These beds are 7'1" in length and either 42½" or 4' wide for a single bed and 6'1" wide for a double bed. 24" is needed at the foot of the bed for a caregiver to move with ease.

At the side of the bed there should be sufficient space—6 feet—for two adjacent wheelchairs to be positioned in order to use a ceiling hoist to transfer from one chair to another.

Position. A bed with the headboard in the center of a wall will provide access on both sides (and this is essential with a double bed for two people), but will restrict wheelchair movement in the bedroom. A single bed adjacent to a wall has the added advantage that the disabled person can reach a wall-mounted light switch. A pull-switch is likely to be difficult to reach and to pull with sufficient strength to turn on or off.

Table for Leisure Activity

Modern management of DMD and other forms of MD tries to maintain walking and standing for as long as possible—sometimes with the use of long leg braces and standing frames. It is unrealistic to expect a child to stand in a frame without an activity in front of him; therefore, it is necessary to provide him with a surface that is suitable for use both from a wheelchair and with a standing frame—to use his computer, stereo equipment, etc. Depending upon space and finances this can be achieved by providing either manual or electrical height-adjustable surfaces.

The surface has an important bearing on both the child's medical management and happiness in the future. Adequate working space is essential for project work, homework, and play. An easily accessible surface will enable the disabled child to slide his forearms on the surface to gain the maximum benefit from his hand function.

An L-shaped adjustable-height system in two separate (but ideally, adjacent) surfaces that can be altered as the child grows is ideal. Height brackets should be positioned on the wall to allow the surface to be adjusted for:

- Wheelchair access: 28–35½ inches
- Standing: 36–43½ inches

As the child grows, if the height needs to be adjusted more than 7½ inches, the bracket position can be raised.

Depth. The front-to-back measurement of the surface must be 23½ inches to allow sufficient depth for the length of the wheelchair including footrests.

Length. The length will be determined by the space available, but ideally should be a minimum of 6' x 4' for the sitting surface and 2' for the standing surface. For the lower surface the aim should be to provide an L-shape so that when the disabled child or adult cannot lift up his arms, the computer keyboard can be placed across the right-angle with the monitor in the corner and the front adjacent surfaces used to support the forearms.

Position. Ideally, the lower surface should be positioned in front of a window and in this case if necessary the maximum height of the surface can be lowered to 33" from the top of the surface to the floor.

Drawers. It is also essential to supply a storage unit, which because the drawers are on runners may be suitable for independent use, and this should be positioned under the standing surface.

Ceiling hoist. A decision needs to be made between a wall-to-wall track in the bedroom or an extended track into the bathroom. If the disabled person is likely to need a ceiling hoist in the future and if it is necessary to strengthen the ceiling, it is prudent for the work to be included in the plans—though the hoist may not be installed for several years. The supplying firm will be happy to advise about both the joists and electrical supply.

Track

Position. The track should be positioned parallel to the wall behind the bed headboard so that the center of the track to the wall is 40 inches.

Length. The track should extend from the wall beside the bed and be long enough to cover the floor area needed for two wheelchairs, to enable the hoist to be used for transfers: total length 9 feet. Unless the room is very wide the track is less noticeable if it extends wall-to-wall. Or, an extended track into the bathroom may be considered.

Control. The control cord must be long enough to allow the switch panel to be positioned on the user's lap and the point where the cord is inserted into the switch should extend to 2' from the floor. If necessary, this length can be altered by adjusting the nut at the top of the cord. Older hoist models that are operated by pull-cords needing a vertical hand movement are not suitable.

Slings. Two universal slings (or an MD sling which includes a head extension, if needed) will be required.

Fused spur outlet. This power socket should be installed on the wall at ceiling height at one end of the length of track. If a hoist is not needed immediately, it is still wise to install the outlet for future use. A rechargeable battery model is recommended as there is no dangling cord between the electrical supply and hoist motor. It is suitable for an extended track, either installed initially or in the future. Anyone with acute hearing may be kept awake by the buzzing sound of the hoist. If the hoist is charged in the bedroom, it is advisable to install a pull-cord or accessible switch to enable the caregiver to turn off the hoist at night.

Model. Recommended models have sensitive light-touch controls and the slings are particularly suitable for people with DMD. In addition the spreader bars are available (either as standard or as a special order) with three sling hooks on the end and with a 360 degree swivel.

Washbasin

Bowl depth. The basin should be shallow enough to enable the user to reach the bottom and—when sitting in his wheelchair—to allow space for his knees underneath.

Mounting. To provide good knee access, a wall-mounted basin is more suitable than either a pedestal model or a basin with vertical supports. An inset basin is ideal as it enables him to slide his arms over the shiny surface to reach his towel, toothbrush, etc. The basin should be positioned so that there is a maximum of 2½ inches between the front of the basin and the front edge of the surface. The top of the basin should be flush with the surface as models with a lip present an obstacle to the user who needs to slide his hands into the water.

Length/width. Ideally 47¼ inches. This allows space at either side of the basin to leave toiletries within reach and provide a surface on which to rest his elbows to comb his hair, etc. If space is limited 32½ inches would be satisfactory. The front corners of the surface may present a hazard to helper's backs and should be rounded off.

Storage. If there is adequate space it is often useful to provide a drawer unit adjacent to the basin for storage.

Height. There is no universally successful height and this will need to be altered as the child grows or when either the child or adult changes his wheelchair. Experience has shown that the only satisfactory solution is a height-adjustable basin with flexible plumbing. If a height-adjustable surface is not possible the recommended height from the bottom of the melamine surface to the floor is 32 inches. A front fascia must be avoided as it will obstruct the joystick control of the powered wheelchair.

Depth. Front-to-back measurement should be 2', to allow adequate depth for the chair plus footrests under the basin. It is important that pipe work under the basin at skirting board level does not reduce the depth and obstruct the wheelchair footrests which are at an approximate height of 13–16 inches.

Chain. The basin should be supplied with a plug and chain as a manual drain lever is too difficult to use. However, an electronic drain plug may be necessary, if the user cannot reach the plug.

Access. There should be a space of at least 36" in front of the basin to allow the disabled person to approach squarely with his wheelchair.

Faucet and Handles

Hot and cold faucet handles are recommended with remote control buttons installed within reach on one side of the basin surface. It is important that the faucet chosen is low, has a handle of at least 6 inches, and the faucet length is sufficient to allow hands to be washed under the outlet. These handles may not be suitable for independent use by a boy with DMD.

Mirror

It is a help to have a mirror on the basin splashback or behind the washbasin, the lower edge at an approximate height of 6" from the surface.

Electric Shaver Outlet

This should be installed adjacent to the washbasin to enable convenient recharging of an electric toothbrush and to allow the use of a corded electric shaver which is lighter than a battery model.

Toilet

A toilet with a standard-height pedestal and long inlet enables a toilet/shower chair to be used over the top. The center of the bowl to the nearest obstruction (including floor level pipes) at the wall side should be 16 inches. Side-entry drainage may obstruct the chair.

The toilet bowl must not be close-coupled as this will not allow a shower chair to be aligned directly over the bowl with the lid and seat raised. The measurement between the front of the tank and the front of the bowl should be 2 feet. To ensure that the equipment lines up correctly, ask the Mermaid Ranger supplier to have a chair in the house when the plumber is ready to install.

Bath

It will be necessary to install a shower unit over the bath as the user may have knee contractures which prevent his legs from being extended forwards. He will be more comfortable with the seat raised up from the bottom of the bath and/or it will be useful for hair washing. The shower should be wall-mounted at the end of the bath opposite the taps. Mounted at the side of the bath makes it more difficult for a helper to reach across the bath to control the shower or lift off the shower head—and the spray of water is more difficult to contain in the bath.

Acrylic bathtubs retain heat better than metal bathtubs; they do not chip when a hoist is used and are resistant enough to withstand an occasional knock. The back of the bath must not be excessively sloped as this obstructs the bath seat—and many helpers find handgrips useful although they may obstruct bath seats.

Shower

A shower must be floor level (without a step down) although shallow floors designed to be used in conjunction with shower chairs are satisfactory provided the access is level. These may be essential in an upstairs installation where there is insufficient floor depth, or recommended where it is vital to contain the water within a very confined area. They may have an advantage over the sloped tiled floor as they are absolutely level, and therefore more stable if a wheelchair needs to be positioned in the shower area. (If the shower area is to be surrounded by carpet it may be advisable to install a single course of tiles around the shower floor).

Shower Curtain. The difficulty of a helper remaining dry can be overcome by the use of a shower guard, either standard or made-to-measure and either portable or fixed to the wall.

Floor. The floor should slope towards a corner outlet to allow the water to be contained within the shower area. The alternative floor coverings are non-slip ceramic tiles or flooring.

Shower Chairs. There are different models available. Features include a variety of footrests, seats, and pressure cushions. There are detachable front arms and straight and splayed height-adjustable side arms—to either increase the seat width or provide trunk support. Made-to-measure models are available.

Electrical Switches

A disabled person with a neuromuscular condition is unlikely to be able to raise his arms and the height of the outlets and light switches must be lower than the height usually accepted for wheelchair use. The ideal height of 28" from the center of the switch to the floor is influenced by the height of the wheelchair arm pads so that he can move his forearm sideways while his elbow is supported on the wheelchair arm pad. One twin switch by the bed should be at skirting-board level to provide power for the bed/turning mattress.

Bathroom. A wall-mounted switch outside the bathroom is easier for anyone with a neuromuscular condition to use than a pull-switch in the room which often requires too much downward pressure. It also enables him to go into a pre-lit room as he cannot maneuver into the room and turn on the switch simultaneously.

Bedroom. In the same way, a switch outside the room will be ideal in addition to two switches in the bedroom.

- *By the bed.* This should be positioned under the hoist track 40" from the wall behind the bed headboard at a height of 30" from the bottom of switch (above the electric bed mattress and bedding).

- *In an accessible position.* This will be necessary for use when he is in his wheelchair in the bedroom. When it becomes dark, it would otherwise mean that as he cannot reach across the bed; he would have to go out of the room to turn on the light.

Electrical Outlets

Outlets with switches should be installed. As a person with a neuromuscular condition will be very dependent upon electrical gadgets, more than the average number of outlets will be needed. Two twin outlets by the bed plus three other twin outlets above the play/equipment surface(s) would be ideal. Where the surfaces are adjustable the outlets should be fitted above the maximum height.

Wheelchair Storage Area

Many disabled people have up to three wheelchairs, and if there is no garage, storage can be a real problem. It is essential to provide space with an adjacent electrical outlet for charging the boy's electric wheelchair. As fumes are given off by some batteries, the chair must not be charged in a bedroom—or in a closet.

Heating

For people with a neuromuscular condition it is necessary to provide a higher than average level of heating, 70–75° F in both bedroom and bathroom. This is particularly important in the bathroom, especially where it has more than one outside wall. A ceiling heat lamp or other auxiliary heat source should be considered.

Smoke Alarm

Building regulations now require a smoke alarm to be wired into the electrical system in all new properties.

Intercom

An intercom for a child to call his parents will be needed. Models which plug into an outlet are more convenient than transmitters and receivers linked with a cord, particularly as the receiver can be moved from one room to another.

Automatic Door Opener

The inability to open either the front or back door is very limiting to a disabled person wanting independence in their outdoor powered wheelchair. An automatic door opener should be considered to increase the independence of all disabled people.

Remodeling

In spite of the care taken by architects to include all details in the plans or job specifications, builders do not always appreciate the need to interpret these instructions precisely. In addition to the work being supervised by the architect, the disabled person or his caregivers need to appreciate the reasons why each recommendation has been made so that they can ensure they are carried out correctly. If possible, the family's occupational therapist should make regular visits while the builder is working.

Kitchen Adaptations

People with neuromuscular conditions usually encounter two major problems which should be taken into account. They are: combined arm and leg weakness and progressive weakness.

Leg Weakness

This can be overcome by using a stool or wheelchair with accessible units that are open underneath, and cupboards with a recess to accommodate the footplates of the chair. Some people will want to use the kitchen both when standing and sometimes from a wheelchair. A muscle wasting condition can mean that for several years a wheelchair is used for part of the day only—when tired or carrying out an activity which is easier from a wheelchair. Then it is necessary to have height-adjustable surfaces.

Arm Weakness

This can make it difficult to lift kitchen utensils and requires a continuous surface along which pans can be slid. Holding pans under a tap or lifting them up from the base of the sink is also difficult. If there are problems in reaching, then kitchen equipment must be positioned properly and at the right height. Poor or diminished hand grip and hand function may also arise. Specialized kitchen equipment can solve these difficulties.

Size of the Kitchen

If the whole kitchen is to be used by the disabled person, it has to be much bigger than usual because units need to be open underneath and storage space must be at an accessible level. The height of appliances and access must be considered. In planning the wall space, think in terms of the size of standard kitchen appliances and cupboards. If the disabled person cannot carry meals into another room, there will have to be space for a table and possibly a rising electric chair.

Layout

An L-shaped or U-shaped kitchen is ideal, but if there is no alternative to a galley kitchen the continuous wheelchair-accessible surface should be on one side, with the kitchen appliances and storage units on the other.

Height Adjustable Units

The height of the units needs to be adjustable to enable the kitchen to be used when standing and sitting; to ensure that the height will be suitable for any wheelchair and seat height; to allow the height to change for different activities; and for disabled and non-disabled users. Height adjustable units can be achieved in three ways:

- Bracket on wall rail: These are usually manually adjusted. Surfaces are fixed to the wall rail with wing nuts. To adjust the surface height you will need to remove the wing nuts manually and shift the surface up or down onto a different level of the bracket. A more expensive bracket is infinitely adjustable and easier to alter simply by turning a nut.

- Hydraulic: A winding handle moves the surfaces, which makes it unsuitable for most people with neuromuscular conditions.

- Electric: Essential when disabled people want to adjust the height themselves.

Surfaces

Because of the need to slide the pans there should be a continuous counter between the stovetop and sink with areas for the preparation of food in between. There must be a space either side of the stovetop to ensure that pan handles can be positioned sideways and not left projecting forwards.

- Food preparation surface: The main area should be between the sink and stovetop with smaller surfaces where useful.

- Surface for microwave: A surface in front of the microwave will enable the user to stabilize their forearms to open the oven—and help to lift/slide the items out.

- Pull-out surfaces below a built-in oven with a sliding door: This surface allows the user to stabilize their forearms to open the oven. If it is necessary to slide food from this surface to another part of the kitchen, an electric height-adjustable trolley can be used.

- Pull-out surface with bowl holes: These may be useful to stabilize a bowl and to provide a surface on which to lean.

Additional Information

Adapt-Ability, Inc.
9355 Dielman Industrial Dr.
St. Louis, MO 63132
Phone: 314-4323-1101
Fax: 314-432-0780
Website: http://www.adapt-ability.org

Jobsite accommodation, home modification, customized wheelchairs, assistive communication, computer access, and training.

Bruno Independent Living Aids, Inc.
1780 Executive Drive
P.O. Box 84
Oconomowoc, WI 53066
Toll-Free: 800-882-8183
Fax: 262-567-4341
Website: http://www.bruno.com

Produces accessibility and mobility products for people with disabilities including battery powered three and four wheeled scooters; automobile, truck, and van lifts to transport scooters; and wheelchairs, power chairs, and stair lifts that allow access to upper and lower levels of buildings.

Maddak, Inc.
661 Route 23 South
Wayne, NJ 07470
Toll-Free: 800-443-4926
Phone: 973-628-7600
Fax: 973-305-0841
Website: http://service.maddak.com/index.asp
E-mail: CustServ@Maddak.com

Maxi-Aids, Inc.
P.O. Box 3209
Farmingdale, NY 11735
Toll-Free: 800-522-6294
Toll-Free TTY: 800-281-3555
Phone: 631-752-0521
Fax: 631-752-0689
Website: http://www.maxiaids.com
E-mail: sales@maxiaids.com

MyMedMart, Inc.
723 Seneca St.
Webster City, IA 50595
Toll-Free: 888-832-7545
Fax: 515-832-4851
Website: http://www.mymedmart.com
E-mail: info@mymedmart.com

Home health care supplies and equipment.

Rehab Designs, Inc.

11700 Commonwealth Drive
Louisville, KY 40299-6303
Toll-Free: 888-889-1114
Phone: 502-266-9061
Fax: 502-266-6251
Website: http://www.rehabdesigns.com
E-mail: info@rehabdesigns.com

Surehands Lift and Care Systems

982 Route One
Pine Island, NY 10969
Phone: 336-427-8765
Fax: 336-427-6969
Website: http://www.gstsdesigns.com/surehands/
surehandsproducts.html
E-mail: service@GSTSDesigns.com

Chapter 33

101 Hints to Help Patients with Muscular Dystrophy

This chapter was written to assist patients with neuromuscular disease in handling their tasks of daily living. All the hints it contains have been field-tested and proven useful. Most were suggested by patients or their families. Only a few have been gleaned from the literature. In this sense, the chapter, like the Heloise books, is truly a do-it-yourself owner's manual. Usually, the hints do not require any special tools or equipment. Most of the gadgets described can be easily made with materials at hand in the ordinary household or purchased at a grocery, hardware, or fabric store or ordered from readily available self-help catalogs.

Hopefully these hints will help you and your caregivers tend to your daily tasks of eating, grooming, dressing, sitting, transferring, communicating, getting around, using the toilet, working, recreating, traveling, shopping, and sleeping.

Dressing

1. Velcro closures make buttoning and donning shoes easier than using buttons, snaps, or shoestrings. Velcro buttons and strips

Reprinted from "101 Hints to 'Help-with-Ease' for Patients with Neuromuscular Disease" with permission from the Muscular Dystrophy Association, www.mdausa.org. © 2003 The Muscular Dystrophy Association. For additional information, call the Muscular Dystrophy Association National Headquarters toll-free at (800) 572-1717. To find an MDA office in your area, look in your local telephone book, or click on "Clinics and Services" on the MDA website.

are available at fabric stores. Velcro tabs can be sewn to shoes at a brace shop or shoe repair shop. Ready-made Velcro closure tennis shoes are usually found at discount department stores.

2. Large bib overalls are excellent garb for young people in wheelchairs. They slip off easily to facilitate using the toilet. A front opening is available in some styles for use with male urinals. Elastic-waist exercise clothing (i.e., sweat pants and running suits) is easier to push down and pull up. A 22-inch zipper can be sewn into the front seam and extended down the leg to allow plenty of room for the use of a urinal.

3. A double bias tape loop (one attached to a belt loop, the other encircling the wrist) makes it easier to lift and lower a pair of trousers when at least one-hand support is needed to stand after using the toilet.

4. Ventilation under plastic braces is improved by wearing fishnet panty hose. This practical apparel is especially useful in the summer.

5. A simple pushing or pulling aid to help bring clothing closer to you from the bed, dresser drawer, or closet without reaching can be made from a wire coat hanger custom bent at either or both ends. Be careful with the sharp end. Wrap the ends with masking tape or slip a soft pencil eraser on the end to help avoid tearing clothing and to provide a better grip.

6. A circular key ring can be attached to a zipper tab that has a hole in it, allowing fingers or thumb to easily grasp the tab and close the zipper. Sticky zippers will slide easily if rubbed with the lead from a lead pencil.

7. Buttoning can be eased by using elastic loops for buttonholes and sewing buttons on with elastic thread. The center of each button (front and back) can be touched with clear nail polish to seal the threads and make the button stay on longer. This works especially well with buttons on cuffs. Buttons can also be fastened to buttonholes for appearance and Velcro patches placed on the back for closure.

8. Although a gentleman's pre-knotted necktie can be adapted with an elastic band, a plastic or metal clip glued or sewn on the back of the knot might be easier to place on a buttoned collar.

9.   Tube socks (socks without heels that stretch to fit the foot) are easy for a child or adult to put on. Socks with a little synthetic fabric in them are also easier to put on for winter wear than socks made of 100 percent wool.

10. A foot that stiffens downward so much that it is hard to get a shoe on can be more easily slipped into a shoe if the back of the shoe is cut vertically and loosely laced. A tennis shoe can be adapted by sewing a zipper down the side. Any shoe repair shop can modify a pair of shoes in this fashion.

11. When a child has difficulty telling the right shoe from the left, draw half an animal on each so the two halves make a whole animal when placed side by side.

12. For the little girl who often puts her dress on backwards, provide a reminder to help her do it right, such as pinning a colorful bow to the front of the dress.

13. Heavy fishing line pulled through zipper tabs and tied in a loop (the knot can be sealed by melting it with the heat from a lighted match) makes it easier to pull the zipper closed. This idea works especially well on men's or women's slacks. The loop is invisible and also washes well.

14. A gastrostomy tube can be covered easily with body-size stockinette tubing. This will protect clothing from getting soiled by the tube. A 10- to 12-inch-wide piece is cut and slipped over the head and arms. Ask your clinic orthotist to give you some.

15. Leaving your leg braces in the shoes provides an instant shoe horn which may help when slipping the shoes and braces onto your feet.

16. Do not try to trim plastic braces by yourself. Even using a sharp tool to carve the plastic can cause it to weaken.

17. Always use shoes that have the same heel height as those worn when your leg braces were fitted. If you don't, your feet and ankles may be tilted up or down, which will throw you off balance. Also check the sole on tennis shoes. Some brands have soft cushion bubbles on the soles that can make you unsteady. Look for firm, flat soles.

18. If one side of the body is weaker, it takes less effort to dress this side first. For example, put the weaker arm into the shirt

sleeve first, the stronger arm next. Whenever possible, sit while dressing so you can safely rest as needed.

19. If you have difficulty buttoning a shirt or blouse, get a larger size, keep it buttoned all the time, and put it on as if it were a pullover shirt.

Communicating

20. When speaking is a problem, a doodle board can be used. Some types are the Magna Doodle, Etch-A-Sketch, and Magic Slate. These handy devices make it unnecessary to carry a pencil and pad. Small electronic models are also available. Look for memory organizers with simple functions that will write out a word, phrase, or sentence on the screen. These instruments are relatively legible, portable, and inexpensive.

21. Large felt tip pens are more easily handled than the average ball-point model. Large-diameter ballpoint pens are available at office supply stores, at checkout counters in many drug stores, discount stores, etc.

22. Pieces cut from a common kitchen sink foam sponge or even some rubber bands wrapped around a pencil/pen make it easier to grip. Many small pen/pencil grips are available at office warehouse stores. These are inexpensive.

23. A small rubber ball can be punctured so a pencil can be forced through. This makes an excellent grip for a pencil or other writing implement. A small lazy Susan turntable on the desk top for pens, tape, paper clips, etc., makes them easier to reach.

24. Many children with poor hand control can learn to write well on a typewriter or computer keyboard. The youngster who is clever with numbers can do many accounting tasks on a small calculator.

25. When hands are too weak to turn the pages of a book, but neck strength and control remain, an excellent head-centered turner can be fashioned by attaching a pencil-thin wooden dowel, approximately 18 inches long, to the center of the brim of a tightly fitting cap or sunshade. A soft pencil eraser

slipped over the end of the dowel can provide friction for turning the page. Mouthsticks and commercial pointers are also available if this does not work.

Sitting, Transferring, and Mobility

26. An effective transfer board can be fashioned from a length of hardwood which is sanded, waxed, and highly polished. Both ends should be beveled. This is a project for someone at your house who likes to work with wood.

27. Transfers and gait can be assisted by using a wide, securely buckled belt around the patient's waist, which is then grasped to support him/her during transfer or steady him/her while walking. However, special gait belts are often inexpensive, usually under $10 at a medical supply store.

28. A king-size satin pillow case is an excellent aid to use as a drawsheet for transfer or turning in bed.

29. Because of its height, a bar stool is a good seat for the patient with weak hip and/or knee extensors. Look for one with a wide leg base. You might also want one with back and arm rests. When rising from a chair with arm covers, the covers can be kept from slipping by laying a sheet of art foam (available at art supply stores) between the cover and the arm rest of the chair. A terry cloth washcloth will also work.

30. Leverage can be increased when moving in bed by using arm elevators constructed with lightweight, wide-based wooded blocks to which dowel handles have been fixed.

31. Football receiver gloves afford a better grip on the handrail when climbing or descending stairs. Baseball or biking gloves are not quite as good.

32. When traveling, an airline wheelchair can be rented for negotiating narrow doors and passageways.

33. Radio waves can cause unintended motion of power wheelchairs or scooters. Take caution using CB radios or cellular phones when your wheelchair power is on. Also be aware of the location of radio transmitters such as radio or TV stations and two-way radios. Try to avoid driving near them.

34.   A heavy rope, knotted at 12-inch intervals and slung from a secure tree branch, can be used for support to help a child with weak legs practice walking outside in the back yard.

35.   Low-cut pile carpeting without padding is safer to walk on than heavy shag or throw rugs and makes wheelchair mobility at home easier to manage.

36.   A lightweight bicycle helmet is comfortable for head protection with children prone to falling. A homemade head protector made of cloth strips filled with closed-cell foam padding sewn to circle and cross the top of the head is also effective.

Recreation

37.   Many libraries will deliver or mail books to your home. Check with your local library for information.

38.   Gardening can be aided by using a length of plastic tubing as a conduit to plant seeds when seated in a wheelchair.

39.   The dimples on a rubber thimble provide friction to help turn the pages of a book or magazine.

40.   For fishermen who have difficulty retrieving a line, several devices are available, including a vest with a lightweight harness which holds the fishing rod in an aluminum tube with a locking feature. Also obtainable is an electronic fishing reel featuring a four-speed control with two manual and two electronic settings.

41.   A spring-loaded billiard cue is available for billiards or pool players who lack strength enough to handle the standard cue.

42.   If you want to play a stringed instrument (guitar, banjo, ukulele, etc.) but have weak hands and wrists, a soft glove can be modified by gluing individual plastic picks onto the fingers, adding a Velcro strap (for quick sizing) at the wrist and opening the thumb area for easy removal. The glove facilitates plucking and strumming stringed instruments by moving the fingers in a clawing manner, either separately or together.

43.   For those who sew, a small magnet glued to the end of a yardstick makes an effective retriever for dropped pins and needles.

44. To find information on the Internet for travelers with physical disabilities, start at http://www.lcweb.loc.gov/nls/reference/ circulars/travel.html.

45. Paddle-minton is a badminton-like game using a short paddle which is easy to handle from a wheelchair. The game's birdie is modified so as not to fly fast or high. The birdie's speed can be adjusted by tying the feathers together for faster play or spreading them apart to slow its flight.

46. The Quad-Bee Frisbee has two adaptive thumb clips allowing someone with upper extremity weakness to hold and throw the device.

47. Hand control in children can be developed with games utilizing rings placed around pegs. Pegs can be made from an old broomstick or other small dowels nailed or glued to a flat board. Rings can be fabricated from the plastic holders found on soda pop or beer cans or cardboard rings can be cut from a cylindrical oatmeal box or a paper towel tube.

48. Wheelchair archery is made easier for persons with weak arms by using a straight arm splint on the arm that holds the bow and a hook fashioned to the other hand to pull the bowstring. Archery may help correct spinal curvature. The arm pulling the string should be on the side that has the more prominent curve of the spine.

49. A secure seat for a small child's use on a seesaw can be fashioned from half of a plastic bucket or a section of an automobile tire. Tape the edges with duct tape for safety.

50. A thick board can be slotted to hold a hand of playing cards for those whose grasp is weak. Ask your handy woodworking friend to make this simple but useful gadget for you.

Housekeeping

51. When bending is a problem in cleaning lower cabinets or appliances, they can be reached with a good spray cleaner. An O'Cedar Light N' Thirsty mop can be used to wipe the surface clean, after allowing the spray to set a few minutes.

52. When fingers are too weak to grasp a broom or mop handle firmly, a leather or cloth loop can be placed over the handle and pulled with the forearm.

Sleeping or Resting

53. Friction is decreased for changing sleep position by using satin or nylon sheets and/or pajamas. But, be careful when sitting on the side of the bed as you will slip quite easily when trying to transfer to your wheelchair or commode.

54. A heavy belt or strap tied to the bedposts or a bed frame is a simple way to gain leverage to turn yourself from side to side.

55. For the couple who want a double bed where only one requires a hospital bed, an extra long (80") twin bed can be attached side by side to an electric hospital bed. Order an electric hospital bed that has no headboard (80"), then a king-size headboard can be attached to both beds.

56. Washable synthetic sheepskin padding or commercial eggcrate foam can be placed under a fitted sheet for more comfort when lying down. Any of a variety of inflatable camping mattresses serve the same purpose.

57. A U-shaped travel neck pillow can be used to support the neck while lying flat or reclining in bed or in a lounge chair.

58. Fiberfill or down comforters are lighter and warmer than wool or acrylic blankets. It is easier to move underneath or to lift them.

59. Covers tented over a straight-back chair at the end of the bed will free your feet and legs while keeping you warm. Using bed corner garters to secure the blanket edges to the mattress is an inexpensive way of keeping them securely tucked. They can be found in the bedding department of discount stores.

60. To easily identify and retrieve a house key from a ring of keys, drill a second hole near the edge of the key so it will hang off center on the key ring or use a plastic key end cover, available at your hardware store.

61. Long body pillows can be used to prop the back for side lying, preventing you from rolling backward. They can also be placed between your knees to decrease pressure and propped to reduce hip contracture.

Grooming

62. An empty half-gallon plastic cylindrical container makes a handy floating support for the head and neck to allow shampooing while the bather is reclined in a tub. Avoid overly hot water when bathing, since it causes fatigue.

63. For a dry shampoo, sprinkle cornstarch or baby powder lightly on oily hair and brush it out. Pull a nylon stocking over the brush bristles and brush vigorously to remove more dirt and restore the sheen to your hair.

64. Cylindrical foam can be purchased in yard lengths and attached or wrapped for extending or enlarging the handle of a razor, comb, toothbrush, or other grooming tool. One end of a flat wooden coat hanger can be drilled to accept a pick-type comb. This device provides a light and easily handled comb extension.

65. Liquid soap containers are convenient to use when attached to the bathroom or shower wall. You do not have to handle a slippery bar of soap, bottle of shampoo, or hair conditioner. Make a slit and pocket in a thick sponge to hold a flat bar of soap. When you wash just squeeze the sponge to get the suds.

66. A toothbrush can be adapted for use by weak hands/wrists by cutting the middle rows of bristles down to half their height. With this modification the front and back of the teeth are brushed by the high front and back bristles while the tops are cleaned by the shortened middle bristles. Such a toothbrush can also be purchased through an appliance catalog, as can an electric-powered model suitable for those lacking the strength or agility to brush their teeth. Look for one with a rotary brush. It is easier to hold in front of your mouth.

67. A washcloth mitten is easier for some folks to use than a regular washcloth for washing oneself or the dishes.

68. A nail clipper and file combination can be mounted on a sturdy board, eliminating the need for thumb or pinch strength when using these implements.

Toileting

69. Use baby wipes instead of toilet tissue. They are easier to hold and you feel (and are) cleaner when you finish using them.

70. Serenity Security Pads worn at night can decrease the number of times you have to use the bathroom. They can also be worn on long car trips.

71. A piece of semi-flexible plastic (like that used to make small pocket rulers) can be employed to fold toilet tissue for use. The tissue is wrapped around two-thirds of the length of the plastic (no sharp edges please), and the remainder used as an extension handle. Another way to provide an extension for cleaning yourself with toilet paper is to wrap the tissue around the working end of a pair of ordinary kitchen tongs.

72. Easy access to and egress from a bathroom can be provided by removing the door (and even part of the door-frame) and hanging an opaque shower curtain instead. This ends the difficulty of opening and closing the door without sacrificing privacy. Offset hinges can also be used to widen the doorway without removing the door.

73. A Texas condom catheter for men or boys who cannot control their urine or are in situations where it is inconvenient to use the toilet can be prescribed by your physician. It is attached with double-sided adhesive tape to avoid leaking and fastened to a leg bag for urine collection. The long connection hose (for the leg bag) can be clamped at the end and placed over a urinal or toilet edge, thus eliminating the need for a leg bag. The condom can be reused if carefully washed in plain soap and water.

Eating

74. A moistened paper towel placed under your plate will keep it from slipping on a tabletop.

75. The diameter of eating utensil handles can be increased with cylindrical foam (available as pipe insulation at the hardware store).

76. Wide-handled plastic mugs are easier to lift when all four fingers can be placed inside the handle. This way a firm grasp is not needed to hold and tip the cup toward the mouth. An inexpensive sip-a-mug can be purchased at most drugstores or supermarkets. This is a light plastic mug with a contoured handle which also serves as a straw.

77. Lightweight plastic bowls are easier to handle than glass or ceramic dishes. A rubber mesh mat will keep them from slipping on the counter or in the lap.

78. A sport-type plastic drink container often has a hole containing a straw in its cover which eases/allows access to its contents.

79. Annoying phlegm can be decreased by limiting the ingestion of dairy foods, but be sure to get your daily calcium quotient in other ways. Citrus juice can cut thick saliva.

80. Suck ice chips before eating if you have difficulty swallowing. It helps desensitize the gag reflex.

81. Chewing licorice just before eating decreases the appetite because it dulls taste buds. Be careful not to overdo this. Too much licorice can decrease your serum potassium level.

82. Where swallowing is difficult, a package of frozen peas placed on the front of the neck may prove of assistance by relaxing muscle spasm.

83. When food gathers in the back of the mouth, tip the chin downward, not upward, to improve ingestion.

84. A little meat tenderizer (MSG) on the back of the tongue will help to break up thick saliva and aid swallowing.

85. A damp dish towel wrapped around the base of a bowl will keep it from slipping on a smooth counter.

86. A simple portable aid to help get the hand to the mouth can be made with any forearm support such as a flat length of wood or even split bamboo (with several slips of Velcro tacked on to secure the arm) and attached in the middle on both sides with a pin to two large dowels which are fixed to a heavy wooden base. This forearm prop can be placed on a table where it acts like a seesaw, lifting the hand to the mouth when the elbow is dropped.

87. A disposable plastic cup with a space cut out along the rim to fit about a child's nose will allow the youngster to drink in a better, more controlled position with his chin forward, rather than having to bend his head back.

88. A child having trouble controlling a cup with one hand can often do better if it is fitted with two handles. This adapted cup

is listed at low cost in ADL catalogs or you can ask a local potter to make one for you if a ceramic mug will not be too heavy to lift.

89. An octopus soap holder which has multiple suction supports makes an effective plate, glass, or cup stabilizer. This gadget can be purchased in most grocery stores.

90. An extra-long plastic straw can be used to eliminate the need to lift a glass when drinking.

Exercising and Managing Contractures

91. Tight heel cords can be treated while a young child rides a rocking horse by fitting the horse with stirrups so that the feet will be stretched up to a more normal position as he/she rocks.

92. Contractures can be measured by folding a piece of paper to match the angle of the joint, tracing the folded edge onto a second sheet, and measuring it with a protractor. By keeping a record of the degree of contracture, the caregiver can see progress, and is more likely to keep working hard at stretching exercises to correct the contractures.

93. Balancing exercises are important because loss of balance can result in a fall with possible injury. Holding on to someone while standing on each foot alone is a simple way to improve balance.

94. A foot board (one-half- to three-quarter-inch plywood padded with a blanket will do) for support at the foot of the bed to keep the feet propped at the ankles during sleep, helps prevent ankle contractures. Of course, this means you must be able to sleep on your back with both feet against the board. You could, however, be side-lying with at least one foot against the board for some effect.

95. If your heels feel sore while you are lying on your back, place a small pillow under your calves to relieve heel pressure. This same technique can be used during the day when you prop up your feet to reduce swelling. Tender heels can be toughened by patting them with a moist tea bag at night. When the tea dries, the tannic acid it contains will act to harden (and

slightly discolor) the skin. Passive stretching of the knee can be accomplished by placing the calves on a pillow supported by a hassock or kitchen chair. In this way, your heels are not resting on the supporting surface and there is no heel pressure that might reduce local vascular circulation.

96. Hand exercises can be fun. Try learning sign language and playing shadow puppets. Or squeeze the poles of a toy that makes an articulated animal loop around. Fingers are exercised comfortably by squeezing a washcloth or sponge in a basin of warm water.

97. Exercising with your child can be made entertaining by strapping a small bell or flag to the arm or leg so that it will ring or flap when the child moves.

98. The easiest way to stretch heel cord contractures is to stand at arm's length from a wall and place your hands on the wall. Lean toward the wall, bending your elbows, while keeping the heels flat on the floor and the knees straight, and attempt to touch the wall with your chest. If this is too hard, you can start with your feet closer to the wall, or bend one knee at a time.

99. When a child is seated, his feet should always be supported. A box or large book will do. Dangling feet are more prone to develop contractures.

100. Simple breathing exercises can be performed by blowing through a straw, blowing up balloons, or blowing a ping pong ball on a tabletop or other flat surface. Playing a harmonica, kazoo, or other wind instrument is a pleasant way to exercise the lungs.

101. Excessive heat will increase symptoms in those with myasthenia gravis. Swimming in a cool pool is the best exercise for these patients. Cool foods and drink are also easier to swallow. Emotional stress, even positive stress, increases weakness in this disease and should be avoided. That's right, you can have too much fun!

Chapter 34

Wheelchairs for Children and Adults with Muscular Dystrophy

What Is a Good Seating Position?

The aim is to achieve:

- A good postural position to minimize the development and severity of deformity and/or to provide support and trunk control. In a progressive disability there is a continual need to review the seating position.

- To maintain function.

- To ensure comfort.

Prioritizing these aims will depend upon the individual person and their importance is likely to vary according to the time of the day, the need to carry out an activity, etc.

This chapter includes "What Is a Good Seating Position?" and "Range of Specifications and Wheelchair Features." Text and figures reprinted with permission from the Muscular Dystrophy Campaign, a United Kingdom charity focusing on all muscular dystrophies and allied disorders © Muscular Dystrophy Campaign. All rights reserved. Additional information is available at www.muscular-dystrophy.org.uk. Figures redrawn for Omnigraphics by Alison DeKleine, January 2004, with permission from the Muscular Dystrophy Campaign. Also, "Treatment for DMD: Wheelchairs FAQ," is reprinted with permission from Parent Project Muscular Dystrophy. © 2003. All rights reserved. For additional information about Duchenne and Becker Muscular Dystrophy, visit the Parent Project website at www.parentprojectmd.org.

Good Postural Position

This is achieved when all parts of the body are supported correctly. As the crucial feature is the maintenance of the correct position of the pelvic girdle, this aspect will be dealt with first.

- All parts of the body must remain in the upright, neutral position, without a posterior tilt that results in sacral sitting or an anterior tilt that throws the spine forwards, although a degree of anterior tilt can be helpful and accepted as balanced posture. The iliac crests must be level, with no pelvic obliquity either to the left or right with associated scoliosis (side curvature of the spine) and no rotation of the pelvis.

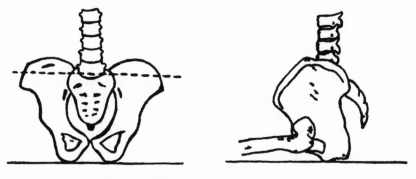

Front (L) and Side (R) neutral position of the pelvis

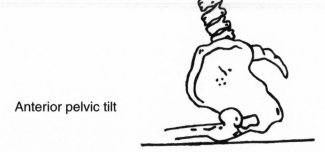

Anterior pelvic tilt

Figure 34.1. Upright Neutral Position of the Pelvic Girdle: Side and Front Neutral Positions of Pelvis and Anterior Pelvic Tilt.

Correct Support for the Whole Body

Correct support for the whole body depends upon the correct size of chair in relation to the following features:

- **Seat width.** This must be wide enough for comfort and yet a snug enough fit to ensure that the pelvis is stabilized. This ensures that the armrests are near enough to the disabled person to eliminate

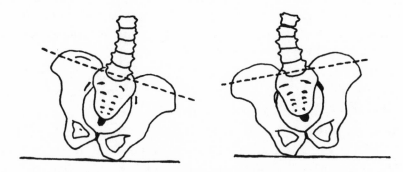

Left and Right pelvic obliquity

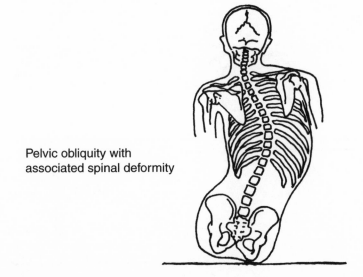

Pelvic obliquity with
associated spinal deformity

Figure 34.2. Obliquity of the Pelvic Girdle and Associated Spinal Deformity

sideways leaning to gain support from the arm pads, and unless the chair is powered, that the propelling wheels are as close to the body as possible.

- If **side pads** are used to reduce the width of the seat, the arm pads of the armrests should be extended inwards over the side pads. This ensures that the disabled person's elbows and forearms are supported without the need to lean sideways.

- **Seat depth.** The seat depth is crucial to ensure that the spine is supported, while at the same time maintaining the pelvis in a neutral position. With the hips at the back of the chair there must be 1"–2" between the front of the seat upholstery and the back of the knee (which is at 90°).

- **Seat surface.** The surface must be firm enough to provide support for the pelvis to keep it level. Good support should be identified initially as it influences comfort.

- **Seat height** in relation to the footrests. The user's thighs must remain parallel to the floor with the ankle joint at a right angle. This is particularly important to prevent plantar flexion (pointing

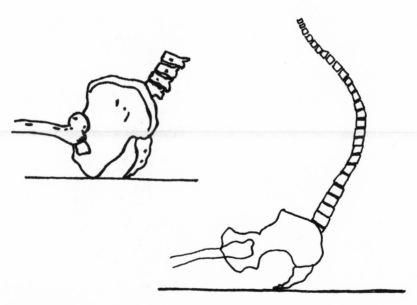

Figure 34.3. Sacral Sitting Causes Spinal Curvature

the foot), which will result in long-term foot deformities and make it very difficult or impossible to wear shoes.

- **Position and angle of the footrests.** Unless a disabled person is in a reclined position in order to relax, most people with neuromuscular conditions need to sit upright to enable them to use their limited ability to reach forward and to maintain head control. To provide stability and to maintain this position, their knee joint should be kept at a right angle. Therefore, the footrests should be parallel to the floor or tipped marginally backwards, ensuring the ankle joint is also kept at a right angle. However, when a wheelchair has large front wheels, the footrest hanger has to be angled to avoid obstruction. But the footrests can be tipped up to achieve the 90° angle at the ankle joint and although the angle at the knee joint will have to be increased, this should be kept to a minimum.

- **Armrest height.** The armrests should be at a comfortable height to ensure the arms are well supported with the shoulders level and not hunched. When the elbows are at the back of the armrests, the elbow joint should be at a right angle.

- **Backrest height.** The backrest should extend to just below the shoulders, for a powered chair and 2" below the axilla for a self-propelled chair. There should be a lumbar pad to ensure good support of the spine and to encourage spinal extension.

- **Headrest.** A headrest should be supplied for anyone with poor head control—and everyone traveling in their wheelchair in a van or mini-bus must use a head support to guard against a whiplash injury. A backrest extension may not lie close enough to the back of the person's head and an adjustable headrest, possibly shaped with side wings, may be better.

- **Position of the wheels on a self-propelled wheelchair or the joystick control of a powered wheelchair.** The position must be considered carefully to ensure that the disabled person is able to maintain an upright position and does not need to lean either towards the wheels or control—or away from them—to gain the correct leverage.

Maintain Functional Ability

Postural support. The seating system must not prevent the user from leaning forwards or reduce function in any way.

Height-adjustable seats. Special feature needed by some adults with neuromuscular conditions.

Comfort

Ability to change seating position. Backache and pain associated with deformity make it essential to be able to alter the pressure on the body, and therefore chairs need:

- Reclining backrests.

- Seats with seat and backrest tilt-in-space that tilt back from the horizontal.

- Leg rests that can be raised and lowered independently of each other.

All these functions should be controlled electrically—to allow the user complete independence to move within his or her chair.

Cost implications. Wheelchairs are used by most people with neuromuscular conditions for all or part of the day. Although comfort is of great importance, this is often compromised because of lack of funds to buy the most comfortable chair.

Wheelchair Specifications and Features That May Be Needed for People with Neuromuscular Conditions

Note: * Most of the features are relevant to all disabled people, but those that are particular (although not exclusive) to people with neuromuscular conditions are highlighted in this section with an asterisk.

Seat Sizes

- **Range of seat width** offered should extend from 10" for the smallest child to 24" for the largest adult.

- ***Adjustable seat width.** This feature appears to be difficult to incorporate into wheelchair design. But it ensures that a chair fits correctly both in the summer when thin clothes are worn and during the winter when extra clothing is needed. Additional width to the chair allows for growth and also helps when a hoist sling is positioned.

- ***Adjustable seat depth** to provide good support to the spine to discourage a posterior pelvic tilt and sacral sitting—and to allow for growth. Although the use of a back support/cushion may help to stabilize the back, the consequential reduction in the seat depth may be contra-indicated in relation to the arm-rest length and the position of the control, etc. It is also important to ensure that support is maintained under the whole length of the femora.

- **Seat height.** The height is important to accommodate the leg length and to provide the optimum level for transfers in and out of the chair. In addition, if a disabled person travels in their wheelchair, the seat height must allow sufficient headroom to enter vehicles.

Seat Height-Adjustability

- ***Seat elevating to a height of approximately 34 inches.** An optional module to allow adults with muscular dystrophy to stand up from the chair or to reach high cupboards, etc.

Upholstery

- **Choice of firm, but comfortable upholstery** for both seat and backrest to provide stability—or a hard base for interfacing a seating system.

- **An attractive appearance and choice of color** are aesthetically important. This helps both children and adults to accept the chairs and aids the psychological adjustment that is needed in deteriorating conditions, not only for a disabled child and adult, but also for their relatives and caregivers.

- ***Seat belt supplied as standard.** This is important to ensure safety from the time the chair is delivered.

Shoulder/Head Support

- **Choice of height of backrest extension**—more often required to cover the needs of tall people and provide shoulder, rather than head, support.

- ***Optional adjustable headrest** with height, forward/backward and sideways adjustment—and optional wings. A headrest extension that follows the angle of the backrest may be too far back to make contact with the person's head. This is particularly true when the person either sits bolt upright or has a forward curvature of their spine. This type of headrest is essential if the wheelchair user travels in a vehicle—to prevent a whiplash injury.

Frame

- **Easy-to-fold or dismantle into small pieces**—light enough to lift into a car with ease.

- **Backrest folds in half** to allow caregivers to lift the disabled person back into the chair, while the base of their spine remains supported. This feature is not always needed, but may be essential where a backrest has been raised—or a backrest extension supplied—to allow for the user's height.

- **Choice of chromium-plated or colored.** Aesthetically, this may be as important to a young person as the color of the upholstery.

- **Suitable for the attachment of an appropriate seating system,** without the need to modify either the frame or the seating system.

- **Provides fixing points** for clamping in a vehicle.

- **Suitable seat height to allow the headroom needed** to access vehicles.

- **Easy-to-grip and height-adjustable pushing handles** for the use of a caregiver when the gears are disengaged.

- **Sturdy, durable, and tamper-proof.**

Armrests

- ***Height-adjustable within 6" range.** This is particularly important following spinal surgery when the disabled person is sitting more upright in the wheelchair.

- ***In/out adjustability.** (See adjustable seat width.)

- **Supplied with side panels** to protect from drafts.

- **Easy-to-remove.**

Arm pads

- ***Width:** Choice of standard, or wide (possibly with side flange) to prevent the user's arm from falling off the arm pad, particularly where the user is unable to lift it on again.

- ***Length:** Standard or extra-long. It is important to provide full-length support which extends under the wrists, in order to control the joystick.

- ***Optional support** behind the elbow, to prevent the arm slipping backwards when maintenance of pressure is needed to power the chair up a pavement curb.

Footrests

- ***Standard flip-up.** It is important for the footrests to move out of the way to allow access for a caregiver and/or to enable the disabled person to stand up from the chair.

- ***Height-adjustability within 6" range.** This is essential to allow various depths of cushions to be used and to adjust the footrest for the individual leg lengths, and at the same time ensure the user's thigh is horizontal.

- ***Forward/backward adjustability.** This is not a standard feature, although some wheelchairs are available with a choice of footrests. However, trunk stability is dependent upon the disabled person having optimum contact of their feet on the footrest. It is therefore important to ensure that their ankles are maintained either at a right-angle or at the most suitable angle to allow for any foot deformities.

- ***Adjustable angle to footrest.** As mentioned, to maintain ankle joint at a right-angle or to allow for plantar flexion foot deformities.

- ***Optional elevating footrests.** This is essential if the backrest reclines and the disabled person has hip contractures.

- ***Electrically retractable.** This is a sophisticated feature that at present is available by special modification only. However, it is often needed because bending down to lift up or swing the footrests to the side may be impossible—yet essential—to allow a disabled person access within restricted spaces and/or to stand up from the chair.

- **Optional heel and calf straps.** These may help a disabled person to retain their feet on the footrest. However, there are occasions when the straps should be removed to allow the optimum position of the feet to be maintained.

Curb Climber

- **Advice on the curb height that the chair will climb comfortably.** The chair's performance needs to be suitable for the surroundings in which it is to be used. Therefore, it is essential that a demonstration and assessment, with good supervision, is carried out in and around the user's home.

- **Large curb-climbing wheels—or a choice of central or side climbers.** It is unlikely that a choice will be available for any particular model of wheelchair, but many users find that if the wheels do not climb the curbs, their choice between central or side climbers will depend upon their line of vision.

Control

- ***Choice of side or center control—or the opportunity to fit the alternative**—if the condition deteriorates. This may be important when considering the user's optimum seating position. It must be balanced, however, against his independence in moving his wheelchair and his ability to gain access under a surface without help to remove or reposition the control or the tray on which the control is fitted. Individual assessment is crucial.

- ***Ability to swing/slide control out of the way** to gain access under desks, tables, and working surfaces.

- ***Forward/backwards and in/out adjustability** to ensure that the disabled person does not have to lean either towards the control—or away from the control—to gain optimum leverage.

- ***Height-adjustability that is independent of the armrest height.** This is a feature that should be available, but is usually a modification.

- ***Sensitive control.** Many people with neuromuscular conditions have severe weakness in their arms and hands and the sensitivity of the control is therefore important.

- ***Sensitive on/off, switch/speed controls that are accessible** on the top of the surface near to joystick. Controls on a sloping raised console may be difficult to reach.

- **Battery charge indicator.** Essential for peace of mind, particularly when undertaking long journeys.

- **High tech shape of remote-control box.** The value of a sharp-looking wheelchair, particularly to young people, cannot be over estimated.

- ***Optional, small remote-control box**—set flush into a tray with no projection below. This option may be necessary for users who need to lean on a tray.

- ***Optional lap-held switches for the control box.** This may be necessary for a disabled person who needs to keep his hands positioned in his lap.

Battery

- **Easy to lift off** in order to fold the chair.

- **Choice of wet or dry**—to cater for the conflicting priorities of superior performance versus ease of maintenance.

- **Charging point must be accessible** to enable a disabled person living on their own to charge the battery independently.

- **Battery range adequate** for the distances likely to be traveled by the disabled person.

Tray

- ***Standard/rectangular or with cut out front**—to ensure optimum support for the disabled person's arms.

- ***Optional, availability in plexiglas**—to allow the disabled person to see the curb climber, when positioning the chair at the edge of the curb.

- **High tech**—not tea tray type. Vital for acceptance.

- **Swings, to store at the side of the chair.** An important practical feature to ensure that the tray is easy to remove and readily available when needed.

- ***Forward/backward adjustability.** The severe muscle weakness in the arms of many people with neuromuscular conditions makes it important that any working surface is placed in the optimum position to ensure maximum hand function—and different activities may require different positions. It may also be useful for the tray to be moved marginally forwards for a helper to gain access—or to allow for the thickness of outdoor clothes.

Price

- **Good value** and as competitive as possible.

- **Inexpensive spare parts that are readily available** to ensure a 48-hour standard service or a 24-hour emergency repair service.

Frequently Asked Questions about Wheelchairs

Will my son stop walking sooner because he has been given a power chair now, while he can still walk?

Having a wheelchair for part time use for the years when walking is becoming more difficult and falls are occurring more frequently, should in no way alter the normal rate of progression of the condition. It will however ensure that he has every opportunity to be involved in as many of his friend's activities as possible, by relieving him of the extra effort of getting there. Use of the chair is usually restricted to long distance, uneven terrain, or times when there is heavy traffic, e.g., in busy school playgrounds when his physical safety is compromised. Remember a boy's social and emotional development is really important, and if his independent mobility is restricted he will feel isolated.

Would it be better for my son to have a self-propelling manual chair so that he gets some exercise?

No. Self-propulsion is really quite hard work and not really the right sort of exercise. Muscles in the arms are undergoing the same cycles of degeneration and regeneration as those in the legs and pushing a wheel chair is not too much fun. Why not save the strength for more enjoyable activities and those which are not likely to cause too much fatigue? Most boys like swimming (great non-weight bearing exercise). It is an activity which can be enjoyed for many years. Bike riding is also beneficial as it is also non-weight bearing and does wonders for coordination and balance. Other forms of exercise that can be enjoyed with the rest of the family may include ball games using lighter balls (puff balls). It is good if interests in activities which can be enjoyed throughout life are fostered and encouraged early. Many boys like remote car or boat clubs.

My son now needs a power chair and I want to buy one that is bigger than the one that our therapist is recommending so that he will not grow out of it too quickly.

Please do not do that. Your therapist will have your best interest at heart and will undoubtedly have recommended a chair that provides some mechanism for expanding the chair in most dimensions as your son grows. It is very important for the chair to be a fairly snug fit; if there is too much room it will not offer adequate support and he will find it necessary to lean down or forwards to gain support. Your therapist will be monitoring his spine very closely for the development of a scoliosis and her attention to your son's posture while in the chair will be to prevent or stall this curvature. A good chair will be narrow in width (but capable of expanding sideways), and the arm rests will always be adjusted to elbow height so that both arms are supported (without leaning) Other modifications will most likely be fitted on the chair to help maintain an upright symmetrical sitting position.

He refuses to use the headrest provided and does not see the need to wear those thoracic pads either.

These two modifications are really important in maintaining a straight spine. The thoracic pads fit him into the right position when he is resting on the back rest, and as he can move in and out of them at will, he will not find them at all restricting. The headrest is very important, as it is a form of protection when traveling, especially up inclines and when stopping suddenly. Most boys with DMD have weak muscles in the front of the neck and also their abdominal muscles, so that they find it difficult to recover forward in these situations. Having the headrest always available gives them a feeling of security and also prevents the leaning forward posture adopted by many older boys who have not had headrest. (They lean forward to prevent backward displacement.)

We were thinking a scooter might be better than a power wheelchair to start off with.

This will depend on your child's needs and your circumstances. A scooter can be good for a part time walker, a boy with Becker MD, or for a family who do not worry about the possibility of needing to re-place the scooter with a chair when more postural support is needed. Good postural modifications are difficult on a scooter, and the good features like electronic tilt in space are not possible on them.

I have heard it is important to swap the joystick from right to left every six months.

This is something often recommended by therapists in the belief most boys lean one way to reach their joy stick. The only problem is that there is a lot of confusion about which way they lean. Is it to-wards the joystick or away from it? Research literature cannot make up its mind. From my experience it is not the joystick's problem, but rather that the chair has not been adjusted or customized to ensure that the boy has no need to lean in any direction. Constant monitor-ing is needed to make sure that:

1. The chair is not too wide (a snug fit) so that he does not have to lean out for arm support).

2. The arm rests are set at elbow height so that he will not lean down for support.

3. The control box or joystick lies immediately under the domi-nant hand, which will ensure that he will not need to lean for-ward to reach it.

Most good chairs come with many possible adjustments to allow the boys to grow and still have good postural support. Your therapist or seating technician will be able to advise on the best chairs for boys with DMD.

If my son sits in a wheelchair all day, won't he become unfit and will his muscles tighten even more?

Yes, it is not good to remain sitting all day. Your physical thera-pist will recommend suitable exercise for your boy, which will be ap-propriate for him at his age and stage. He will undoubtedly spend time out of the chair. Most boys enjoy swimming or hydrotherapy, which is a wonderful way of stretching out and moving freely without too much effort. It is also provides good respiratory exercise, but most of all it will allow him to have some fun with family and friends out of his chair. Stretching out his tighter tendons is done in many ways and will depend on your particular circumstances. Some boys spend time in long leg braces, others stand for a time in a standing frame or supine stander, while some may lie flat on their stomachs with weights over bottom and ankles to give a good stretch to hips, knees, and ankles.

My son is six and loves to come shopping, but gets tired and cranky. His therapist wants me to have a wheelchair to use on these occasions, but I want a stroller or preferably a buggy. What should I do?

This is a difficult decision for many parents especially for newly diagnosed boys. A wheelchair so early is such a horrible reality check. Boys do tire however and they do need help over the long distances. An infant's stroller does fill the bill for a very short time, but not for a six year old as his peers would most definitely regard it as babyish. A larger buggy which would him fit better is really not suitable for long, and is still not age appropriate. A smart little folding wheelchair for occasional use is really the best solution. For trips to the park, etc., he could ride a bike or tricycle (some have a push handle on the back) or he could be pushed or pulled in a wagon.

Chapter 35

Home Health Care

They come under many names: personal care attendants, certified nursing attendants, home health care workers, and personal assistants. Some are trained in the medical profession, while others are simply students or other able-bodied folks willing to take on some tough but possibly rewarding work.

They can be a positive boon to people who have physical disabilities and who require regular help getting ready for work or school or other daily routines. Many people affected by the neuromuscular diseases in MDA's program have benefited from employing home health care workers, and have been able to pursue active lifestyles with their help.

The position of home care attendant requires an odd mix of attributes. Physical strength is important if lifting and transferring are required. A lack of squeamishness about the human body is essential if help is required with bathing, dressing, and toileting. Medical knowledge is, of course, a plus, but not all attendants have it. Other qualities such as patience, a sense of humor, and a level head in times of emergency can be equally crucial.

Reprinted from "Home Health Care: Home Is Where the Help Is" by Phil Ivory, *QUEST*, Volume 8, Number 1, February 2001. Reprinted with permission from the Muscular Dystrophy Association, www.mdausa.org. © The Muscular Dystrophy Association. For additional information, call the Muscular Dystrophy Association National Headquarters toll-free at (800) 572-1717. To find an MDA office in your area, look in your local telephone book, or click on "Clinics and Services" on the MDA website.

Family: Too Close to Home

Some people whose mobility has been limited by neuromuscular disorders may be able to rely on family members to provide home health care. But in some cases the kind of daily help that is required may be too much to ask, even of a loved one. What is more, in such cases it can be hard for the person receiving care to complain if the quality of care seems inadequate. And having one's spouse help with bathing and toileting on a daily basis could take the ardor out of the most passionate love life.

Hiring a professional may be preferable. However, the economy affects the hiring of home health care aides. The better the job market, the fewer people willing to accept difficult, demanding, and underpaid positions—which unfortunately is how most home care positions can accurately be described.

Finding and Hiring the Right Person

In screening and hiring home health care aides, a home care center or hospital could be a good starting point for information. It may be necessary to place an ad in a local newspaper, on the Internet, or in a visible public place, providing broad information about the work schedule, type of help needed, and wages offered. For the interview process, the employer should be totally honest about the most difficult or embarrassing aspects of the job. This is the only way to give applicants a fair chance to ponder the realities of the position before accepting. It is also an opportunity to talk about the nature of the disease and the specific care necessitated by it.

Writing a job description and discussing it in detail with applicants is a good idea, too. A description could include detailed entries for such topics as bathing, dressing, exercise, bowel and bladder management, transferring, meal preparation, housekeeping, laundry, shopping, and assistance with transportation. Another important topic of discussion is the aide's time off.

The interviewer should take notes after each interview, or the applicants may begin to blur together. It is highly advisable to seek and check references; if a home care agency is referring the applicants, the agency should be able to help with background checks.

Unfortunately, it is not unusual for trusting employers to learn too late that the person they welcomed into their home has a troubling past, possibly including a criminal record.

Cordial Relations

Once an attendant has been hired, a cordial, professional working atmosphere is essential. Much of the responsibility for setting the right tone rests on the employer. But what if an attendant becomes ill, or there is a sudden blowup resulting in a severing of relations, leaving the employer stranded at home without care?

It is a good idea to prepare in advance a list of backup attendants before they are needed. It should include people who can be counted on to provide essential care, not necessarily the full scope of services provided by the regular attendant. A backup list could include friends, family members, or former attendants.

Following are accounts of several families and individuals affected by neuromuscular diseases and their experiences hiring home health care workers.

Needing Help in Paradise

Tamara Moore lives in Paradise, California. She's 32 and is affected by several debilitating conditions, including carnitine palmityl transferase deficiency, a metabolic disorder.

Tamara Moore uses a wheelchair part of the time. Her symptoms, which can be exacerbated by numerous factors including exercise and stress, come and go unpredictably and often involve severe bouts of pain and weakness. Tamara and her husband, Rob, who is 41, have been married for 13 years and have two children. "Usually, we bring in a CNA [certified nursing assistant] three times a week to help her bathe," says Rob. "And then, depending on whether she's going through a lot of symptoms at the time, we can have a nurse come in daily. Otherwise, it's a physical therapist or CNA that would come in three times a week."

"We live in a retirement community even though we are not retired, and there are a lot of home health care aides in this area," he says. Rob, who provides some of Tamara's care himself, is largely responsible for managing the home care. Unfortunately, the time when Tamara most needs home care is the time when she is least able to take a hand in management.

"Usually when I am in need of their assistance, I am in rather bad shape and not always completely aware of what's going on," she says. "It's a very vulnerable time for me, being so sick and sometimes unable to move, and it's important for me to feel that the home health worker helping me is competent, sensitive, and really cares."

Attitude Is Crucial

Moore feels it is important that attendants be empathetic enough to be able to imagine what it is like to be "in my situation and in their hands." Her husband agrees that attitude is paramount.

"We have people that come in and are pretty negative, who sometimes have a worse outlook on life than patients do," he says. "I've heard people come in and say things like: 'Wow, you are really lucky to be alive.' Things you just wouldn't normally say. Most of the CNAs that come in are simply nursing assistants that require an eight-week course," he says. "They're not real high-tech people or anything like that. They're pretty low paid."

The hospital that provides the home care workers does background checks, but Rob has his own list of questions for each applicant. "I screen them pretty well. I ask them how long have they been doing this, what are their qualifications. I ask them if they know about my wife's disease and what are they willing to learn about it. I also go a lot on what Tamara feels," he says. "If she is uncomfortable with somebody, then I have to act on what she says."

"Most of the time, the problem is just their attitudes. 'I don't get paid much for this job, so that's how I'm going to act.' That sort of thing."

Developing Bonds

Rob says it is natural, even expected, that a closeness or intimacy develops between the caregiver and the person being cared for. "It gets close. When you are working closely with somebody, you need to have some kind of relationship and I would expect that. The first year was kind of crazy because it's very, very hard to find good, reliable, dependable people out there."

What about transferring and lifting? "Most of the time I'll just do that myself, unless my back is out," says Rob. "My wife just prefers me to do it."

Rob doesn't think the aides are being paid enough. "We are asking somebody to take care of somebody's life, and they've got to do a lot of dirty stuff, and I don't think they are being compensated enough for it. I think that's the problem, but then again they need more training, too. It's pretty much an unregulated field. You have to regulate it yourself. Leave no stone unturned," says Rob about the rigors of checking and selecting aides.

"Just because they are a nurse or health care provider doesn't automatically conclude that they are necessarily competent, sensitive, or even caring," Tamara says. "I have come to meet many home health workers, though, who are everything that I could hope for in a person who is caring for me during such a difficult time. In fact, one of them is my husband!" she says.

Ready for School

Kim Clark, 38, of Toledo, Ohio, has a 13-year-old son with Duchenne muscular dystrophy, Jordan. Jordan uses a motorized wheelchair and needs help in the morning getting dressed and ready for school.

"I have somebody come in every morning, Monday through Friday," Clark says. "He gets him up and dressed and in his wheelchair and gives him breakfast and gets his book bag together, while I pack his lunch and then he gets him on the school bus and then I sign his paperwork and he leaves for the day."

The aide, Richard McInrow, also comes in the evenings sometimes to provide respite care. He has been helping the Clarks for several years. "We hope to hold on to Richard as long as we can," Clark says. But they have not been happy with all the aides they have hired. "The first year was kind of crazy because they would send people and it's very, very hard to find good, reliable, dependable people out there. They come and go a lot," Clark notes.

"First of all, I don't think they are trained to properly lift these patients because I would ask them, 'Didn't you get training before you had to go into somebody's house? Didn't you have enough training in this?' And they would say: 'No.' Periodically they will be tested on things and they give certain classes, but I don't think it's in-depth enough."

High Achiever in St. Paul

Judy Guerin, 50, is a Minnesota native and lives in St. Paul. For many years, she believed she had limb-girdle muscular dystrophy. In 1995, her diagnosis was amended to spinal muscular atrophy. She uses a motorized wheelchair and has a limited range of physical motion.

Guerin lives alone and works as an office manager for the state in the Division of Rehabilitation Services. Being part of the work force has always been very important to her. She requires assistance with bathing, dressing, and other tasks in order to maintain her career.

In 1988, a change in legislation made it necessary for her to use her own earnings to pay for her home care. Ironically, if she had chosen to quit working, her home care would have been paid for by the state. "The system was taking $1,000 out of my pay to help pay for the aides, which left me less than $800 a month to live off of, and that included rent and everything else. So out of my paycheck, I saw less than half."

"I could have lived off general assistance, SSI, and everything else, and not had to worry," she says. "Besides, Social Security does not consider me disabled, so every year I need to prove that I am disabled." Although Guerin has received a diagnosis of a severe neuromuscular disorder, the Social Security Administration ties its definition of disability to a person's inability to work. Guerin's 40-hour work week flies in the face of their definition.

"They said my brother wasn't disabled, and my brother is more disabled than I am, and he finally just gave up. He got tired of the fight." Her brother stopped working so he could have home care costs paid by the state. Fortunately, in 1999 a legislative change corrected the situation so that she could keep working and still receive benefits to pay for her care.

Due Recognition

Guerin's decision to keep working despite the financial disadvantage the situation imposed on her was one of the reasons she was recognized with MDA's 2000 Personal Achievement Award for Minnesota. The award honors outstanding individuals who are affected by the neuromuscular diseases in MDA's program. Guerin currently has two aides, one hired through a welfare-to-work program. The other started right out of high school and has no training at all. It's a tremendous challenge, she says, training the aides and hanging on to the good ones. "To train good people, you need to be very verbal. You need to tell them what you need. They are there to help you."

"It's not an easy thing to do, finding somebody to get you up at 6:15 in the morning and be around all the time. I have my aides for nine hours during the day, during which time I use them four times. They come back and forth four times to take care of me. They come in the morning to get me up and get me to work. One of them meets me at noon and I go to the bathroom. And then they meet me again at 4:30 when I'm finished with work. And then they come again at night to put me to bed."

Low pay, she says, is one reason why good aides move on to other jobs or become nurses. "In my opinion, they should be paid $20 an hour. Unfortunately, they only make about $8. Who wants to work for $8.50 an hour? Not many people that I know."

Getting Tough When Needed

Guerin learned how unpleasant it is to be robbed by someone you've hired to help you. "I've had aides steal money out of my purse," says Guerin. "I've had them steal my credit cards. It's a royal pain."

What do you do when faced with that kind of betrayal? "Basically you fire them, and you keep very close tabs on everything you own. Your trust toward the people is very hard. It takes a long time to build that up."

Guerin has not experienced verbal or physical abuse from aides, mostly, she says, because she would not tolerate it. "I have an extremely sharp tongue and I can give as well as I can take. So if anybody does get abusive, they are immediately fired, at which point they are beaten with my tongue!"

She relies to a large extent on instinct when screening applicants. "You learn from experience. I can tell within the first time or two that they do me if they are going to be any good at all. Depending on how they move your arms and legs, or how careful they try to be, or how embarrassed they are. Bathing is a part of it—so how embarrassed are they going to be seeing a naked body?" She generally finds that people who are training to go into nursing are better prepared for the challenges of the job. "They know what they're getting themselves into."

What if an aide doesn't show up? "I have my own back-up. My brother is also disabled so my sister-in-law can take care of me. I have other friends that will come and take care of me, but not on a real regular basis. If I have an attendant that is sick and the other attendant can't make it, then, yes, there are people I can fall back on." She adds, "To train good people, you need to be very verbal. You need to tell them what you need. They are there to help you."

Chapter 36

Feeding Tubes

What is a feeding tube or gastrostomy?

This is a tube that goes into the stomach through the stomach wall. It enables a person to be given food and drink if they are unable to eat all they need by mouth by passing food directly into the stomach via the tube.

Why might I need one?

Some people with neuromuscular conditions find that they can only eat very slowly due to the shape of their mouths or weakness affecting their chewing and swallowing muscles. Mealtimes can take a long time and eating can become a chore that takes up too much of their day. It can also lead to arguments between children and their parents. Many families describe mealtimes as stressful rather than enjoyable. The use of a gastrostomy tube (g-tube) can reduce these problems and ensure that the person is always well fed without it taking too much time and effort.

Some people with neuromuscular conditions have specific problems with swallowing. Food or drink may go down the wrong way, so that instead of going down to the stomach, it goes down the wrong tube into the lungs. This is called aspiration. If this happens often, the

387

person is prone to chest infections and finds it hard to put on weight. A g-tube is a simple and very effective way of avoiding these problems as the food can go straight into the stomach.

How do they put in a g-tube?

This depends on each individual and the team will decide the best way depending on how old the person is, how good their breathing is, and what sort of tube they are going to have.

Fitting the g-tube usually requires a short surgical operation that lasts about 30 minutes and usually requires a general anesthetic. During the surgery, a hole (stoma) about the diameter of a small pencil is cut in the skin and into the stomach. The stomach is gently attached to the abdominal wall. The g-tube is then fitted into the stoma. It is a special tube held in place by a disc or water filled balloon that has a valve inside allowing food to go in, but nothing to come out.

The hole can be made in two ways. One way uses a tube with a light on the end (endoscope). This is put into the mouth and fed down the gullet (esophagus) into the stomach. The light shines through the skin showing the surgeon where to make the hole. The other way does not use an endoscope, instead a small opening is made in the abdomen so the surgeon can see to put the tube in the right place. This results in a small scar next to the g-tube. Both of these are classed as minor operations.

Will it hurt?

There will be slight discomfort after the operation, but this can be dealt with using ordinary painkillers. Once it has healed you will hardly feel it is in there.

What is inside my stomach?

The tube needs either a disc or water filled balloon to keep it in place. This is attached to the tube and sits just inside your stomach. The g-tube can be easily removed by a trained person.

What does a g-tube look like?

There are different types of g-tubes. The two main ones are a PEG (percutaneous endoscopic gastrostomy) or a button. The PEG is a length of tubing with a valve at the end. Sometime this is put in first until the stoma site has healed well. It can then be replaced with a button. A button looks very much like the small valve that is used to inflate a child's beach ball. It is made of clear, soft plastic and sits right next to the skin. A length of tubing is connected at feed times to pass food in.

Can I eat some normal food or drink?

It depends on why the tube was inserted. If it was because of slow mealtimes or poor weight gain only, it is okay to continue eating and drinking as usual. In this way your mealtimes can be as long or short as you wish as you know you can top up enough calories via the tube. Some people use the g-tube mainly as insurance so that the person can always be sure of getting food and drink even if they do not feel like eating by mouth.

However, if the reason for having the tube is that the person has swallowing problems and aspirates on food or drinks, it is important to have advice on what is safe to take by mouth. The team may recommend that only certain amounts or types of food or drink are safe by mouth. Sometimes it is the safest option to stop taking food by mouth altogether. This is not a forever decision and the swallowing will be monitored so alterations can be made as things change.

What food can I put in the g-tube?

It is recommended that a commercially available food is used. This will provide a balanced diet including all the essential vitamins and minerals needed. Some of these foods contain fiber so that regular bowel movement can be maintained even if you are unable to eat fruit, vegetables, and other high fiber foods. Specific advice with respect to the type of food and the quantity required will be provided by a dietitian.

It is advisable to stick to these foods to avoid the tube getting blocked. Liquid medicines can also be put down the tube.

What if I am thirsty?

In some cases it is okay to drink normally. If the team has said that you cannot drink by mouth then fluids added via the g-tube will reduce thirst.

Will I use the g-tube at normal mealtimes?

The g-tube can be used at anytime that suits the individual. The food can be given by attaching a syringe to the tube and pouring in the food or by using an electric pump. This way food can be given without the person or helper needing to do anything during the meal. Some people choose to stick to regular mealtimes while others use a pump and continuous food to allow feeding to be done mainly at night. Some families find that it is nice to sit down to eat together even though one of them is getting their main meal through the g-tube. The person can sometimes be having a light snack at the same time or just a drink. Each person's routine is individual and is decided on with all their needs in mind.

Will people know that I have a g-tube?

The tube is very small and is hidden by clothing, so nobody will notice it unless you show them. When a person is undressed, for example for swimming, the tube may be seen and people have come up with a variety of methods to help conceal it. For children, especially girls, a one-piece swimsuit is enough to cover the tube. For older children and adults, a slightly larger than usual adhesive bandage will disguise the tube quite well.

Can I have a bath and go swimming?

Yes. You can return to normal activities. In fact, swimming is encouraged. Just make sure the feeding port is closed.

Will it catch on my clothes and fall out?

This is unlikely as the tube is secured either by a little water filled balloon or a small plastic disc. As the hole is only a fraction of this size, the tube cannot pull out until the balloon is deflated, which is only normally done to renew the tube. If the tube ever does come out—don't panic. Place a clean dry towel over the stoma to absorb drainage. Contact nursing staff to help you or change the tube if you have been shown what to do. If in doubt, go to the emergency room. The stoma can close up quite rapidly so it is important to get it replaced relatively quickly to avoid another general anesthetic. It is worth having a plan of action before the event so you know what to do if it happens.

Will it be there forever?

This is a decision that the person and their medical team should make together depending on the person's weight, health, and eating abilities including swallowing. A g-tube can just be there as a backup and does not have to be used every day.

If a g-tube is removed, the hole in the stomach will heal over extremely rapidly—as fast as 45 minutes, so the fitting of the g-tube can be reversed very quickly with just a small scar remaining.

How much time will I need to spend taking care of my gastrostomy?

Usually g-tubes need very little maintenance. They need to be kept clean, but a bath or shower does most of this for you. They will need to be replaced if the balloon inside the stomach gets old and punctures—this can happen every 6 months or so, but varies with different types. The tube can be replaced by a professional helper, such as a home healthcare nurse, but many parents or caregivers quickly learn to do it themselves. Replacing a g-tube takes about a minute and is not as messy or unpleasant as many people fear.

Will it leak?

Most g-tubes leak a small amount, but this is easily taken care of with a little damp cotton wool. The fluid that leaks out from the stomach can irritate the skin around the tube so it is important to clean any leaks and to apply a little protective cream.

Normally, the degree of leakage is very small, and it will not be enough to mark or stain clothes. A tube that leaks more than a little probably needs replacing because the balloon is leaking or it is not the correct size. In either case, the doctor or nurse will give advice and help solve the problem.

What other complications might there be?

Occasionally, the skin around the stoma can become sore, or infected, or it can get a bit hardened. It is therefore important to look at the stoma when cleaning it, and ask your nurse or doctor to look at it if you are concerned.

Stomach ache, bloating, or diarrhea can occur if too much food is put into the stomach too quickly. This may happen if the stomach is not used to large volumes. A feeding regime should be discussed with a dietitian or nurse so that tolerance can be gradually built up.

What stops the food coming back out?

The g-tube has a one-way valve fitted to keep stomach contents in and air, etc., out.

Will I taste anything?

A person's taste-buds are on their tongue, so they will not taste food that is given via the g-tube, although some say they can taste food a bit if they burp after a feeding. Some people will still be able to take food and drink by mouth so will still taste food. One advantage of a g-tube is that unpleasant tasting medicines can be taken via the tube instead of by mouth, and in the case of children, this can ensure they always get a full dose of medicine on time.

What will it feel like while I am being fed?

Most people do not notice anything at all. If an attempt is made to feed a person too quickly, they will soon complain of feeling sick just as they would if they ate too much, too quickly. If this happens, then the rate of feeding is easily reduced or stopped.

Will I still feel hungry, and then full after a feed?

Yes. The stomach will still fill and empty in the normal way, giving the usual sensations of hunger and satisfaction.

Can I still be sick?

Yes, in most cases a g-tube will allow a person to vomit as they normally would, and this can be a useful reaction when they are unwell and their body needs to reject something from their stomach.

In some cases, the doctor may recommend an operation called a Nissen's fundoplication to tighten the muscles at the top of the stomach to make it harder for food to flow back up from the stomach into the food pipe (gastro esophageal reflux). This is usually done when there is a risk of refluxed food coming up and going into the lungs.

To determine if a person needs a fundoplication, the doctor may ask for a pH study which will show how prone they are to acids coming up from the stomach. A person with a fundoplication finds it harder to vomit, so if you have a gastrostomy, stomach contents can be emptied out through the gastrostomy when you feel sick. Occasionally, the placement of a gastrostomy can cause gastro-esophageal reflux, and some children may have to return to have a fundoplication later.

Chapter 37

Managing Toileting and Hydration

When you've gotta go, you've gotta go. But if you are away from home for business or pleasure, many people with neuromuscular diseases say you could also be out of luck when nature calls. From cupboard-sized airplane restrooms, to inaccessible public facilities, to challenges involved in transferring independently, active people who have limited mobility face numerous obstacles in emptying their bladders away from home.

In some cases, the issue is accessibility. Not all public bathrooms labeled handicapped are easily reached by people using wheelchairs, such as those located on a different floor in a building without an elevator. The stalls may be too small for a chair or too snug for self-transfer. Maybe the bathroom or stall doors are hung awkwardly, creating a barrier to a person in a wheelchair.

Then there are situations in which the bathroom is accessible, but it is impossible to transfer without assistance from a co-worker or a total stranger, neither of which is usually a desirable option.

Reprinted from "When You've Gotta Go, You've Gotta Go" by Jennie Borodko Stack, *QUEST*, Volume 8, Number 1, February 2001. Reprinted with permission from the Muscular Dystrophy Association, www.mdausa.org. © The Muscular Dystrophy Association. For additional information, call the Muscular Dystrophy Association National Headquarters toll-free at (800) 572-1717. To find an MDA office in your area, look in your local telephone book, or click on "Clinics and Services" on the MDA website. And "Dehydration," reprinted with permission from the Muscular Dystrophy Campaign, a United Kingdom charity focusing on all muscular dystrophies and allied disorders. © 2003 Muscular Dystrophy Campaign. All rights reserved. Additional information is available at www.muscular-dystrophy.org.uk.

As for airplane restrooms: Tiny and often inaccessible to begin with, those facilities are usually viewed by people with physical disabilities as more trouble than they are worth. And considering the consequences, that is saying a lot. Leaving home for a few hours or more typically requires tough choices, and can result in some unpleasant realities from holding it in until it hurts, to being dropped by unskilled attendants during a transfer. Choosing greater involvement in life also may require tradeoffs that limit independence in other ways, such as asking for transfer assistance when you would rather not. Other choices can be embarrassing (just wear adult diapers); painful (just use a catheter); and even unhealthy (just say no to water).

To help find practical solutions to this difficult problem, *Quest* interviewed product suppliers, health care practitioners, and several people with neuromuscular diseases. There is probably no single solution that will work for everyone, but these ideas may prove useful, either as presented or when adapted to individual situations.

Ask for the Help You Need

Occupational therapist Vicki Pollyea of Tampa, Florida, has Charcot-Marie-Tooth disease, which has weakened her extremities and caused her to use a wheelchair. She can transfer herself, but fatigues easily. Pollyea works as a writer and speaker on a part-time, freelance basis. When she leaves home on errands or personal matters, she frequently obtains needed restroom help from her husband.

"I don't hesitate to ask for assistance when I need it, but obviously I'd rather do these things independently," she says. "If all else fails and I can't get into the bathroom, I will go and lock the door to stop anyone else from coming in, and then have my husband come in and help me transfer." On those occasions when help is not available, Pollyea says she makes other choices. "I very often do lose a bit of privacy on some of these things, but you have to decide which is the easiest. Sometimes it's an energy-saving thing: There is a bathroom, but it would require going from your vehicle to your chair and getting in there. Maybe using a [portable] urinal in the vehicle with a blanket around the shoulders would save some energy."

Plan Ahead

Some people deal with the accessibility issue by choosing to wear special clothing, such as pants with open sides or seams, kept closed with Velcro. Corrections counselor Gail Ableman of Cheney, Washington, finds those unacceptable. Ableman has Friedreich's ataxia, which affects her balance. She uses a wheelchair and can stand briefly to transfer. At work, she helps place female prisoners in a work-release program, and the nature of her position requires that she convey a strong, professional image. "I can't let them know [my limitations]. I'm always telling them, 'Don't make me get out of this chair!' I think they wonder if I can," she chuckles.

To maintain an authoritative image, she chooses to wear regular work clothing, which makes it more time-consuming and difficult to urinate. Ableman admits, "I've had to sit and ache many, many times. I guess it might be a pride thing. There are times where I think, 'I can't do this anymore,' but I don't want to use special clothing." To minimize her need to urinate away from home, she reduces caffeine and other fluid intake and uses the bathroom before leaving the house "whether I have to or not."

Extreme Measures

Strategies that work well for the semi-ambulatory may be of little use to those with more extensive muscle involvement. While an internal catheter or adult diapers are not very satisfactory solutions, those are two of the most common suggestions, notably from people who are not using them. Medical supply companies offer options that include a variation on an internal catheter. It features the usual tubing attached to a plastic collection bag, but the tip inserted into the urethra is pre-lubricated, which is said to be easier to insert and more comfortable to wear. However, many women with neuromuscular diseases say they prefer not to run the risk of infection or experience the discomfort that often results. Also, since self-catheterization requires a certain amount of flexibility and fine motor skill, those with limited upper-body mobility may require assistance with the procedure.

A Man's World

"For a guy who's got sensation, it's probably the last place a guy would go," says Jerry Ferro of internal catheterization. With a master's degree in rehabilitation counseling, Ferro runs a private counseling practice and leads a general support group for the Orlando, Florida, MDA chapter. Men, for obvious anatomical reasons, have a somewhat easier time of it than women when the bladder needs to be emptied away from home.

Ferro has SMA and uses a power wheelchair; he also uses a more comfortable urinary-collection device called an external or condom catheter. "Men that I know who can't go to the bathroom themselves find that this is very helpful," he says.

External collectors are available through medical suppliers and, unlike internal catheters, do not require a doctor's prescription. Mike Lee of DS Medical says, "Basically, they're a condom with a hole in the end of it attached to a tube that runs to a leg bag concealed under the pants. It's completely concealed, so you could theoretically go for a long period of time before you drain the leg bag."

However, during extended periods away from a toilet, even a large leg bag can fill up. If there is no acceptable place to empty the leg bag, a typical solution would be to use a portable plastic urinal as a temporary receptacle. But for those who do not have room to conceal the device, a little creativity makes a big difference. "In public, we don't use a standard urinal because it's so obvious. We've found that with the Big Gulp-size cups [from convenience stores], you can pretty well hide them and nobody knows what they're for," says Ferro. In a private place such as a vehicle, he empties the leg bag into the cup, and then leaves the cup hidden until he can dispose of it in a bathroom.

A Female What?

For women who have ruled out catheterization and absorption products, there are two kinds of urinary devices that might help. Those with some upper-body strength or who have trusted assistants might be able to use female urinals modified from the more familiar styles used by men. They are designed to fit feminine anatomy and can be sterilized and reused. Most are priced under $15, and can be used with or without assistance, as long as the user can be positioned at the edge of a chair, with the device held in place as it fills.

"It's designed ergonomically so that when it is pressed up against the perineal area it seals. As long they have minimal control they can use it," says Linda Asta, inventor of the Feminal, a urinal designed for women. "It holds 1,000 cubic centimeters [about a quart] and it's also designed for women who have limited hand mobility as well. We do have patients who are bedridden. They can hold it themselves or a caregiver can hold it for them."

Another type of aid is collect-and-deflect items that either shunt urine directly into the toilet or send it to a tube that empties into the commode or a container. The abilities they require range from having a trusted assistant help guide the device into position to being able to stand briefly. For example, OnTheGo is a soft, reusable plastic cup connected to tubing. "If you're able to hold onto it and fit it snugly against the body, it does create a seal so that there is no spillage when one is urinating. You would simply have to be able to sit on a chair and have the tube hanging over the chair," says Kathleen Farrell, inventor of OnTheGo.

For those who can stand, but who experience difficulty with the up-down movement of sitting and rising, a disposable paper trough called a Whizzy might help. Created by Janis Wagner, who is affected by muscular rheumatism, the sturdy, nonflushable product is designed for urinating from a standing position. To use it, women need to be able to hold the lightweight funnel in place and to stand long enough to void. Users face the toilet in a standing position.

"I designed it specifically so that if someone does not have grip strength, she can literally just let it rest on her fingers. I made it so that you don't have to move your legs at all. You can keep them in a natural position. There is no bending of any sort that's necessary," says Wagner.

Daily Living Devices

Many people with neuromuscular disease find it useful to combine medical equipment with strategies and independent-living aids. For those with some arm strength, a sling-type device can be positioned under one leg, then used to lift it out of the way before placing a urinary collector. Other adaptive tools include a pair of plastic-coated tongs or a longer-handled reach extender to add range of motion for wiping.

To leave hands free to aid in transfer and keep clothing accessible, some use a large set of clips connected by a cord similar to the ones used to keep a bag of potato chips closed. One clip attaches to the top of the pants, while the other fastens to the shirt.

Be Healthy, Don't Dehydrate

While dealing with the need to urinate away from home may require careful timing of fluids and selection of foods, it is essential to make up for liquid loss as soon as possible. Going without fluids for eight or more hours a day is dangerous.

"Dehydration leads to dry mouth, cramps, and physical discomfort because your electrolyte balance gets thrown off. Then the kidneys are not getting flushed, so that the medications you are taking are not being flushed properly," says Maura Del Bene, a registered nurse who is clinical administrator of the Division of Neuromuscular Disease at Columbia University in New York. "Women are at risk for urinary tract infections for holding their urine for a very long period of time."

Other possible risks of dehydration extend to cancer of the bladder, which is believed to arise from irritation of the bladder lining triggered by a buildup of chemicals. In a recent study by Harvard University of nearly 48,000 men, those who consumed 88 ounces of liquid per day had half the incidence of bladder cancer of that reported by men who drank 40 ounces per day or less. The conclusion was that drinking plenty of fluids may help prevent the disease by diluting the urine, said the researchers.

It is recommended that average-sized adults (a 140-pound woman or 175-pound man) consume eight to twelve 8-ounce glasses of non-caffeinated liquid daily. Do not wait until you feel thirsty; by then, dehydration has already begun. Healthy urine output is about 30 ounces, or nearly a quart, a day. Another way to tell if you are getting enough water is by checking the color of the urine. Liquid intake is adequate when the urine is pale yellow in color, but when the body is deprived of needed fluid, the output decreases and the urine turns much darker.

Dehydration

Some disabled youngsters are prone to dehydration because they restrict their drinking. In this section, the reasons behind this are reviewed and ways to encourage children to keep up their fluid intake are suggested.

As they get older, children assume more independence; they begin to dress, wash, and feed themselves. A potty trained toddler learns to get to the bathroom and to use the toilet, but this natural progression can be more complicated for a child whose muscles are weak. Running to the bathroom might have been easy as a 3-year-old boy with Duchenne MD, but by 4 or 5 the child may be getting slower and start to have the occasional accident on the way. This can be embarrassing for the child, especially in the public forum of a nursery or primary school.

The problems that a youngster has in getting to the toilet do not end at school or in the nursery. Car journeys, holidays, even playtime with friends can be daunting if an accessible toilet is not available. If going to the restroom causes a fuss on family outings, is an embarrassment in front of friends, and a chore for caregivers, the child reasons that it would be easier to avoid having to go to the toilet at all in these situations—and the way to do that would be to cut down on drinking.

A teenager has even stronger reasons for not drinking: parties, pubs, school, and college (especially if the person is in a mainstream environment surrounded by able-bodied friends) all become hazardous when this private function becomes more like a public performance.

Why Is It Important to Keep Up Fluid Intake?

About 75% of our body consists of water; it has a vital role to play in keeping our bodies functioning properly. If our water content drops, several things can happen:

- **Constipation.** Water is used by the body to soften feces, and therefore helps to keep the bowel movements regular. With insufficient water, the feces become hard and impacted in the colon causing stomach pain, distension, and constipation. Although this can be treated with laxatives, these do not solve the cause of the constipation. Severe cases can mean that a child has to go to the hospital for treatment (usually an intervenous drip to rehydrate the body, and an enema to relieve pain).

- **Toxins.** The water we drink is processed by the kidneys and expelled by the body along with various toxins, as urine. If we do not flush the toxins away, they remain in our body.

- **Kidney damage.** It is possible that kidney damage might occur in the long run due to chronic dehydration. This problem is currently being investigated.

- **Hypotension and postural symptoms.** These result from the reduced volume of blood in the body because of its lower water content. They could lead to tiredness, irritation, and dizziness, especially on standing up. Young people who use wheelchairs could also experience dizziness when transferring from a bed to the chair, or when using a standing frame.

- **Kidney stones.** Chronic dehydration is known to be a contributory factor in kidney stone formation in susceptible individuals, particularly in hot climates. It causes severe recurrent stomach pains and impairment of the kidney function due to repeated infection and obstruction.

- **Aches and pains, sunken eyes, and dry skin.** All are physical manifestations of dehydration.

How Can You Encourage a Child or Teenager to Drink?

1. **Start from a very early age.** Try to make it as easy as possible for the child to get to a toilet. If the bathroom at home is upstairs, a young child could use the potty downstairs. The child may need reassurance about this, and will need to know that he or she is not naughty, or abnormal, even if the occasional accident still happens. If a child starts to wet the bed, it is worth considering whether this could be due to the physical problems of getting out of bed and to a toilet—rather than assuming that the bedwetting has a purely psychological basis.

2. **Check out the facilities at the nursery or school.** Are the toilets accessible?

3. **Explain to teachers and caregivers** why it is important that the child needs to keep up a normal fluid intake, and why they might be reluctant to go to the toilet unless the process is made as uncomplicated as possible. Is the child comfortable with their caregiver? If a child does not like, or is embarrassed with a caregiver, then they will keep toilet visits to a minimum.

   - Letting a child keep a drinking bottle close at hand during the day can be a good idea.

   - Try to check on toilet facilities before you embark on a journey.

4. **Aids and equipment.** There are many products on the market which can make toileting simpler:

   - Portable urinals for males and non-spill adaptors can be obtained as soon as getting to a toilet is difficult, or for use in a car. There is also a wide choice of urinals for females.

   - If sitting on the toilet is proving uncomfortable or balancing on it is difficult, a toilet chair superimposed over the pan may be the solution. It is essential to assess the chair with an occupational therapist to ensure that it can be used safely and provides correct support. The choice of chair will depend on whether it is also to be used in the shower or bath.

- A variety of toilet trainer seats or covers are available to give comfort and security to small children who find the toilet opening too large.

If a person cannot press against the ground with their feet when sitting on the toilet, it makes the process more difficult, especially when the muscles are weaker than normal. Footplates can be used here.

Where to Find Urinary Devices

DS Medica
2105 Newpoint Place, Suite 600
Lawrenceville, GA 30043-5561
Toll-Free: 800-633-1565
Phone: 770-407-4400
Fax: 888-633-1565
Website: http://www.medshipdirect.com
E-mail: customerservice@medshipdirect.com

Internal and external catheters for males and females. Components such as catheter condoms, leg bags.

A-Plus Medical
International Sani-fern, Inc.
P.O. Box 4117
Downey, CA 90241
Toll-Free: 800-542-5580
Phone: 562-928-3435
Fax: 562-862-4373
Website: http://www.freshette.com

The Freshette, a female urine-collection device.

New Angle Products
Box 25641
Chicago, IL 60625
Phone: 773-478-6779
Website: http://www.whizzy4you.com
E-mail: whizzy4you@aol.com

The Whizzy, a disposable paper trough.

R.D. Equipment
230 Percival Drive
West Barnstable, MA 02668
Phone/Fax: 508-362-7498
Website: http://www.rdequipment.com
E-mail: info@rdequipment.com

Electric Leg Bag Emptier, a device for draining leg bags.

Mobility Transfer Systems
P.O. Box 253
Medford, MA 02155
Toll-Free: 888-854-4687
Website: http://www.bedhandle.com
E-mail: info@mtsmedequip.com

SpillProof URSEC male urinal

OnTheGo
316 21st Avenue N.E.
St. Petersburg, FL 33704
Phone: 727-533-9184
Website: http://www.womenstandtogo.com

OnTheGo, a soft plastic cup and tube.

Rochester Medical Corporation
One Rochester Medical Drive
Stewartville, MN 55976-1647
Toll-Free: 800-615-2364
Phone: 507-533-9600
Fax: 507-533-9740
Website: http://www.rocm.com
E-mail: info@rocm.com

Internal and external catheters for men and women. Supplies and components such as tubing, collection bags and condoms for catheters.

Part Seven

Parenting Children
with Muscular Dystrophy

Chapter 38

You Are Not Alone: Dealing with a Muscular Dystrophy Diagnosis

When parents learn that their child has a disability or a chronic illness, they begin a journey that takes them into a life that is often filled with strong emotion, difficult choices, interactions with many different professionals and specialists, and an ongoing need for information and services. Initially, parents may feel isolated and alone, and do not know where to begin their search for information, assistance, understanding, and support.

For Parents When They Learn Their Child Has a Disability

If you have recently learned that your child is developmentally delayed or has a disability (which may or may not be completely defined), this message may be for you. It is written from the personal perspective of a parent who has shared this experience and all that goes with it.

When parents learn about any difficulty or problem in their child's development, this information comes as a tremendous blow. The day my child was diagnosed as having a disability, I was devastated — and so confused that I recall little else about those first days other than the heartbreak. Another parent described this event as a "black sack" being pulled down over her head, blocking her ability to hear,

"You Are Not Alone," by Patricia McGill Smith, *News Digest*, ND20, 3rd Edition, National Dissemination Center for Children with Disabilities (NICHCY), 2003.

see, and think in normal ways. Another parent described the trauma as "having a knife stuck" in her heart. Perhaps these descriptions seem a bit dramatic, yet it has been my experience that they may not sufficiently describe the many emotions that flood parents' minds and hearts when they receive any bad news about their child. Many things can be done to help yourself through this period of trauma. That is what this chapter is all about. In order to talk about some of the good things that can happen to alleviate the anxiety, let us first take a look at some of the reactions that occur.

Common Reactions

On learning that their child may have a disability, most parents react in ways that have been shared by all parents before them who have also been faced with this disappointment and this enormous challenge. One of the first reactions is denial—"This cannot be happening to me, to my child, to our family." Denial rapidly merges with anger, which may be directed toward the medical personnel who were involved in providing the information about the child's problem. Anger can also color communication between husband and wife or with grandparents or significant others in the family. Early on, it seems that the anger is so intense that it touches almost anyone, because it is triggered by the feelings of grief and inexplicable loss that one does not know how to explain or deal with.

Fear is another immediate response. People often fear the unknown more than they fear the known. Having the complete diagnosis and some knowledge of the child's future prospects can be easier than uncertainty. In either case, however, fear of the future is a common emotion: "What is going to happen to this child when he is five years old, when he is twelve, when he is twenty-one? What is going to happen to this child when I am gone?" Then other questions arise: "Will he ever learn? Will he ever go to college? Will he or she have the capability of loving and living and laughing and doing all the things that we had planned?"

Other unknowns also inspire fear. Parents fear that the child's condition will be the very worst it possibly could be. Over the years, I have spoken with so many parents who said that their first thoughts were totally bleak. One expects the worst. Memories return of persons with disabilities one has known. Sometimes there is guilt over some slight committed years before toward a person with a disability. There is also fear of society's rejection, fears about how brothers and sisters will be affected, questions as to whether there will be any more brothers or sisters in this family, and concerns about whether the husband or wife will love this child. These fears can almost immobilize some parents.

Then there is guilt—guilt and concern about whether the parents themselves have caused the problem: "Did I do something to cause this? Am I being punished for something I have done? Did I take care of myself when I was pregnant? Did my wife take good enough care of herself when she was pregnant?" For myself, I remember thinking that surely my daughter had slipped from the bed when she was very young and hit her head, or that perhaps one of her brothers or sisters had inadvertently let her drop and did not tell me. Much self-reproach and remorse can stem from questioning the causes of the disability.

Guilt feelings may also be manifested in spiritual and religious interpretations of blame and punishment. When they cry, "Why me?" or "Why my child?" many parents are also saying, "Why has God done this to me?" How often have we raised our eyes to heaven and asked: "What did I ever do to deserve this?" One young mother said, "I feel so guilty because all my life I had never had a hardship and now God has decided to give me a hardship."

Confusion also marks this traumatic period. As a result of not fully understanding what is happening and what will happen, confusion reveals itself in sleeplessness, inability to make decisions, and mental overload. In the midst of such trauma, information can seem garbled and distorted. You hear new words that you never heard before, terms that describe something that you cannot understand. You want to find out what it is all about, yet it seems that you cannot make sense of all the information you are receiving. Often parents are just not on the same wavelength as the person who is trying to communicate with them about their child's disability.

Powerlessness to change what is happening is very difficult to accept. You cannot change the fact that your child has a disability, yet parents want to feel competent and capable of handling their own life situations. It is extremely hard to be forced to rely on the judgments, opinions, and recommendations of others. Compounding the problem is that these others are often strangers with whom no bond of trust has yet been established.

Disappointment that a child is not perfect poses a threat to many parents' egos and a challenge to their value system. This jolt to previous expectations can create reluctance to accept one's child as a valuable, developing person.

Rejection is another reaction that parents experience. Rejection can be directed toward the child, toward the medical personnel, or toward other family members. One of the more serious forms of rejection, and not that uncommon, is a "death wish" for the child—a feeling that many parents report at their deepest points of depression.

During this period of time when so many different feelings can flood the mind and heart, there is no way to measure how intensely a parent may experience this constellation of emotions. Not all parents go through these stages, but it is important for parents to identify with all of the potentially troublesome feelings that can arise, so that they will know that they are not alone. There are many constructive actions that you can take immediately, and there are many sources of help, communication, and reassurance.

Seek the Assistance of Another Parent

There was a parent who helped me. Twenty-two hours after my own child's diagnosis, he made a statement that I have never forgotten: "You may not realize it today, but there may come a time in your life when you will find that having a daughter with a disability is a blessing." I can remember being puzzled by these words, which were nonetheless an invaluable gift that lit the first light of hope for me. This parent spoke of hope for the future. He assured me that there would be programs, there would be progress, and there would be help of many kinds and from many sources. And he was the father of a boy with mental retardation.

My first recommendation is to try to find another parent of a child with a disability, preferably one who has chosen to be a parent helper, and seek his or her assistance. All over the United States and over the world, there are Parent to Parent Programs. The National Dissemination Center for Children with Disabilities (NICHCY) has listings of parent groups that will reach out and help you. If you cannot find your local parent organization, write to NICHCY to get that local information.

Talk with Your Mate, Family, and Significant Others

Over the years, I have discovered that many parents do not communicate their feelings regarding the problems their children have. One spouse is often concerned about not being a source of strength for the other mate. The more couples can communicate at difficult times like these, the greater their collective strength. Understand that you each approach your roles as parents differently. How you will feel and respond to this new challenge may not the same. Try to explain to each other how you feel; try to understand when you do not see things the same way.

If there are other children, talk with them, too. Be aware of their needs. If you are not emotionally capable of talking with your children or seeing to their emotional needs at this time, identify others within your family structure who can establish a special communicative bond with them. Talk with significant others in your life—your best friend, your own parents. For many people, the temptation to close up emotionally is great at this point, but it can be so beneficial to have reliable friends and relatives who can help to carry the emotional burden.

Rely on Positive Sources in Your Life

One positive source of strength and wisdom might be your minister, priest, or rabbi. Another may be a good friend or a counselor. Go to those who have been a strength before in your life. Find the new sources that you need now.

A very fine counselor once gave me a recipe for living through a crisis: "Each morning, when you arise, recognize your powerlessness over the situation at hand, turn this problem over to God, as you understand Him, and begin your day."

Whenever your feelings are painful, you must reach out and contact someone. Call, write, or get into your car and contact a real person who will talk with you and share that pain. Pain divided is not nearly so hard to bear as is pain in isolation. Sometimes professional counseling is warranted; if you feel that this might help you; do not be reluctant to seek this avenue of assistance.

Take One Day at a Time

Fears of the future can immobilize one. Living with the reality of the day which is at hand is made more manageable if we throw out the *what ifs* of the future. Even though it may not seem possible, good things will continue to happen each day. Worrying about the future will only deplete your limited resources. You have enough to focus on; get through each day, one step at a time.

Learn the Terminology

When you are introduced to new terminology, you should not be hesitant to ask what it means. Whenever someone uses a word that you do not understand, stop the conversation for a minute and ask the person to explain the word. Go to those who have been a strength before in your life. Find the new sources that you need now.

Seek Information

Some parents seek virtually tons of information; others are not so persistent. The important thing is that you request accurate information. Do not be afraid to ask questions, because asking questions will be your first step in beginning to understand more about your child.

Learning how to formulate questions is an art that will make life a lot easier for you in the future. A good method is to write down your questions before entering appointments or meetings, and to write down further questions as you think of them during the meeting. Get written copies of all documentation from physicians, teachers, and therapists regarding your child. It is a good idea to buy a three-ring notebook in which to save all information that is given to you. In the future, there will be many uses for information that you have recorded and filed; keep it in a safe place. Again, remember always to ask for copies of evaluations, diagnostic reports, and progress reports. If you are not a naturally organized person, just get a box and throw all the paperwork in it. Then when you really need it, it will be there.

Do Not Be Intimidated

Many parents feel inadequate in the presence of people from the medical or educational professions because of their credentials, and sometimes, because of their professional manner. Do not be intimidated by the educational backgrounds of these and other personnel who may be involved in treating or helping your child. You do not have to apologize for wanting to know what is occurring. Do not be concerned that you are being a bother or are asking too many questions. Remember, this is your child, and the situation has a profound effect on your life and on your child's future. Therefore, it is important that you learn as much as you can about your situation.

Do Not Be Afraid to Show Emotion

So many parents, especially dads, repress their emotions because they believe it to be a sign of weakness to let people know how they are feeling. The strongest fathers of children with disabilities whom I know are not afraid to show their emotions. They understand that revealing feelings does not diminish one's strength.

Learn to Deal with Natural Feelings of Bitterness and Anger

Feelings of bitterness and anger are inevitable when you realize that you must revise the hopes and dreams you originally had for your child. It is very valuable to recognize your anger and to learn to let go of it. You may need outside help to do this. It may not feel like it, but life will get better and the day will come when you will feel positive again. By acknowledging and working through your negative feelings, you will be better equipped to meet new challenges, and bitterness and anger will no longer drain your energies and initiative.

Maintain a Positive Outlook

A positive attitude will be one of your genuinely valuable tools for dealing with problems. There is, truly, always a positive side to whatever is occurring. For example, when my child was found to have a disability, one of the other things pointed out to me was that she was a very healthy child. She still is. The fact that she has had no physical impairments has been a great blessing over the years; she has been the healthiest child I have ever raised. Focusing on the positives diminishes the negatives and makes life easier to deal with. Do not be afraid to ask questions, because asking questions will be your first step in beginning to understand more about your child.

Keep in Touch with Reality

To stay in touch with reality is to accept life the way it is. To stay in touch with reality is also to recognize that there are some things that we can change and other things that we cannot change. The task for all of us is learning which things we can change and then set about doing that.

Remember That Time Is on Your Side

Time heals many wounds. This does not mean that living with and raising a child who has problems will be easy, but it is fair to say that as time passes a great deal can be done to alleviate the problem. Therefore, time does help.

Find Programs for Your Child

Even for those living in isolated areas of the country, assistance is available to help you with whatever problems you are having. NICHCY's State Resource Sheets list contact persons who can help you get started in gaining the information and assistance you need. While finding programs for your child with a disability, keep in mind that programs are also available for the rest of your family.

Take Care of Yourself

In times of stress, each person reacts in his or her own way. A few universal recommendations may help: Get sufficient rest; eat as well as you can; take time for yourself; and reach out to others for emotional support.

Avoid Pity

Self-pity, the experience of pity from others or pity for your child is actually disabling. Pity is not what is needed. Empathy, which is the ability to feel with another person, is the attitude to be encouraged.

Decide How to Deal with Others

During this period, you may feel saddened by or angry about the way people are reacting to you or your child. Many people's reactions to serious problems are caused by a lack of understanding, simply not knowing what to say, or fear of the unknown. Understand that many people do not know how to behave when they see a child with differences, and they may react inappropriately. Think about and decide how you want to deal with stares or questions. Try not to use too much energy being concerned about people who are not able to respond in ways you might prefer.

Keep Daily Routines as Normal as Possible

My mother once told me, "When a problem arises and you don't know what to do, then you do whatever it was that you were going to do anyway." Practicing this habit seems to produce some normalcy and consistency when life becomes hectic.

Remember That This Is Your Child

This person is your child, first and foremost. Granted, your child's development may be different from that of other children, but this does not make your child less valuable, less human, less important, or in less need of your love and parenting. Love and enjoy your child. The child comes first; the disability comes second. If you can relax and take the positive steps just outlined, one at a time, you will do the best you can, your child will benefit, and you can look forward to the future with hope.

Recognize That You Are Not Alone

The feeling of isolation at the time of diagnosis is almost universal among parents. In this chapter, there are many recommendations to help you handle feelings of separateness and isolation. It helps to know that these feelings have been experienced by many others, that understanding and constructive help are available to you and your child, and that you are not alone.

Additional Information

National Dissemination Center for Children with Disabilities (also known as NICHCY)
P.O. Box 1492
Washington, DC 20013
Toll-Free: 800-695-0285 (V/TTY)
Fax: 202-884-8441
Website: http://www.nichcy.org
E-mail: nichcy@aed.org

Chapter 39

Discussing Muscular Dystrophy with Family and Friends

This information relates particularly to Duchenne muscular dystrophy and discussions involving the affected child, siblings, friends, and interested/responsible adults.

Initial Reactions

When parents find that a child has a severe illness, they experience a sense of shock. When the illness is severe, prolonged, debilitating, and associated with a restricted life expectancy as with muscular dystrophy, the shock is most likely to be severe.

Shock reactions include a sense of unreality, numbness, disbelief, denial, and grief. These become associated quite rapidly with feelings of guilt, anger, frustration, depression, rapid mood swings, intense searching for a cause or cure, and heightened feelings of protectiveness towards the child. There may also be feelings of hopelessness and total helplessness. Questioning of the purpose of life and the value of going on living for both parent and child are common. From feelings of desolation and destructiveness, parents search for hope. Goals for the future and optimism about possible opportunities can provide bases for structuring current living. Gradually, out of these phases, parents evolve a more or less effective style of coping which suits them and their situation.

Learning to Cope

A major issue for parents, and a responsibility with which they must learn to cope, is what and how to tell other people including the child. In part this depends on the severity of the illness and the age of the child at the time of diagnosis. If the child is obviously unwell and has a restricted or decreasing level of physical functioning at the time of diagnosis, then he/she requires clear direct responses to their questions about what is wrong with them. In some instances these may be appropriately provided by the medical personnel concerned. However, parents need to discuss the sort of information which medical personnel would give. Usually the initial discussion is best between parent and child, followed by joint discussion with doctors and others. Because muscular dystrophy is uncommon, it should not be assumed that medical personnel could engage in such discussion without an opportunity for thought and preparation. However, a caring and thoughtful doctor with an approachable manner is likely to be more helpful than one specialist who is remote and abrupt however well informed.

Often diagnosis occurs at a time when the child is physically weak, but has not yet lost obvious functioning. Then, as always, explanations given will be affected by the child's age and stage of thinking.

Guidelines for Discussion

Professionals associated with work with children and families affected by muscular dystrophy (MD) disease recommend the following guidelines for discussion.

Listen carefully to the child's questions. If necessary, ask further questions in order to respond clearly to what is being asked, and do not respond to what is not being asked. In general, it is best to create a situation in which the child feels free to ask what they need or want to know, rather than giving them information based on what you think they should ask or should know.

There are no right responses. Questions from children will vary substantially depending on their age, ability, and emotional state. Responses should be directed by your knowledge of the individual child and the questions asked.

In the pre-school years most children with MD will need to understand that their muscles are not as strong as those of other children,

416

and that while they can and should try hard, there are some things that they may find more difficult to do than some other children. When they ask why they have muscle weakness, it may be appropriate to say that the weakness is called muscular dystrophy. However, it may be appropriate especially initially to explain the muscle strength on the basis of individual differences, i.e., people are different, some are black, some are white, some are well, some are ill, some are strong, some are not so strong, etc.

Using the words muscular dystrophy means that the child needs to be told something about the condition, or else he/she is likely to find out from others. If muscular dystrophy is present in other family members, explanations about the difference between this child and others will be appropriate.

Physical skills and strength are very important to children at this age. They are becoming more independent emotionally, and often measure their relations with other children in terms of their ability to keep up. The most physically able children often are group leaders at this stage. It is very important to allow the children the opportunity to keep trying, not too be too protective or negative.

In the pre-school or early primary years many children will become aware that they cannot do some things as easily as they could before. When they talk about this it should be confirmed, and the sorts of practical difficulties they are having must be discussed. This may lead to suggestions about other ways to do things to achieve what they want. Discussion about feeling frustrated and angry is likely to be appropriate at this stage. Helping the child to label their emotional reactions, to understand them, and then to find ways to manage them, is a major test for all parents and children in this age bracket.

There is a need for a balance at all stages between practical realism and acceptance of what is happening, understanding and sharing the negative emotional reactions, and still allowing everyone space for optimism, hope, and encouragement. This can be built by encouraging the child to express emotional reactions, but also to build patience and perseverance with physical activities. Valuing these temperamental characteristics in these children is particularly important. At the same time, helping them to develop skills in sedentary activities and leisure pursuits from early in their lives is realistic forward planning, which enables them to build and maintain competence for as long as possible. These provide long term areas of self reliance, and social and recreational outlets.

Feelings of the child's physical vulnerability, as well as the parents' emotional vulnerability can lead to protectiveness towards both. The parents may feel unable to discuss some topics or aspects of a topic with the child or siblings. If this is the case, they should seek counseling to help them build their ability to handle such situations.

Feelings of protectiveness towards the child may be a natural consequence of concern about the extreme effects of possible injury, but it adds to the child's burden. The child needs to be as independent as possible, and able to engage in activities for as long as possible. Parents need to help children to determine acceptable and unacceptable risks. Excessive or unnecessary restrictions on activities will be likely to produce feelings of frustration, anger, and depression in the child.

However, very young children do not know or want to be told of restrictions or risks. Parents may find themselves being seen as excessively protective by the child and possibly other adults, as they attempt to defend them against falls, etc.

Mortality

The two key issues which children with MD need to understand gradually are the reductions in physical functioning with age and the probable restricted life span.

Concepts of death alter throughout childhood. Between the ages of 10–13, children begin to develop something like an adult concept of death. Awareness of death is dependent on experiences and on discussions with other people. Even though television represents evidence of death daily, many children do not experience death at close quarters through awareness of the death of relatives or friends. The death of animals or pets can be a helpful time to foster discussion of this topic which adults may otherwise tend to avoid.

Children aged 2–5 years become aware of death and tend to have a magical notion of it as a temporary state which involves coming alive again. It is seen somewhat like sleeping and waking. Younger school age children tend to regard death as more permanent, but as something which happens to others, especially the elderly, rather than themselves.

Response to questions about mortality and MD are most likely to be required by school age children. In response to a question about MD and death, a parent may find a reply along the following lines helpful. "Everyone dies. People who had MD in the past used to live very short lives, but that is not so much the case now. Your life is likely to be shorter than some others, but we do not know how much shorter. People with MD now live into their thirties. Medical science is finding more ways to prevent the restrictions that affect people with MD, and there are likely to be more."

Acknowledgment of distress and sadness as appropriate reactions to such news is important. Discussions might then gradually move to accidental death and the advantage of knowing that your life span may be short in enabling planning to occur. Parents should react naturally when telling a child of these matters. Parents should feel free to express some sadness and to weep. While they may hide from the child the full burden of their own distress, they should not hide it completely. Sharing tears and cuddles provides comfort for both to pursue the discussion further later.

- If a child is suddenly very ill and death is imminent, then little discussion is usually required. Confirmation of what is happening is mostly all that is required. Children may hesitate to discuss topics if they feel that adults cannot cope with the discussion or will be too upset. They usually show relief when discussion is out in the open.

Others

It is important to point out to other people that children with MD have a right to learn about MD at their own pace without others forcing the realization on them. If parents are following the principles outlined, they will need to consider restricting the number of people that they tell about the child's condition in order to give the child time to find out gradually. This does mean that a number of responsible adults will learn of the condition as the child does. It will be necessary to explain to each person being told who they can discuss the matter with and why few people know. Otherwise, they are likely to discreetly go against parent's wishes in order to unburden themselves, and out of feelings that the parents are being excessively secretive.

As adults are told of the condition, they will need also to be briefly informed about the parent's plans for helping the child to realize the nature of the condition. They have to be asked specifically not to discuss the subject with others or the child until the parents indicate it is appropriate to do so. This may necessitate the parents holding a discussion with some or all of the child's teachers to outline what is occurring and what judgment is appropriate. It will be helpful to have a school nurse or the child's doctor present at such a discussion.

Discussion with older siblings may be necessary before the child with MD is ready to hear the explanations. If this is the case, it is likely to involve explanations along the lines described earlier with the provision that they will need to keep their understanding secret between them and the parents until the younger child is ready to understand. This can prove very difficult to achieve as the older child is likely to be very upset and protective towards the sibling. Practical explanations to siblings may be all that is appropriate or practical until the child with MD is ready to understand.

Conclusion

Resilience, a positive attitude, and optimism are characteristics of childhood which require particular nurturing in these circumstances. After the initial shock, parents should assert themselves to take an active informed role in dealing with the emotional as well as the physical of this illness. Recognition of this fact is a major step along the way.

Chapter 40

Daily Life with Muscular Dystrophy

General Care Guidelines

Bones

When bones are not subjected to the normal stresses of everyday living (such as occurs during walking, running, and jumping), they lose calcium and become soft or brittle. Soft bones fracture more easily than normal bones. This is not often a problem until well into the wheelchair phase when accidents, such as falling from the chair or during transfers to or from the chair, may cause a fracture. Sometimes it is not very obvious that a fracture has occurred until an x-ray is taken because of persisting pain or increasing swelling.

If most of the weight of the body is put onto one buttock for long periods while sitting in a wheelchair, there may be discomfort in that area or even sciatica (pain down the back of the leg) if there is pressure on the sciatic nerve.

Bowel Management

Good diet and a regular bowel routine are essential, and these habits can be established early in a child's life. It is important that the person with muscular dystrophy avoids becoming constipated, particularly as his ability to move around decreases. Constipation may lead to abdominal discomfort and pain, and may also result in what appears to be diarrhea. This paradoxically occurs when liquid bowel material flows around the accumulated hard fecal material.

If constipation does become a problem, regular enemas or bowel washouts may be required. If a boy attends a school for the physically disabled, it is usually possible to arrange for these treatments to be given at school. Usually, an oral medication is also started. When the bowel is emptied the enemas can be stopped and control maintained with the oral medication.

Sleeping

During sleep most people toss and turn without realizing that they are doing it. When weakness is moderate to severe, it is not possible for boys with Duchenne muscular dystrophy to turn or move about much to make themselves comfortable. Parents often have to help the boys move or turn so that they can get back to sleep. This is difficult for parents as they too need to have good sleep. Medical attendants or therapists will be able to offer advice about various mattresses that can sometimes help.

It has been the experience of many parents that water beds significantly assist the comfort levels of children affected by MD. In many instances the number of night turns has been reduced from 6–8 times per night down to 1–2 per night. It should be noted that bladder type water beds have been found to be generally not suitable. The preferred type being the waveless, baffled bladder which offers the highest degree of comfort and stability.

Dietary Advice

As weakness increases and mobility decreases, particularly when a person is limited to a wheelchair, energy requirements are less, and less food is required. Therefore, it is important to monitor food intake. The problems caused by excessive weight gain cannot be over emphasized. Not only is obesity bad for the health of the child, it also increases difficulties for caregivers who are required to assist with everyday activities such as dressing, bathing, and toileting.

Dietitians are able to advise on the level of food intake required and on the appropriate balance of the various components of the diet. Good dietary advice plays an important role for the older person with

Duchenne muscular dystrophy, but the basis for good care lies in the appropriate attitude of parents to diet in the early stages of the disease.

Specific Issues of Daily Life

Living with a Duchenne muscular dystrophy (DMD) diagnosis in your family will likely make daily life more difficult. But by making some adjustments and educating yourselves on issues like education, diet, mobility, and exercise will help you see that there are ways to maintain many of the day-to-day activities to which you are accustomed.

Environmental Accessibility

As with any disability, certain everyday needs and routines will change. DMD is no different in this aspect, especially once mobility decreases and a wheelchair is introduced into daily life.

At Home

Ask yourself "how accessible is my home?" Your son will need to get around within your house and remain as independent as possible once he cannot climb stairs or is confined to a wheelchair. Ask yourself:

- Will he be able to get around this house with ease?
- Will he be able to get in and out of the house with ease?

There are solutions to these kinds of problems. Keep in mind that special equipment or additions to your home may be necessary. Wider doorways and ramps can make your life easier. They can help your son get in, out, and around your house.

At School

Most young men with DMD can attend their local pre-school and elementary school with little difficulty. Keep open communications with your school and provide them with as much information as you can about DMD and how it will affect your son. You can work with your school to collaborate and develop your child's talents and help him learn how to take on the tasks he finds difficult.

Once walking becomes difficult; many schools will make special arrangements or even structural additions in order to help make his daily activities easier. Even transportation to and from school can be arranged. Keep in mind that there are some cases where a school may be unsuitable for your son and an alternative or specialized school may be better.

Education Needs

About 33% of young men who have DMD are learning disabled in some capacity, although few cases are serious. Many doctors believe that there are abnormalities in the brain due to the lack of a working dystrophin gene. These abnormalities are thought to be the cause of subtle cognitive and/or behavioral deficits. The main areas affected are attention span, verbal learning, memory, and emotional interaction.

Speech Difficulties

For young men who suffer from both DMD and learning disabilities, language and communication skills are typically the main concern. But manual skills, visual skills, and creativity are often excellent in young men with DMD, which is perhaps why many become very good artists.

Learning Difficulties

If you suspect that your son has a learning disability, he should be evaluated by a developmental or pediatric neuropsychologist either through your school system's special education department or through your child's own pediatrician. If a learning disability is diagnosed, there are educational and psychological therapies that can be started right away. The specialist may also prescribe exercises that can help you interact with your child which may help improve these disabilities. His school should also provide him with special help if necessary.

Diet

Unfortunately, there are no special dietary additions or regiments that are proven to help slow the progression of DMD. It is known that weight gain will cause additional burden for muscles. Some physicians recommend a diet high in protein and low in carbohydrates and fat. For young men taking steroids (prednisone or Deflazacort), sodium-restricted diets are often recommended.

Caloric Intake

Steroid regimens often cause an increase in appetite. Families need to be concerned about weight gain as obesity causes increased burden on muscle. In the event parents choose to have their sons begin steroid therapy, diet management should be addressed from the start. Although steroid therapy may not be suitable for every child, initiating a sound diet may allow longer use of steroids while avoiding excess weight gain. As mobility decreases, calorie burn also decreases. Caloric intake should be monitored in order to keep weight at a healthy level.

Foods

The combination of immobility and weak abdominal muscles in young men with DMD may cause constipation. A diet high in fluid fiber including fresh fruits and vegetables should help the digestion process.

Mobility

Mobility can come in many forms—strollers, bikes (if able), unassisted walking, walking with a brace, electric scooters, and manual or electric chairs. Whatever the means, getting from place to place (assisted or not) is essential to a DMD child just as it is to any child. Parents should consider that while it may be painful for them to take the next step for their child to use an alternate method to get around, it is a far better choice than a child feeling stuck.

Physical Therapy

Physical therapy (PT) is one of the ways to help your son because it can increase and prolong mobility. Keep in mind that insurance will not usually cover daily physical therapy. Families should consult with their own physical therapist in order to develop a comprehensive routine that is manageable and fun.

Stretching Tendons

Daily stretching exercises of three specific tendons (Achilles, hamstring, and iliotibial bands) will extend ambulation.

The Achilles tendon (ankle joint) often becomes tight in young men with DMD. A tight Achilles tendon may result in toe walking. Prolonged stretching of the Achilles tendon can prevent this condition.

As muscle degeneration progresses and the child spends more time sitting, the hamstring (muscle behind the knee) gets tighter and tighter. It is important to stretch the hamstring in order to prolong movement and maintain a higher level of comfort.

You may notice that when your child is sitting, he draws up his legs and allows his knees to spread. This indicates tightening of the iliotibial bands (hip flexors) and can interfere with ambulation. These important tendons need to be stretched. In order to stretch properly, the child will usually require instruction from a physical therapist. In addition, sitting in long leg braces may assist with proper positioning and lessen knee contractures that may develop.

Swimming

Experts agree that a regimen of swimming and other water exercises (also known as aquatic therapy) is a good way to keep muscles as lean as possible without causing additional stress to the body. Floating the body in water helps prevent muscle strain and injury that might occur otherwise. Equally important is the benefit of swimming to respiratory mechanics (how parts of your body's respiration system work together to function properly). A cardiac evaluation is recommended before beginning any form of swim therapy. Also, never swim alone.

Horseback Riding

Therapeutic horseback riding (also called hippotherapy) allows young men with DMD to stretch and work muscles that they would normally not be able to use on land.

Exercise

Exercise can help young men with DMD in the same way that it helps everyone else: to build skeletal muscles, keep the body healthy, and make you feel better in general. But keep in mind that too much exercise can do more harm than good. Therefore, a person with DMD should never go to the point of exhaustion. Please consult your physician before beginning any exercise regimen.

Types of Exercise

Most experts agree that a regimen of swimming and other water exercises (also known as aquatic therapy) is a good way to keep muscles as lean as possible without causing additional stress to them. The flotation of the body in the water helps prevent muscle strain and injury that might occur otherwise. As with anyone, please consult a physician before beginning any new exercise program.

Sleeping

Young boys diagnosed with Duchenne MD typically do not have problems with sleep (although their parents often experience significant problems due to stress). However, as the disorder progresses, boys with Duchenne MD will begin to experience problems with sleeping.

Some boys on steroid regimens experience difficulty sleeping. Please consult with the physician if this is the case. Sometimes changing the regimen slightly or alternating the type of steroid may decrease sleeping problems.

With increasing weakness, young men often get restless at night and complain of headaches in the morning. Restlessness and early morning headaches may be a first sign of weakening respiratory muscles. It is very important to monitor pulmonary function and be attentive to signs of respiratory problems. Please discuss any issues that come up with your doctor.

Additional Information

Parent Project Muscular Dystrophy (PPMD)
1012 North University Blvd.
Middletown, OH 45042
Toll-Free: 800-714-KIDS (5437)
Phone: 513-424-0696
Fax: 513-425-9907
Website: http://www.parentprojectmd.org
E-mail: info@parentprojectme.org

Chapter 41

Age and Mobility Stages

The information required to assist you with everyday needs depends on the age of your child and his mobility. However, some services are relevant irrespective of age or mobility and have been described in the first part of this chapter. They include:

- Occupational therapists and physiotherapists
- Muscular Dystrophy Association
- Respite care

Occupational Therapists and Physiotherapists

Occupational therapists, along with physiotherapists, are skilled in assessing and solving the physical problems encountered in everyday living.

Everyone needs to be independent and the problems encountered by boys with Duchenne muscular dystrophy are shared by many people with physical disabilities. Stairs, rough or hilly school grounds, and access to the toilet and bathroom facilities are a few of the difficulties to be overcome. These problems are not only experienced by boys with Duchenne muscular dystrophy. They are shared by many people with physical disabilities.

Excerpted with permission from "A Guide for Parents: Section 5–Everyday Living," by the Muscular Dystrophy Association (MDA)–Australia, www.mda.org.au. © 2003 MDA–Australia. All rights reserved.

For most families, the use of a few aids and some minor home modifications are all that are required to allow as much independence as possible. Occupational therapists can advise on ramps, handrails, and equipment such as shower chairs, extended shower hoses, bottles for toileting, pick-up tongs, levers on taps, height adjustable tables, and other aids. They can offer advice on techniques for transferring and lifting and the availability of hoists. They can visit the school or home to assess what is required to promote access and independence.

Some families will find that their family home, in the long term, will be unsuitable for wheelchair access or will not be appropriate for things like bathing or toileting. If it is necessary to renovate or to move, it is vital that the advice of an appropriate occupational therapist be sought before proceeding.

The Muscular Dystrophy Association

As a result of ongoing contact with families, the Muscular Dystrophy Association has wide experience in dealing with problems that families encounter. The association often provides a good first point of contact. They can direct you to organizations offering different skills, information, and support appropriate to your son's age and stage of development.

Respite Care

Respite care provides families with a break from the pressure of caring for a child with a disability. It also allows the child contact with new friends and experiences. Respite care is available from a number of organizations.

Age and Mobility Stages

There are many other services to support day to day living that parents may want to contact depending on the age and mobility of their child. The following information is presented according to five different age and mobility stages.

- Pre-school age children
- Walking primary school age children
- Non-walking primary school aged children
- Secondary school aged children
- Post secondary school young adults

Preschool Aged Children

This stage includes the period of diagnosis. There is a great need for general information about the disease. For some families, professional counseling is useful. It is a very important time for establishing priorities and establishing a plan which will enable the family to lead as normal a life as possible. Planning for primary education is important at this stage.

Some families may question the appropriateness of the diagnosis at this stage because they observe their son to be gaining in strength. The diagnosis however, remains correct. Usually, between the ages of three and six, normal muscle growth and development is not being outstripped by the continuing muscle weakness associated with the disease. The net effect is that the child appears to be getting stronger.

Walking Primary School Age Children

This stage sees mobility decline. Children have a fear of falling and the subsequent struggle to get up again. It may be the time to investigate wheelchairs. Sometimes a large stroller is used for outings as an interim measure before a wheelchair is required.

Because the child is losing mobility, this is an important time to learn correct lifting and transferring techniques from a physiotherapist. First, it is necessary to protect your own back from injury, and second, the person being lifted needs to feel secure during the lifting process. This security is possible if the correct lifting procedure is used. It is also important that your son can instruct others on the lifting techniques most suitable to him.

Physiotherapy exercises need to be built into an everyday routine. Disharmony over this task is wasted energy. Sometimes a brief rest from the physiotherapy program may help the whole family, and it is important to recognize that all members of the family have needs.

Many children are extremely frustrated by their loss of independence. Signs of this frustration may occur as disruptive behavior, a decline in work performance, or general apathy. Although it is premature to discuss the prognosis of the illness at this age, it is not too early to begin to establish a pattern of communicating feelings with your child. The walking child can still participate in community recreational programs. Contact with other families with a child of a similar age with Duchenne muscular dystrophy is also helpful.

Parents cover new ground with the beginning of school. In many instances, problems related to schooling can be overcome with the support of an integration aide. Some boys experience learning difficulties as a direct result of the disease and require specialized teaching.

Non-Walking Primary School Age Children

Often when a child acquires an electric wheelchair, he enjoys renewed enthusiasm for life. He now feels safe from the dangers of falling and has a guaranteed and independent means of mobility. Parents on the other hand can find this time difficult, as it is an obvious indicator of their son's declining strength and mobility. Families now have to deal with staring and public curiosity when moving in the community.

The use of the wheelchair may require home and school modifications, but there is considerable expert advice available to assist with these changes.

Recreational programs may also need development at this time. Community activities previously enjoyed may no longer be appropriate. It is worth embarking on new activities which can accommodate decreased mobility in the future.

Education planning for secondary school is important. Educational goals established for primary school may need revision. Sometimes it is valuable to devote special time to other children in the family. Your son's needs are obvious. Other children in the family may feel they are less important because they have less of your time.

Transport issues also need to be addressed. Public transportation in the form of bus, train, and the use of taxi cabs is the most relevant for wheelchair use. Many families find it necessary to change the family car at this time, using vans that accommodate wheelchairs.

Secondary School Aged Children

At this stage, the child becomes very much aware of his own individuality and must face his shortened life expectancy. Continuing contact with other boys of similar age is important.

In a climate of declining strength and increasing school demands, it is valuable to consider issues such as quality of life versus academic achievement. Despite the obvious physical decline, parents need to face their child's need for independence and demonstrate a willingness to let go. As with any child at this age, sexual development needs to be recognized. Parents should be mindful that difficult behavior manifested at this time may simply be typical adolescent behavior associated with exploring increasing maturity.

Employment opportunities and prospects for independent living can be explored at the latter part of this stage. Computers are offering great potential for work opportunities.

Post Secondary School Young Adults

The most fundamental issue is deciding on the most meaningful use of time. Both educational and philosophical choices made up until now will significantly influence what will be pursued. Further study, employment, and independent living accommodations are areas for consideration. Some will wish to satisfy the desire for an independent source of income. Adult relationships outside the family are also important. The physical demands of caring for a person increase. In particular, your son will require turning during the night, lifting, and other nursing management.

This stage of development sees an adult person becoming increasingly dependent. However, a person who is physically dependent is still capable of making their own decisions.

Education

Intellectual and social development is important to any child. However, it is perhaps most important to the physically disabled child. As the child with muscular dystrophy loses physical strength, he will find that more of his pleasure and feelings of achievement come from the development of verbal, intellectual, and social skills.

Some boys with Duchenne muscular dystrophy have delays in their mental or speech development and require assessment and advice from a psychologist, speech pathologist, or other professionals working in these areas. Some may have come to medical attention because of these problems. While poor language skills and learning difficulties are more common in Duchenne muscular dystrophy than in the population as a whole, this does not mean that all boys are affected and most progress through school normally. However, if a boy is having problems an assessment by an educational psychologist may be needed to make recommendations on what remedial help may be required. Parents should be aware that while the muscle problem is progressive, any language or educational difficulties that occur do not get worse as time goes on.

Deciding on the type of schooling that is most appropriate for your child and your family situation, is a decision which needs careful thought. Do you choose a regular school or do you choose an alternative school? The decision is one only you can make, but there are some issues which when considered, will make that decision a little easier.

The first step is to decide what you want from education and then allocate priorities to these objectives. The objectives may change. When your child is young, you have sole responsibility to determine these goals. As your child matures his particular needs become clearer, and he will also have his own opinion to take into consideration.

The education objectives to consider include:

- academic achievement
- independence
- the development of social skills
- quality of life
- employment opportunities

Having decided which of these goals is most important for you, the decision on the school that best meets your son's needs becomes much easier. Be flexible; allow these priorities to change with the flux of time.

Generally, at primary school age, children with Duchenne muscular dystrophy see themselves as able bodied and do not see their needs as any different to anyone else's.

Specific Educational Considerations

Accessibility: This is an important consideration particularly as mobility becomes more difficult and especially important when your child is using a wheelchair. For example, a multi-story building makes participation in classes difficult. Toileting is another consideration.

Physical environment: Alternative schools are built with access in mind. They have rooms and facilities designed to teach people with disabilities. For example, a kitchen with specialized cooking equipment and aides, and a heated swimming pool for hydrotherapy may be provided.

Learning Climate: An alternative school provides greater opportunity for a one to one learning situation. In addition, both the pace of the school day and the pace of learning are tailored to individual needs.

You Are Not Alone

At the time when a child is diagnosed as having Duchenne muscular dystrophy his parents feel very alone, especially those who have never heard of muscular dystrophy. They feel that they are the only people in the world with a child with this disease. They worry about how they will cope, how they will tell other members of the family, and how everyone will deal with the situation. Parents can find it very helpful to share these challenges with another parent who has a child with muscular dystrophy, particularly if that child is at the same stage as their child.

The Muscular Dystrophy Association can link parents with another family for this kind of support. Both the association and other families with a child with Duchenne muscular dystrophy have a very good idea of how parents feel and will not impose themselves. Help is available when it is required.

Chapter 42

Education Rights and Responsibilities of Parents of Children with Muscular Dystrophy

Chapter Contents

Section 42.1—Individuals with Disabilities Education
      Act (IDEA) 438
Section 42.2—Your Rights in the Special Education
      Process 465
Section 42.3—Integration of the Student with Muscular
      Dystrophy into a School Physical Program 471

Section 42.1

Individuals with Disabilities Education Act (IDEA)

"Related Services for School-Aged Children with Disabilities," NICHCY
News Digest 16, 2nd Edition, 2001, National Dissemination Center for
Children with Disabilities (NICHCY).

The Individuals with Disabilities Education Act Amendments of
1997 (IDEA '97) mandates that "...all children with disabilities have
available to them a free appropriate public education [FAPE] that
emphasizes special education and related services designed to meet
their unique needs and prepare them for employment and independent living" [Section 601(d)(1)(A)]. In accordance with the IDEA '97
and other federal laws, more than 5.9 million children with disabilities (ages 3 through 21) across the nation received special education
and related services in the 1997-98 school year (U.S. Department of
Education, 1999b).

What, precisely, are related services, and why are they an important part of educating children with disabilities? Who is eligible for
related services, and how are related services delivered? This section
briefly examines the answers to these and other questions.

An Overview of Related Services under IDEA

Several important federal laws address the educational needs of
children and youth with disabilities. One such law, passed in 1975, is
the Education of All Handicapped Children Act, otherwise known as
EHA or Public Law (P.L.) 94-142. This law mandated that special
education and related services be made available to all eligible school-
aged children and youth with disabilities. Since the time of EHA's
enactment, Federal funds have been provided to help State and local
educational agencies provide special education and related services
to children with disabilities.

In 1990, as part of its reauthorization by Congress, the EHA was
renamed the Individuals with Disabilities Education Act, or IDEA
(P.L. 101-476). The law was again amended in June 1997 as P.L. 105-17.

The 1997 law is called the Individuals with Disabilities Education Act—referred to hereafter as IDEA '97.

Finding Specific Sections of the Regulations

As you read the explanations about the law, you will find references to specific sections of the Federal regulations (such as Section 300.24) implementing the IDEA '97. You can use these references to locate the precise sections in the Federal regulations that address the issue being discussed. For example, following the list of related services, you are given the reference Section 300.24(a). This reference tells you that, if you wanted to read the exact words the regulations use, you would look under Section 300.24(a) of the Code of Federal Regulations (CFR) for Title 34 (sometimes referred to as 34 CFR).

What Are Related Services?

In general, the final regulations for IDEA '97 define the term related services as "transportation and such developmental, corrective, and other supportive services as are required to assist a child with a disability to benefit from special education..." [Section 300.24(a)]. The following are included within the definition of related services:

- speech-language pathology and audiology services;
- psychological services;
- physical and occupational therapy;
- recreation, including therapeutic recreation;
- early identification and assessment of disabilities in children;
- counseling services, including rehabilitation counseling;
- orientation and mobility services;
- medical services for diagnostic or evaluation purposes;
- school health services;
- social work services in schools;
- parent counseling and training; and
- transportation [Section 300.24(a)].

Who Is Eligible for Related Services?

Under IDEA '97, a student must need special education to be considered eligible for related services (unless the related service needed by the child is considered special education rather than a related service under State standards) [Section 300.7(a)(2)(ii)]. A child must have a full and individual evaluation to determine:

- if he or she has a disability as defined under IDEA '97, and
- if, because of that disability, he or she needs special education and related services.

For the purposes of this publication on related services, however, it is useful to know that the law requires that a child be assessed in all areas related to his or her suspected disability. This includes, if appropriate, evaluating the child's:

- health,
- vision,
- hearing,
- social and emotional status,
- general intelligence,
- academic performance,
- communicative status, and
- motor abilities [Section 300.532(g)].

A variety of assessment tools and strategies must be used to gather relevant functional and developmental information about the child [Section 300.532(b)]. The evaluation must be sufficiently comprehensive so as to identify all of the child's special education and related services needs, whether or not those needs are commonly linked to the disability category in which he or she has been classified [Section 300.532(h)].

If the evaluation shows that the child does have a disability, and that because of that disability he or she needs special education and related services, then he or she meets the criteria for special education and related services.

How Do People Know What Related Services a Child Needs?

The evaluation process is intended to provide decision makers with the information they need to determine: (a) if the student has a disability and needs special education and related services, and, if so, (b) an appropriate educational program for the student. It also allows them to identify the related services a student will need.

Following the child's evaluation and the determination that he or she is eligible for special education and related services, a team of individuals called the IEP team—which includes the parents and, where appropriate, the student—sits down and writes an Individualized Education Program (IEP) for the student. The IEP team looks carefully at the evaluation results which show the child's areas of strength and need. The team decides what measurable annual goals (including benchmarks or short-term objectives), among other things, are appropriate for the child. Part of developing the IEP also includes specifying "the special education and related services and supplementary aids and services to be provided to the child, or on behalf of the child, and a statement of the program modifications or supports for school personnel that will be provided" for the child:

- to advance appropriately toward attaining the annual goals,

- to be involved and progress in the general curriculum (that is, the curriculum used by nondisabled students),

- to participate in extracurricular and other nonacademic activities, and

- to be educated and participate with other children with disabilities and nondisabled children [Section 300.347(a)(3)].

Thus, based on the evaluation results, the IEP team discusses, decides upon, and specifies the related services that a child needs in order to benefit from special education. Making decisions about how often a related service will be provided, and where and by whom is also a function of the IEP team.

It is important to recognize that each child with a disability may not require all of the available types of related services. Moreover, as Attachment 1 accompanying the regulations to IDEA '97 points out, "As under prior law, the list of related services is not exhaustive and may include other developmental, corrective, or supportive services (such as artistic and cultural programs, art, music, and dance therapy) if they are required to assist a child with a disability to benefit from special education in order for the child to receive FAPE" (U.S. Department of Education, 1999a, p. 12548). As States respond to the requirements of Federal law, many have legislated their own related service requirements, which may include services beyond those specified in IDEA '97. Further, "if it is determined through the [IDEA's] evaluation and IEP requirements that a child with a disability requires a particular supportive service in order to receive FAPE, regardless of whether that service is included in these [Federal] regulations, that service can be considered a related service...and must be provided at no cost to the parents" (p. 12548).

It is useful to note that IDEA '97 does not expressly require that the IEP team include related services personnel. However, if a particular related service is going to be discussed in an IEP meeting, it would be appropriate for such personnel to be included or otherwise involved in developing the IEP. IDEA '97 final regulations state that, at the discretion of the parent or the public agency, "other individuals who have knowledge or special expertise regarding the child, including related services personnel as appropriate" may be part of a child's IEP team [Section 300.344(a)(6)]. Appendix A of the regulations specifically states (at Question 30) that, if a child with a disability has an identified need for related services, the public agency responsible for the child's education should ensure that a qualified provider of that service either:

- attends the IEP meeting, or

- provides a written recommendation concerning the nature, frequency, and amount of service to be provided to the child (U.S. Department of Education, 1999a, p. 12478).

Once the IEP team has determined which related services are required to assist the student to benefit from his or her special education; these must be listed in the IEP. The IEP also must include a statement of measurable annual goals (including benchmarks or short-term objectives) related to:

- meeting the child's needs that result from his or her disability to enable the child to be involved in and progress in the general curriculum (or for preschool children, as appropriate, to participate in appropriate activities), and

- meeting each of the child's other educational needs that result from the disability [Section 300.347(a)(2)].

In addition to this key information, the IEP must also specify with respect to each service:

- when the service will begin; and

- the anticipated frequency (how often), location (where), and duration (how long) of the service [Section 300.347(a)(6)].

The IEP is a written commitment for the delivery of services to meet a student's educational needs. A school district must ensure that all of the related services specified in the IEP, including the amount, are provided to a student.

Changes in the amount of services listed in the IEP cannot be made without holding another IEP meeting. However, if there is no change in the overall amount of service, some adjustments in the scheduling of services may be possible without the necessity of another IEP meeting.

Do the Parents Have to Pay for the Related Services the Child Receives?

No. School districts may not charge parents of eligible students with disabilities for the costs of related services that have been included on the child's IEP. Just as special and regular education must be provided to an eligible student with a disability at no cost to the parent or guardian, so, too, must related services when the IEP team has determined that such services are required in order for the child to receive FAPE and have included them in the student's IEP.

A Closer Look at Specific Related Services

Perhaps the best way to develop an understanding of related services is to look at each in more detail. Because there are quite a few services that can be considered as related services, the information presented about each of the following related services is intended only as an introduction. It is not the intent of this document, just as it is not the intent of the law, to exhaustively describe each related service. It may be helpful, however, to read further about the services in order to know what related services are most commonly provided to students with disabilities and, in some situations, their families. The related services described below are organized in alphabetical order.

Artistic/Cultural Programs

Artistic/cultural programs are specifically mentioned in Attachment 1 of the Federal regulations for IDEA '97 as "other developmental, corrective, or supportive services (such as artistic and cultural programs, art, music, and dance therapy) if they are required to assist a child with a disability to benefit from special education in order for the child to receive FAPE" (U.S. Department of Education,

1999a, p. 12548). Artistic and cultural programs are designed by art therapists, dance therapists, and music therapists to address the individual needs of students with disabilities. These professionals:

- assess the functioning of individual students;

- design programs appropriate to the needs and abilities of students;

- provide services in which music, movement, or art is used in a therapeutic process to further the child's emotional, physical, cognitive, and/or academic development or integration; and

- often act as resource persons for classroom teachers.

Art therapy provides individuals with disabilities with a means of self-expression and opportunities to expand personal creativity and control. By involving students with art and the creative art process, art therapists work to help students address their unique needs, which may include resolving emotional conflicts, developing self-awareness or social skills, managing behavior, solving problems, reducing anxiety, and improving self-esteem (American Art Therapy Association, 2000).

Dance/movement therapy uses movement as a means for promoting personal growth and furthering the emotional, cognitive, and physical integration of an individual (American Dance Therapy Association, 1998). Dance therapy can develop and promote good posture, discipline, concentration, coordination, agility, speed, balance, strength, and endurance.

Music therapy uses music and music-related strategies to assist or motivate a student to reach specific educational goals as well as address his or her physical, psychological, cognitive, behavioral, and social needs (American Music Therapy Association, 2000). Music and music learning are often used to strengthen nonmusical areas such as academic skills, physical coordination, communication, sensory-motor development, expression of emotions, and stress reduction.

Assistive Technology Devices and Services

Assistive technology (AT) refers to various types of devices and services designed to help students with disabilities function within their environments. Many areas are covered under the umbrella of assistive technology, including computers, adaptive toys and games, devices to improve positioning and mobility, devices designed to help individuals with disabilities communicate (called augmentative communication devices), and electronic aids to daily living (RESNA Technical Assistance Project, 1992).

An assistive technology device means "any item, piece of equipment, or product system, whether acquired commercially off the shelf, modified, or customized, that is used to increase, maintain, or improve the functional capabilities of a child with a disability" (Section 300.5). Assistive technology devices may be used for personal care, sensory processing of information, communication, mobility, or leisure. For young children, assistive technology may involve adaptive toys or simple computer software games to stimulate eye-hand coordination (Derer, Polsgrove, & Rieth, 1996). For other children, it may involve adaptive eating utensils, electronic augmentative communication devices, or a voice-activated word processing software program.

An assistive technology service means "any service that directly assists a child with a disability in the selection, acquisition, or use of an assistive technology device" (Section 300.6). School districts are responsible for helping individuals with disabilities select and acquire appropriate assistive technology devices and train them in their use, if doing so is necessary for them to receive FAPE (Section 300.308). Such services include:

- evaluating a child's needs, including a functional evaluation in the child's customary environment;

- purchasing, leasing, or otherwise providing for the acquisition of assistive technology devices by children with disabilities;

- selecting, designing, fitting, customizing, adapting, applying, maintaining, repairing, or replacing assistive technology devices;

- coordinating and using other therapies, interventions, or services with assistive technology devices (such as those associated with existing education and rehabilitation plans and programs);

- training or technical assistance for a child with a disability or, if appropriate, the child's family; and

- training or technical assistance for professionals (including individuals providing education or rehabilitation services); employers;

or other individuals who provide services to, employ, or are substantially involved in the major functions of that child (Section 300.6).

Rothstein and Everson (1995) suggest several guidelines for decision making regarding assistive technology, including:

- look for simple solutions;
- consider the learning and work style of the student;
- consider the long-range implications of the student's disability and the device;
- look at each device for ease of use and maintenance, timeliness, adaptability, portability, dependability, durability, and technical support needed;
- investigate all options;
- compare similar devices from different manufacturers, and
- purchase devices only after consulting with a professional.

Consideration of a child's need for assistive technology devices and services occurs on a case-by-case basis in connection with the development of a child's IEP. Thus, when an IEP of a student with a disability is being developed, reviewed, or revised (if appropriate), the IEP team must determine his or her need for an assistive technology device or service, determine those devices that will facilitate the student's education, and list them in the IEP. The public agency must then provide them to the student at no cost to the parents.

May a child use a school-purchased AT device in his or her home or other setting? According to the IDEA '97's final regulations, the answer to this question would be determined on a case-by-case basis. Such use in nonschool settings would be "required if the child's IEP team determines that the child needs access to those devices in order to receive FAPE" [Section 300.308(b)]—for example, to complete homework. Question 36 of Appendix A of the regulations adds that "the parents cannot be charged for normal use, wear and tear. However, while ownership of the devices in these circumstances would remain with the public agency, State law, rather than Part B [of IDEA], generally would govern whether parents are liable for loss, theft, or damage due to negligence or misuse of publicly owned equipment used at home or in other settings in accordance with a child's IEP" (U.S. Department of Education, 1999a, p. 12479).

Audiology

Audiology includes:

- identifying children with hearing loss;

- determining the range, nature, and degree of hearing loss, including referral for medical or other professional attention for the habilitation of hearing;

- providing habilitative activities, such as language habilitation, auditory training, speech reading (lip-reading), hearing evaluation, and speech conservation;

- creating and administering programs for prevention of hearing loss;

- counseling and guidance of children, parents, and teachers regarding hearing loss; and

- determining children's needs for group and individual amplification, selecting and fitting an appropriate aid, and evaluating the effectiveness of amplification [Section 300.24(b)(1)].

Some schools have hearing screening programs and staff trained to conduct audiologic screenings of children. Others may participate in regional cooperatives or other arrangements that provide audiological services. Those school districts that do not have diagnostic facilities to evaluate students for hearing loss and related communication problems or central auditory processing disorders may refer students to a clinical setting, such as a hospital or audiology clinic, or make other contractual arrangements (American Speech-Language-Hearing Association, personal communication, August 1, 2000).

Counseling Services

Counseling services, according to the American School Counselor Association (1999), focus on the needs, interests, and issues related to various stages of student growth. School counselors may help students with personal and social concerns such as developing self-knowledge, making effective decisions, learning health choices, and improving responsibility. Counselors may also help students with future planning related to setting and reaching academic goals, developing a positive attitude toward learning, and recognizing and utilizing academic strengths. Other counseling services may include parent counseling and training and rehabilitation counseling (that is, counseling specific to career development and employment preparation) (Maag & Katsiyannis, 1996).

Counseling services are services provided by qualified social workers, psychologists, guidance counselors, or other qualified personnel [Section 300.24(b)(2)]. A school counselor is a certified professional who meets the State's certification standards. In some schools, the counselor may also perform some functions similar to those of the school psychologist as described under Psychological Services.

Medical Services

Medical services are considered a related service only under specific conditions. By definition, the term "means services provided by a licensed physician to determine a child's medically related disability that results in the child's need for special education and related services" [Section 300.24(b)(4)]. Thus, medical services are provided (a) by a licensed physician, and (b) for diagnostic or evaluation purposes only.

Occupational Therapy

Occupational therapy (OT) services can enhance a student's ability to function in an educational program. These services are "provided by a qualified occupational therapist" and include:

- "improving, developing, or restoring functions impaired or lost through illness, injury, or deprivation;
- improving [a child's] ability to perform tasks for independent functioning if functions are impaired or lost; and
- preventing, through early intervention, initial or further impairment or loss of function" [Section 300.24(b)(5)].

Occupational therapy services in schools may include such services as:

- self-help skills or adaptive living (e.g., eating, dressing);
- functional mobility (e.g., moving safely through school);
- positioning (e.g., sitting appropriately in class);
- sensory-motor processing (e.g., using the senses and muscles);
- fine motor (e.g., writing, cutting) and gross motor performance (e.g., walking, athletic skills);

- life skills training/vocational skills; and

- psychosocial adaptation.

Parent Counseling and Training

Parent counseling and training is an important related service that can help parents enhance the vital role they play in the lives of their children. When necessary to help an eligible student with a disability benefit from the educational program, parent counseling and training can include:

- "Assisting parents in understanding the special needs of their child;

- Providing parents with information about child development; and

- Helping parents to acquire the necessary skills that will allow them to support the implementation of their child's IEP or IFSP" [Individualized Family Service Plan] [Section 300.24(b)(7)].

The last aspect—that of helping parents acquire necessary skills to support the implementation of their child's IEP or IFSP—is new in IDEA '97 and was added to:

recognize the more active role acknowledged for parents...[as] very important participants in the education process for their children. Helping them gain the skills that will enable them to help their children meet the goals and objectives of their IEP or IFSP will be a positive change for parents, will assist in furthering the education of their children, and will aid the schools as it will create opportunities to build reinforcing relationships between each child's educational program and out-of-school learning (U.S. Department of Education, 1999a, p. 12549).

Physical Therapy

Physical therapy means "services provided by a qualified physical therapist" [Section 300.24(b)(8)]. These services generally address a child's posture, muscle strength, mobility, and organization of movement in educational environments. Physical therapy may be provided to prevent the onset or progression of impairment, functional limitation, disability, or changes in physical function or health resulting from injury, disease, or other causes. Qualified providers of these services may:

- provide treatment to increase joint function, muscle strength, mobility, and endurance;

- address gross motor skills that rely on the large muscles of the body involved in physical movement and range of motion;

- help improve the student's posture, gait, and body awareness; and

- monitor the function, fit, and proper use of mobility aids and devices.

Psychological Services

Psychological services are delivered as a related service when necessary to help eligible students with disabilities benefit from their special education. In some schools, these services are provided by a school psychologist, but some services are also appropriately provided by other trained personnel, including school social workers and counselors. Under IDEA '97 regulations, the term psychological services includes:

- "administering psychological and educational tests and other assessment procedures;

- interpreting assessment results;

- obtaining, integrating, and interpreting information about a student's behavior and conditions relating to learning;

- consulting with other staff members in planning school programs to meet the special needs of children as indicated by psychological tests, interviews, and behavioral evaluations;

- planning and managing a program of psychological services, including psychological counseling for students and parents; and

- assisting in developing positive behavioral intervention strategies" [Section 300.24(b)(9)].

IDEA '97 requires that, in the case of a child whose behavior impedes his or her learning or that of others, the IEP team consider, if appropriate, strategies (including positive behavioral interventions, strategies, and supports) to address that behavior [Section 300.346(a)(2)(i)]. These interventions and strategies may focus not only on the result of an absent, inadequate, inconsistent, or negative behavior blocking learning, but also on the curricular and instructional issues that may trigger problems (Dwyer, 1997). Positive behavioral interventions and supports involve a comprehensive set of strategies aimed at providing a student with a disability an improved lifestyle that includes reductions in problem behaviors, changes in social relationships, an expansion of prosocial skills, and an increase in school and community inclusion (Fox, Vaughn, Dunlap, & Bucy, 1997).

Psychologists and school social workers may be involved in assisting in developing these positive behavioral intervention strategies. However, as the U.S. Department of Education (1999a) notes: "[T]here are many other appropriate professionals in a school district who might also play a role...These examples of personnel who may assist in this activity are not intended to imply either that school psychologists and social workers are automatically qualified to perform these duties or to prohibit other qualified personnel from serving in this role, consistent with State requirements" (p. 12550).

Recreation

Recreation services generally are intended to help students with disabilities learn how to use their leisure and recreation time constructively. Through these services, students can learn appropriate and functional recreation and leisure skills (Schleien, Green, & Heyne, 1993). According to the IDEA '97 final regulations, recreation as a related service includes:

- assessment of leisure function;
- therapeutic recreation services;
- recreation programs in schools and community agencies; and
- leisure education [Section 300.24(b)(10)].

Recreational activities generally may fall into one or more of the following classifications: (1) physical, cultural, or social; (2) indoor or outdoor; (3) spectator or participant; (4) formal or informal; (5) independent, cooperative, or competitive; or (6) sports, games, hobbies, or toy play (Moon & Bunker, 1987). Recreational activities may be provided during the school day or in after-school programs in a school or a community environment. Some school districts have made collaborative arrangements with the local parks and recreation programs or local youth development programs to provide recreational services.

451

As part of providing this related service, persons qualified to provide recreation carry out activities such as:

- assessing a student's leisure interests and preferences, capacities, functions, skills, and needs;

- providing recreation therapeutic services and activities to develop a student's functional skills;

- providing education in the skills, knowledge, and attitudes related to leisure involvement;

- helping a student participate in recreation with assistance and/ or adapted recreation equipment;

- providing training to parents and educators about the role of recreation in enhancing educational outcomes;

- identifying recreation resources and facilities in the community; and

- providing recreation programs in schools and community agencies.

Rehabilitation Counseling Services

Rehabilitation counseling services are "services provided by qualified personnel in individual or group sessions that focus specifically on career development, employment preparation, achieving independence, and integration in the workplace and community.... The term also includes vocational rehabilitation services provided to a student with disabilities by vocational rehabilitation programs funded under the Rehabilitation Act of 1973, as amended" [Section 300.24(b)(11)].

The role of the rehabilitation counselor, according to the Council on Rehabilitation Education (1996), is to provide students with disabilities "assistance to their vocation, social, and personal functioning through the use of professionally recognized interaction skills and other appropriate services" (p. 36). To this end, rehabilitation counseling services generally may include:

- assessment of a student's attitudes, abilities, and needs;

- vocational counseling and guidance;

- vocational training; and

- identifying job placements in individual or group sessions.

School Health Services

School health services under the IDEA '97 final regulations means "services provided by a qualified school nurse or other qualified person" [Section 300.24(b)(12)]. These services may be necessary because some children and youth with disabilities would otherwise be unable to attend a day of school without supportive health care. School health services may include interpretation, interventions, administration of health procedures, the use of an assistive health device to compensate for the reduction or loss of a body function (Rapport, 1996), and case management.

Typically, school health services are provided by a qualified school nurse or other qualified trained person who is supervised by a qualified nurse. In some instances, if a school nurse is not employed by a school district, health services may be provided and/or coordinated by a public health nurse, a pediatric home care nurse, or a hospital- or community-based pediatric nurse practitioner or specialist. States and local school districts often have guidelines that address school health services. State agency guidelines that address school health services for special health care needs may address staffing requirements, infection control, medication administration, nursing procedures, classroom modifications, transportation, and policies (Porter, Haynie, Bierle, Caldwell, & Palfrey, 1997).

Possible school health services include:

- special feedings;
- clean intermittent catheterization;
- suctioning;
- the management of a tracheostomy;
- administering and/or dispensing medications;
- planning for the safety of a student in school;
- ensuring that care is given while at school and at school functions to prevent injury (e.g., changing a student's position frequently to prevent pressure sores);
- chronic disease management; and
- conducting and/or promoting education and skills training for all (including the student) who serve as caregivers in the school setting.

Social Work Services in Schools

Issues or problems at home or in the community can adversely affect a student's performance at school, as can a student's attitudes or behaviors in school. Social work services in schools may become necessary in order to help a student benefit from his or her educational program. Social work services in schools include:

- "preparing a social or developmental history on a child with a disability;

- group and individual counseling with the child and family;

- working in partnership with parents and others on those problems in a child's living situation (home, school, and community) that affect the child's adjustment in school;

- mobilizing school and community resources to enable the child to learn as effectively as possible in his or her educational program; and

- assisting in developing positive behavioral intervention strategies" [Section 300.24(b)(13)].

Speech-Language Pathology Services

Speech-language pathology services are provided by speech-language professionals and speech-language assistants in accordance with State regulations, to address the needs of children and youth with communication disabilities. Under the IDEA '97 final regulations, these services include:

- identification of children with speech or language impairments;

- diagnosis and appraisal of specific speech or language impairments;

- referral for medical or other professional attention necessary for the habilitation of speech or language impairments;

- provision of speech and language services for the habilitation or prevention of communicative impairments; and

- counseling and guidance of parents, children, and teachers regarding speech and language impairments" [Section 300.24 (b)(14)].

Transportation

Transportation as a related service is included in an eligible student's IEP if the IEP team determines that such a service is needed. Transportation includes:

- travel to and from school and between schools;

- travel in and around school buildings; and

- specialized equipment (such as special or adapted buses, lifts, and ramps), if required to provide special transportation for a child with a disability [Section 300.24(b)(15)].

Public school districts must provide transportation to students with disabilities in two situations. These are:

- if a district provides transportation to and from school for the general student population, then it must provide transportation for a student with a disability; and

- if a school district does not provide transportation for the general student population, then the issue of transportation for students with disabilities must be decided on a case-by-case basis if the IEP team has determined that transportation is needed by the child and has included it on his or her IEP (Office of Special Education Programs, 1995).

If the IEP team determines that a student with a disability needs transportation to benefit from special education, it must be included in the student's IEP and provided as a related service at no cost to the student and his or her parents (Office of Special Education Programs, 1995).

Not all students with disabilities are eligible to receive transportation as a related service. As Attachment 1 of the Federal regulations for IDEA '97 points out:

> It is assumed that most children with disabilities will receive the same transportation provided to nondisabled children, unless the IEP team determines otherwise. However, for some children with disabilities, integrated transportation may not be achieved unless needed accommodations are provided to address each child's unique needs. If the IEP team determines that a disabled child requires transportation as a related service in order to receive FAPE, or requires accommodations or

modifications to participate in integrated transportation with nondisabled children, the child must receive the necessary transportation or accommodations at no cost to the parents. This is so, even if no transportation is provided to nondisabled children (U.S. Department of Education, 1999a, p. 12551).

A student's need for transportation as a related service and the type of transportation to be provided must be discussed and decided by the IEP team. Whether transportation goals and objectives are required in the IEP depends on the purpose of the transportation. If transportation is being provided solely to and from school, in and around school, and between schools, no goals or objectives are needed. If instruction is provided to a student to increase his or her independence or improve his or her behavior during transportation, then goals and objectives must be included in the student's IEP (Office of Special Education Programs, 1995).

Delivering Related Services

As was described in Part I, once a child has been evaluated and found eligible for special education and related services, the IEP team develops an individualized education program (IEP) for the child. This will include specifying the special education and related services that the child will receive as part of his or her free appropriate public education (FAPE). Beyond specifying the related services, however, is the delivery of the services. This section looks briefly at how school districts typically provide children with disabilities with related services.

Who Provides Related Services?

Providers of related services in the schools typically include (but are not limited to) professionals such as: school counselors, school psychologists, school social workers, school health professionals, speech-language pathologists, and occupational and physical therapists. The training and credentialing of these professionals will vary from State to State.

IDEA requires that related services are provided by qualified personnel. However, neither the law nor the regulations specify the levels of training that an individual needs in order to be considered qualified. It is the State that establishes what constitutes "suitable qualifications for personnel providing special education and related services" [Section 300.136(a)(1)(ii)]. This includes establishing the "highest entry-level academic degree needed for any State-approved or -recognized certification, licensing, registration, or other comparable requirements that apply to a profession or discipline" in which a person is providing special education and related services [Section 300.136(a)(2)].

The IDEA also permits, but does not require, the use of paraprofessionals and assistants who are appropriately trained and supervised to assist in the provision of special education and related services. The use of paraprofessionals and assistants is contingent upon State law, regulations, or written policy giving States the option of determining whether paraprofessionals and assistants can be used to assist in the provision of special education and related services, and, if so, to what extent their use would be permissible (U.S. Department of Education, 1999a, pp. 12561-12562).

Apart from the requirements of the IDEA '97 and standards of training that individual States establish as "suitable qualifications" for their various related services providers, a number of professional organizations exist and publish standards as well. These groups can be a valuable source of information to parents and professionals alike. Contact information is available at the end of this section.

While States may consider the recognized standards of professional organizations in deciding what are "appropriate professional requirements in the State," there is nothing in the statute or the regulations that requires States to do so (U.S. Department of Education, 1999a, p. 12560; see also [Section 300.136(b)(3)].

How Are Related Services Generally Delivered?

A school district must ensure that all of the related services specified in the student's IEP are provided, including the amount specified. The district usually decides how the services listed in the IEP will be delivered to the student. For example, the district may provide the services through its own personnel resources, or it may contract with another public or private agency, which then provides the services. Contracted service providers must meet the same standards for credentialing and training as public agency service providers do.

Generally, there are two basic kinds of related services interventions offered by schools to meet the range of student needs. These are:

1. **Direct Services.** Direct services usually refer to hands-on, face-to-face interactions between the related services professional and the student. These interactions can take place in a

variety of settings, such as the classroom, gym, health office, resource room, counseling office, or playground. Typically, the related service professional analyzes student responses and uses specific techniques to develop or improve particular skills. The professional should also:

- monitor the student's performance within the educational setting so that adjustments can be made to improve student performance, as needed, and

- consult with teachers and parents on an ongoing basis, so that relevant strategies can be carried out through indirect means at other times.

2. **Indirect Services.** Indirect services may involve teaching, consulting with, and/or directly supervising other personnel (including paraprofessionals and parents) so that they can carry out therapeutically-appropriate activities. For example, a school psychologist might train teachers and other educators how to implement a program included in a student's IEP to decrease the child's problem behaviors. Similarly, a physical therapist may serve as a consultant to a teacher and provide expertise to solve problems regarding a student's mobility through school (Dunn, 1991). Good practice is generally thought to include the following aspects:

- The intervention procedure is designed by the related service professional (with IEP team input) for an individual student.

- The related service professional has regular opportunities to interact with the student.

- The related service professional provides ongoing training, monitoring, supervision, procedural evaluation, and support to staff members and parents.

One type of service intervention is not necessarily better than the other (American Occupational Therapy Association, 1999) as long as the safety of the student is not compromised. In most school systems student needs are addressed through a combination of direct and indirect services (Smith, 1990). The type of service provided depends upon the individual needs of the student and his or her educational goals. Decisions about direct or indirect service delivery, therefore, are made on an individual, case-by-case basis.

It is not uncommon for districts to employ certified or trained assistants—such as a physical therapy assistant, a certified occupational therapy assistant, or a speech-language pathology assistant—to assist in the delivery of related services. In fact, in recent years there has been an increased emphasis on team members (e.g., teacher, therapist, and family member) delivering services under the supervision of an expert rather than only having an expert deliver direct services to a child (American Occupational Therapy Association, 1999). As stated previously, the final regulations for IDEA '97 make clear that nothing in the statute or regulations prohibits the use of paraprofessionals and assistants who are appropriately trained and supervised to assist in the provision of special education and related services, in accordance with State law, regulations, or written policy [Section 300.136(f)].

Where Are Related Services Provided?

In recent years, there has been a significant shift in where related services are provided. Rather than providing services in a separate room, as was the more common practice in years past, schools are emphasizing providing some services to students in natural activities and environments. Today it is not unusual to find speech-language services integrated into instructional activities in the regular education classroom, or occupational or physical therapy provided during physical education classes in gyms. As an example, asthma medication or glucose monitoring (as a school health service) may be done in the classroom or wherever the student with a disability happens to be. Thus, services may be delivered in a regular education class, a special education class, a gym, a therapy room, or in other locations in the school, home, or community.

Of course, there may be some services that need to be delivered in a separate setting such as a counseling room or office in order to assure confidentiality for the student and family. Such services may include individual and group counseling, parent counseling, and, frequently, consultation with staff and parents about individual students.

It is interesting to note that this shift in location accompanies a lesser focus on the traditional medical model of related services and greater attention given to an educational-results model. The medical model, typically found within a hospital or clinical setting, focuses on identifying and treating the particular illness, trauma, or deficit in a clinical setting. The educational model stresses the importance of the student's attaining IEP goals and objectives as well as addressing the capabilities and challenges presented by the particular disability (Hanft & Striffler, 1995).

How Are Related Services Coordinated?

Depending on the nature and type of related services to be provided, many professionals may be involved with, or on behalf of, the student with a disability. This may include one or more therapists, a special educator, a regular educator, counselor, a school psychologist, social workers, the school nurse or other health services staff, paraprofessionals, or the school principal. Clearly, there must be communication between the IEP team and the related service provider(s) to ensure that services are being delivered as specified in the IEP and that the student is making progress. If the student is not progressing as expected, adjustments in his or her program may be needed. The IEP team would need to make any such decisions.

When a student's IEP includes related services, it may be appropriate for related services professionals to be involved in the review of student progress and any decision to modify instruction or reevaluate the student's needs. Furthermore, if adjustments are made in the IEP, each teacher, related service provider, and other service provider who is responsible for implementing the revised IEP must be informed of:

- his or her specific responsibilities related to implementing the child's IEP; and

- the specific accommodations, modifications, and supports that must be provided to the child in accordance with the IEP [Section 300.342(b)(3)].

The IEP team may determine that it is highly desirable that related services be delivered in educational settings through a team approach. As mentioned, related services are not isolated from the educational program. Rather, they are related to the educational needs of students and are intended to assist the child in benefitting from the educational program. In order to ensure the integrated delivery of services, some school systems use a case management approach in which a team leader coordinates and oversees services on behalf of the student. In some schools, this person might be the child's special education teacher. In other schools, supervisory school district personnel may assume this responsibility.

References

American Art Therapy Association. (2000). *Art therapy: Definition of a profession* [On-line]. Available: www.arttherapy.org/definitions .htm

American Dance Therapy Association. (1998). *Dance/movement therapy: Frequently asked/answered questions (FAQ)* [On-line]. Available: www.adta.org/education.html

American Music Therapy Association. (2000). *Frequently asked questions about music therapy* [On-line]. Available: www.musictherapy.org/faqs.html

American Occupational Therapy Association (1999). *Occupational therapy services for children and youth under the Individuals with Disabilities Education Act* (2nd ed.). Bethesda, MD: Author.

American School Counselor Association. (1999). *The role of the professional school counselor* [On-line]. Available: www.schoolcounselor .org

Council on Rehabilitation Education. (1996). *Accreditation manual for rehabilitation counselor education programs.* Rolling Meadows, IL: Author.

Derer, K., Polsgrove, L., & Rieth, H. (1996). A survey of assistive technology applications in schools and recommendations for practice. *Journal of Special Education Technology*, XIII(2), 62-80.

Dunn, W. (1991). *Consultation as a process: How, when and why?* In C. Royeen (Ed.), *School-based practice for related services.* Bethesda, MD: American Occupational Therapy Association.

Dwyer, K. (1997, November). School psychology and behavioral interventions. *Communique*, 26(3), 1, 4-5.

Fox, L., Vaughn, B., Dunlap, G., & Bucy, M. (1997). Parent-professional partnership in behavioral support: A qualitative analysis of one family's experience. *Journal of the Association for Persons with Severe Handicaps*, 22(4), 198-207.

Hanft, B., & Striffler, N. (1995). Incorporating developmental therapy in early childhood programs: Challenges and promising practices. *Young Children*, 8(2), 37-47.

Hill, E., & Snook-Hill, M. (1996). Orientation and mobility. In M. C. Holbrook (Ed.), *Children with visual impairments: A parent's guide.* Bethesda, MD: Woodbine House.

Maag, J., & Katsiyannis, A. (1996). Counseling as a related service for students with emotional or behavioral disorders: Issues and recommendations. *Behavioral Disorders,* 21(4), 293-305.

Moon, M., & Bunker, L. (1987). Recreation and motor skills programming. In M. Snell (Ed.), *Systematic instruction of the moderately and severely handicapped* (pp. 214-244). Columbus, OH: Charles E. Merrill.

Office of Special Education Programs, U.S. Department of Education. (1995, July 12). *Letter to Smith.* Washington, DC: Author.

Porter, S., Haynie, M., Bierle, T., Caldwell, T., & Palfrey, J. (1997). *Children and youth assisted by medical technology in educational settings: Guidelines for care.* Baltimore, MD: Paul H. Brookes.

Rapport, M. (1996). Legal guidelines for the delivery of special health care services in schools. *Exceptional Children,* 62(6), 537-549.

RESNA Technical Assistance Project. (1992). *Assistive technology and the individualized education program.* Arlington, VA: RESNA Press.

Rothstein, R., & Everson, J. (1995). Assistive technology for individuals with sensory impairments. In K. Flippo, K. Inge, & J. Barcus (Eds.), *Assistive technology: A resource for school, work, and community* (pp. 105-129). Baltimore, MD: Paul H. Brookes.

Schleien, S., Green, F., & Heyne, L. (1993). Integrated community recreation. In M. Snell (Ed.), *Instruction of students with severe disabilities* (4th ed.) (pp. 526-555). New York: Macmillan.

Smith, P. (1990). *Integrating related services into programs for students with severe and multiple handicaps.* Lexington, KY: Kentucky Systems Change Project, Interdisciplinary Human Development Institute.

U.S. Department of Education. (1999a, March 12). Assistance to states for the education of children with disabilities and the early intervention program for infants and toddlers with disabilities; final regulations. *Federal Register,* 64(48), 12406-12671.

U.S. Department of Education. (1999b). *To assure a free appropriate public education: 21st annual report to Congress on the implementation of the Individuals with Disabilities Education Act.* Washington, DC: Author.

Organizations

Alliance for Technology Access
1304 Southpoint Blvd., Suite 240
Petaluma, CA 94954
Phone: 707-778-3011
TTY: 707-778-3015
Fax: 707-765-2080
Website: http://www.ataccess.org
E-mail: ATAinfo@ATAccess.org

American Academy of Audiology
11730 Plaza America Drive, Suite 300
Reston, VA 20190
Toll-Free: 800-AAA (222)-2336
Phone: 703-790-8466
Fax: 703-790-8631
Website: http://www.audiology.org/index.php

American Occupational Therapy Association
4720 Montgomery Lane
P.O. Box 31220
Bethesda, MD 20824-1220
Toll-Free: 800-377-8555 (TTY)
Phone: 301-652-2682
Fax: 301-652-7711
Website: http://www.aota.org

American Physical Therapy Association
1111 N. Fairfax St.
Alexandria, VA 22314-1488
Toll-Free: 800-999-2782
Phone: 703-684-2782
TTY: 703-683-6748
Fax: 703-684-7343
Website: http://www.apta.org
E-mail: practice@apta.org

American School Counselor Association
1101 King Street, Suite 625
Alexandria, VA 22314
Toll-Free: 800-306-4722
Phone: 703-683-2722
Website: http://www.schoolcounselor.org/
E-mail: asca@schoolcounselor.org

American Speech-Language-Hearing Association
10801 Rockville Pike
Rockville, MD 20852
Toll-Free (Public): 800-638-8255
Toll-Free (Professionals/Students): 800-498-2071
Phone (TTY): 301-571-0457
Website: http://www.asha.org
E-mail: actioncenter@asha.org

American Therapeutic Recreation Association
1414 Prince Street, Suite 204
Alexandria, VA 22314
Telephone: 703-683-9420
Fax: 703-683-9431
Website: http://www.atra-tr.org/atra.htm
E-mail: atra@atra-tr.org

National Consortium for Physical Education and Recreation for Individuals with Disabilities (NCPERID)
School of Physical Education, Wellness, and Sport Studies
University of South Florida
4202 E. Fowler Ave. PED 214
Tampa, FL 33620-8600
Phone: 813-974-3443
Fax: 813-974-4979
Website: http://ncperid.usf.edu

National Institute of Art and Disabilities (NIAD)
551 23rd Street
Richmond, CA 94804
Phone: 510-620-0290
Fax: 510-620-0326
Website: http://www.niadart.org
E-mail: admin@niadart.org

RESNA
Rehabilitative Engineering & Assistive Technology of North America
1700 N. Moore Street, Suite 1540
Arlington, VA 22209-1903
Phone: 703-524-6686
TTY: 703-524-6639
Fax: 703-524-6630
Website: http://www.resna.org
E-mail: natloffice@resna.org

National Dissemination Center for Children with Disabilities (also known as NICHCY)
P.O. Box 1492
Washington, DC 20013
Toll-Free (V/TTY): 800-695-0285
Fax: 202-884-8441
Website: http://www.nichcy.org
E-mail: nichcy@aed.org

Section 42.2

Your Rights in the Special Education Process

"Rights and Responsibilities of Parents of Children with Disabilities:
Update 1999," ERIC Clearinghouse on Disabilities and Gifted Education.

Parents of Children with Disabilities

Parents of children with disabilities have a vital role to play in the education of their children. This fact is guaranteed in federal legislation that specifies the right of parents to participate in the educational decision-making process. As your child progresses through educational systems, knowing and following through on your rights and responsibilities ensures that you are a contributing partner with professionals who will influence your child's future. This section provides you with an introduction to your rights and responsibilities in the special education process.

What Are Your Rights in the Special Education Process?

Public Law 101-476 (IDEA) clearly defines the rights of children with disabilities and their parents. A basic provision of the law is the right of parents to participate in the educational decision-making process. Your rights, more specifically, include the following:

- Your child is entitled to a free, appropriate public education, meaning it is at no cost to you as parents, and it meets the unique educational needs of your child.

- You will be notified whenever the school wishes to evaluate your child, wants to change your child's educational placement, or refuses your request for an evaluation or a change in placement.

- You may request an evaluation if you think your child needs special education or related services.

- You should be asked by your school to provide "parent consent" meaning you understand and agree in writing to the evaluation and initial special education placement for your child. Your consent is voluntary and may be withdrawn at any time.

- You may obtain an independent evaluation if you disagree with the outcome of the school's evaluation.

- You may request a reevaluation if you suspect your child's current educational placement is no longer appropriate. The school must reevaluate your child at least every 3 years, but your child's educational program must be reviewed at least once during each calendar year.

- You may have your child tested in the language he or she knows best. For example, if your child's primary language is Spanish, he or she must be tested in Spanish. Also, students who are hearing impaired have the right to an interpreter during the testing.

- The school must communicate with you in your primary language. The school is required to take whatever action is necessary to ensure that you understand its oral and written communication, including arranging for an interpreter if you are hearing impaired or if your primary language is not English

- You may review all of your child's records and obtain copies of these records, but the school may charge you a reasonable fee for making copies. Only you, as parents, and those persons directly involved in the education of your child will be given access to personal records. If you feel any of the information in your child's records is inaccurate, misleading, or violates the privacy or other rights of your child, you may request that the information be changed. If the school refuses your request, you then have the right to request a hearing to challenge the questionable information in your child's records.

- You must be fully informed by the school of all the rights provided to you and your child under the law.

- You may participate in the development of your child's Individualized Education Program (IEP) or, in the case of a child under school age, the development of an Individualized Family Service Plan (IFSP). The IEP and IFSP are written statements of the educational program designed to meet your child's unique needs. The school must make every possible effort to notify you of the IEP or IFSP meeting and arrange it at a time and place agreeable to you. As an important member of the team, you may attend the IEP or IFSP meeting and share your ideas about your child's special needs, the type of program appropriate to meeting those needs, and the related services the school will provide to help your child benefit from his or her educational program.

- You may have your child educated in the least restrictive school setting possible. Every effort should be made to develop an educational program that will provide the greatest amount of contact with children who are not disabled.

- You may request a due process hearing to resolve differences with the school that could not be resolved informally.

What Are Your Responsibilities in the Special Education Process?

Parental responsibilities to ensure that a child's rights are being protected are less clearly defined than are parental rights. These responsibilities vary depending on the child's disabling condition and other factors. Some of the following suggestions may be helpful:

- Develop a partnership with the school or agency. You are now an important member of the team. Share relevant information about your child's education and development. Your observations and suggestions can be a valuable resource to aid your child's progress.

- Learn as much as you can about your rights and the rights of your child. Ask the school to explain these rights as well as the regulations in effect for your district and state before you agree to a special education program for your child. Contact disability organizations for their publications on special education rights.

- Ask for clarification of any aspect of the program that is unclear to you. Educational and medical terms can be confusing, so do not hesitate to ask.

- Make sure you understand the program specified on the IEP or IFSP before agreeing to it or signing it. Ask yourself if what is planned corresponds with your knowledge of your child's needs.

- Consider how your child might be included in the regular school activities program. Do not forget areas such as lunch, recess, art, music, and physical education.

- Monitor your child's progress. If your child is not progressing, discuss it with the teacher and determine whether the program should be modified. As a parent, you can initiate review of your child's educational program.

- Discuss with the school or agency any problems that may occur with your child's assessment, placement, or educational program. It is best to try to resolve problems directly with the agency or school. In some situations, you may be uncertain as to how you should resolve a problem. All states have advocacy agencies that can usually provide you with the guidance you need to pursue your case.

- Keep records. There may be many questions and comments about your child that you will want to discuss, as well as meetings and phone conversations you will want to remember. It is easy to forget information useful to your child's development and education if it is not written down.

- Join a parent organization. In addition to the opportunity to share knowledge and support, a parent group can be an effective force on behalf of your child. Many times parents find that as a group they have the power to bring about needed changes that strengthen special services.

What Can You Offer the IEP or IFSP Process?

In the final analysis, parents of children with disabilities should be involved in the IEP or IFSP process as much as they want to be and as much as they can be. The following are suggestions for ways parents can become involved:

- Before attending an IEP or IFSP meeting, make a list of things you want your child to learn.

- Bring any information the school or agency may not already have to the IEP or IFSP meeting. Examples include copies of medical records, past school records, and test and medical evaluation results.

- Discuss what related services your child may need. Your child may need to be involved with many other specialists and professionals besides his or her teacher, including occupational therapists, physical therapists, or speech-language pathologists.

- Discuss what assistive technology devices or services your child may need and have these listed in your child's IEP or IFSP.

- Ask what you can do at home to support the program.

- Make sure the goals and objectives listed in the IEP or IFSP are specific and measurable.

- Periodically, ask for a report on your child's progress.

- Regard your child's education as a cooperative effort. If, at any point, you and the school cannot reach an agreement over your child's educational and developmental needs, ask to have another meeting. Remember, compromise on your part and the school's or agency's part may be important in resolving conflicts and maintaining a good working relationship. If, after a second meeting, there is still a conflict over your child's program, you may wish to ask for a state mediator or a due process hearing.

What Resources Are Available?

Many organizations have information to help guide you through the special education process. Since the specific criteria and procedures used by school districts vary, it is important to familiarize yourself with the information provided by state and local agencies. You will find your local school district's director of special education and his or her staff helpful in accessing such information and guiding you through the process.

Additional resources are available from national disability organizations. Some of them have state and local chapters that can provide more locally based support. All states now have federally supported parent information and training centers. The contacts cited may be able to help you locate such a center in your state:

The Council for Exceptional Children (CEC)
1110 North Glebe Road
Suite 300
Arlington, VA 22201
Phone: 703-620-3660
TTY: 866-915-5000 (text only)
Fax: 703-264-9494
Website: http://www.cec.sped.org/

National Dissemination Center for Children with Disabilities (also known as NICHCY)
P.O. Box 1492
Washington, DC 20013-1492
Toll-Free: 800-695-0285
Phone: 202-884-8200 (V/TTY)
Fax: 202-884-8441
Website: http://nichcy.org
E-mail: nichcy@aed.org

Sources

National Information Center for Children and Youth with Disabilities (1993). "Individualized Education Programs (IEPs): Federal Regulations and Appendix C to Part 300." NICHCY Briefing Paper. Washington, DC.

National Information Center for Children and Youth with Disabilities (1993). "Questions and Answers about the IDEA." NICHCY *News Digest*, Volume 3, Number 2. Washington, DC.

Section 42.3

Integration of the Student with Muscular Dystrophy into a School Physical Program

All students, whether disabled or not, have a need to feel part of their peer group. Sports are a great way that students can get involved with each other in a fun and active way. Self esteem is also increased when they feel they are making a worthy contribution. It is easy for MD students to miss out on this opportunity. This is where you can help. In the PE program, by modifying game rules or using different equipment, you can involve the MD student physically in part of your session. This is important as they are particularly at risk of becoming socially isolated. If play is not possible, they should be encouraged to be part of the group by umpiring, scoring, or coaching.

Schools are in a unique position, to introduce students to a variety of sports from which they can make decisions as to which community sports they wish to pursue. This should be true for MD students too. There are sporting clubs for individuals with MD where games are designed for them and competition is between MD players only. However, if MD students are not introduced to these sports at school they may never discover the enjoyment that can be experienced through playing them.

Modified Games

Sporting games are listed that form a part of the secondary school curriculum and suggested changes that can be made to include the MD student. Remember that the emphasis should be on enjoyment and play rather than competition for the MD student and the others involved.

Softball

Set up a tee (normally used in tee ball) and have a lightweight bat and ball for the MD student when it is his turn to bat. (Use a plastic bat, a foam ball, a large rubber ball or plastic ball with holes). These can be purchased from service stations, toy shops, or sports stores. This equipment should only substitute normal playing equipment for the MD student. Also give him an opportunity to hit a ball thrown to him (The ball should be bigger and the throw should be much softer).

To overcome weakness in shoulder movements, advise MD students to hold the bat with one hand and swing their wheelchair around. The force of the swing to hit the ball will come from the wheelchair momentum, not the strength of their arm. To make it possible for him to reach first base rule that the ball must be thrown to two people before it reaches first base.

When fielding, attach a piece of foam to the wheelchair in front of the student's legs so that they can move around the outside of the diamond and stop the ball. A bike basket could also be attached to the side of the wheelchair so he can move into positions under the ball for a catch. If the ball touches the bike basket on the full the batter is out.

Soccer

Include the student in the soccer drills with a big balloon soccer ball or physio ball. MD students can practice head butting, and kicking using his wheelchair, to other students or the aide.

Half field balloon soccer can be played for about 20 minutes to involve the MD student for part of the session. It can also utilize skills the other students have learned in an easy and fun way. Another option is to divide the class into those who want to play a fun game of balloon soccer with the MD student and those who want to play a full field game of soccer.

Hockey

To modify hockey to suit an MD student, quite a few changes need to be made and special equipment must be used. The game can be played in a similar way to soccer. It is played on an indoor or outdoor tennis or basketball court, with five players in each team. Each has a lightweight hockey stick. A plastic ball with holes is used and cones can mark the goal area at each end.

Golf

For a higher functioning MD student position him forward in a wheelchair to make access to hitting the ball possible. Support his arms to make shoulder movement easier for him, and if necessary allow him to use lightweight hockey stick.

For a lower functioning student limit golf to putting only. Use the practice green at the beginning of the golf course or put the ball at the edge of each putting green and score the amount of hits it takes him to get the ball into the hole (so he does not have to drive it down the range).

Orienteering

This is a great sport for MD students to be involved in because it does not require much modification. Because of this MD students are made to feel a part of the group and can compete against the other students on the same level

Prepare well. Organize the course so that a wheelchair can get around it. Have simple codes at each checkpoint that can be copied by the MD student.

Have students go out in pairs. This is safer for all the students, but particularly for the MD student. Encourage the MD student's partner to allow him to do as much as possible. A compass can be fixed to the arm of his wheelchair. The map can be laid flat and stuck to his table that fits into his wheelchair.

It is understood that modifying games may take away a sense of competition for the other students. Therefore games will need to be played without the MD student being physically involved. However, when this occurs engage him in other ways. Encourage him to know the rules well and become a good umpire.

Teaching Umpire Skills

Take time to teach the MD student the rules of each sport. This can be done while explaining the rules to the other students. Give them a set of rules and go through these with the student to make sure he understands.

Video replays of the television coverage of sports are another way of teaching sporting skills to students and umpiring skills to the MD student. Student's learn by example so while the MD student is learning what is required to be a good umpire, his classmates are learning specific skills such as footwork and racket swing.

Umpire with the MD student until he is confident. Give encouragement and praise.

An alarm (for example, a self defense alarm) may need to be used if the MD student cannot use a whistle comfortably as he may find it difficult to continually bring it up to his mouth.

Warm Up Activities

If it is not possible for the MD student to participate in the whole PE session, it is important for him to be involved for a short time in pre-game activities. Therefore a few activities that specifically involve the MD student and so help teach skills to the other students have been suggested. However, these are only examples of how activities can be modified.

Beanbag Hockey

This game should be played indoors on a wooden court. Divide the group into 2 teams and give each student a number. Use rolled up newspaper for 3 hockey sticks, a beanbag, and 2 chairs for goals. Place the beanbag and 2 hockey sticks in the middle of the chairs and then call a number. The people from each team with that number run to the middle and aim to score a goal for their team by hitting the beanbag under their chair.

Allow the MD student to hold a hockey-stick so that he does not have to reach down and pick one up when his number is called.

Balloon Volleyball

This game should be played indoors on a wooden volleyball court. Divide the group into 2 teams and have each team stand down their side line except 1 player who stands in the center of the court with a badminton racket. Play starts when 1 player hits a balloon over the net. After playing he runs to the end of the line and the person at the beginning of the line runs on to the court to play next. Meanwhile the player of the side must try to hit the balloon back over the net. If that player does not get if over, the next person in line tries. The side has 3 chances to hit the balloon over. Play continues until one side scores 11 points.

Obstacle Course

An obstacle course can be set up by using cones, chairs, gym mats, landmarks and anything else in the sports storeroom. Two similar courses can be set up and the class can be divided into two teams. The MD student can be one team and an able-bodied student in a manual wheelchair on the other team. using this method, the competition between the teams will be equal. All the players on each team must complete the obstacle course. The team that finishes first is the winner.

The obstacle course can be modified to teach a number of different skills. An example is to hit a ball with a hockey stick or kick a soccer ball around the course.

Safety Issues

Some games could possibly be modified for the MD student, but because he is in a wheelchair it would be dangerous to have him on the field competing against other students for the ball. Therefore safety of the other children must be considered.

Safety of the MD student is also important. Remember that:

- Balance is easily lost.
- Fatigue is a serious hazard. Only moderate exercise should be done.
- No strain should be exerted.
- Strength exercises are contraindicated.
- Consultation with the student's doctor or parents is recommended to ensure that activities and planned modifications will have no adverse effects.
- Although safety of the MD student is essential, it does not mean that he should be over protected. All MD students are likely to fall at some stage, but like other individuals recover quickly.

Further Guidelines for Teachers

As integration into normal sport for the MD students is relatively new, you will need to discover their interest and work with them to make participation appealing and accepting. Praise and encouragement are essential in motivating them to be involved.

It is important to have an understanding of which muscle groups are more severely affected and which movements are possible. This allows you to concentrate on what they can do rather than on what they cannot do. Through this, their abilities will be strengthened and realistic goals will be obtained.

Do not underestimate what they can do.

Motivate the MD student to participate as much as possible. When the other students go for a jog around the oval or run a cross country event, encourage the MD student to drive around in his wheelchair with them.

Put some thought into how you can modify further sporting activities to allow some types of participation of the MD student with the group. This is important because as his peers are expanding their experiences and skills in sport, he is progressively becoming limited in his movement, experiences, and skills.

The whole class can also be involved in setting the rules so the MD student can participate. In this way competition can still be maintained and the MD student will be accepted by his peers.

Muscular dystrophy progresses at different rates in each MD student, therefore each child will have a different degree of muscle weakness. Using the information will give you an understanding of how to integrate them into a normal sport program; however, it is by no means comprehensive. Sport programs must be planned on an individual basis according to the child's abilities and limitations.

Chapter 43

Estate Planning Issues When Parents Have a Disabled Child

Chapter Contents

Section 43.1—Overview of Estate Planning 478
Section 43.2—The Letter of Intent 486
Section 43.3—The Special Needs Trust 493

Section 43.1

Overview of Estate Planning

"Overview of Estate Planning Issues," by Lawrence A Frolik, J.D.,
L.L.M., National Dissemination Center for Children with Disabilities
(NICHCY), updated 1994. reviewed 2004.

When parents have a son or daughter with any type of disability, they must plan their estates carefully to best benefit that child. How parents leave their assets after death may greatly affect the quality of life for their son or daughter with special needs. This section presents basic information to help parents begin considering the very important issues involved in developing an estate plan when the future of a son or daughter with a disability must be taken into account.

Many families believe that they have so few assets that an estate plan is not necessary. This is not true. We often have more assets than we realize, although some assets may become important only after our death. The most notable asset of this type is life insurance. Therefore, whether you consider yourselves a family of substantial means or with little or no assets, estate planning should be done.

How the Type of Disability Affects Estate Planning

Disabilities, of course, can take many forms and have varying degrees of severity. The nature and severity of your child's disability will affect the nature of the estate plan that you, as parents, develop.

Physical disabilities or health impairments. Many individuals have physical disabilities or health impairments that do not affect their ability to manage financial or other affairs. If your son or daughter has such a condition, how to leave your estate depends on a number of factors. The primary factor will be whether or not your son or daughter receives (or may one day need to depend on) government benefits such as Supplemental Security Insurance (SSI), subsidized housing, personal attendant care, or Medicaid. If your child does receive (or may one day need to depend on) government benefits, then it is most important to create a special estate plan that does not negate his or her eligibility for those benefits.

On the other hand, you may have a son or daughter with a physical disability or health impairment who is not eligible for or who is not receiving government benefits. In this case, you may be able to dispense with elaborate planning devices and merely leave your child money outright, as you would to a nondisabled child. If you believe that the disability may reduce your son or daughter's financial earning capability, you may want to take special care to leave a greater portion of your estate to this child than to your nondisabled children.

There are some exceptions to this simplified approach, of course. One exception is when parents are somewhat fearful of their son or daughter's financial judgment. If you are concerned that your son or daughter with a disability may not responsibly handle an inheritance, then you can utilize a trust, just as you would for a nondisabled heir. Another exception is if your child's disability or health impairment involves the future possibility of deteriorating health and more involved health care needs. While your son or daughter may be capable of earning money and managing an inheritance at present or in the immediate future, in twenty or thirty years time deteriorating health may make it difficult for him or her to maintain employment or pay for health care. Government benefits might then become critical to your child's security. Remember, benefits include much more than money; your child may also be eligible for valuable services such as health care, vocational rehabilitation, supported employment, subsidized housing, and personal attendant care. If, however, he or she acquires too many assets through inheriting all or part of your estate, he or she may be ineligible for these benefits. Therefore, in order to protect your son or daughter's eligibility for government benefits at some point in the future and to provide for his or her long-range needs, you may need to consider establishing a special estate plan.

Cognitive disabilities or mental illness. If your son or daughter's disability affects his or her mental capability, the need to create a special estate plan is more clearcut. Mental illness and cognitive disabilities often impair a person's ability to manage his or her own financial affairs while simultaneously increasing financial need. As a result, you must take care to ensure that there are assets available after your death to help your son or daughter, while also providing that the assets are protected from his or her inability to manage them. More information will be given later in this section about various ways to accomplish this. First, however, let us take a look at some basic information about wills and why a will is so important.

Writing a Will

All parents, but particularly parents of individuals with disabilities, should have a will. The object of the will is to ensure that all of the assets of the deceased parent are distributed according to his or her wishes.

If at death you have no will, your property will be dispersed according to the law of the state in which you live at the time of your death. This law is called the state's law of intestacy. Although laws of intestacy vary from state to state, in general they provide that some percent of assets of the decedent passes to the surviving spouse and the rest is distributed to the children in equal shares. Writing a will is highly recommended, since the laws of intestacy are rarely the most desirable way to pass property to one's heirs.

Although it is theoretically possible for any individual to write a will on his or her own, it is unwise to do so. Because of the technical nature of wills, it is highly advisable to have a lawyer prepare one. Parents of individuals with disabilities particularly need legal advice because they often have special planning concerns. If you do not have a lawyer, you can call the local bar association which will provide you with the name of an attorney in your vicinity. It is preferable, however, to contact a local disabilities group which may be able to put you in contact with an attorney familiar with estate planning for parents of persons with disabilities. Not all lawyers are familiar with the special needs associated with caring and providing for individuals with disabilities. Before you hire a lawyer, be sure to find out if he or she has ever prepared estates for other parents who have sons or daughters with disabling conditions. If the lawyer has not, it is best to find a more experienced attorney. The cost of an attorney varies according to the attorney's standard fee and the complexities of the estate. The attorney can quote you a price based upon an estimation of the work. If the price quoted is beyond your immediate means, it may be possible to negotiate a payment plan with the attorney whereby you pay over time.

When making a will, however, remember that not all the assets you control are governed by a will. Joint property with right of survivorship, for example, passes independently of a will. If, for example, Tim and Sarah own a house as joint owners with rights of survivorship, upon Tim's death Sarah automatically inherits the house without regard to what Tim's will might say. Similarly, life insurance is paid out to the named beneficiary without regard to the will. The insurance is a contract between the owner and the insurance company, and the insurance company must pay the insurance to whomever the owner states. Many individuals have death benefits under an employer-provided pension plan. These, too, are not governed by the will, but are paid to whomever the employee has designated. (Note: If you create a special estate plan to provide for your child with a disability—in particular, if you set up a special needs trust—review any life insurance policies you have purchased, and be sure that you have not designated your child as a beneficiary. The same is true for relatives who may have designated your child as the beneficiary of their policies.)

Personal property, such as clothing, furniture, and household effects, should be distributed by the will independently of the often more valuable assets such as stocks, bonds, and real estate. Personal property is often of great sentimental importance, but may have little financial value. To avoid disharmony after the death of the last parent, it is generally a good idea to make an equal division of the personal property among the children. In some cases, the parents may wish not to include the child with the disability in the division, particularly if that might disqualify this person from government benefits. However, in most cases it is advisable to leave the person with a disability a share of the personal property so that he or she does not feel excluded.

Remember, a will goes into effect only upon the death of the person who created it. Until death, the creator of the will can freely revoke, alter, or replace it.

How to Start Planning Your Estate: What to Consider

When parents have a son or daughter with a disability, they should give careful consideration to developing an estate plan that provides for that person's future best interests. Here are some suggestions that can help parents approach planning their estate when a son or daughter with a disability must be taken into consideration.

First: Realistically assess your son or daughter's disability and the prognosis for future development. If necessary, obtain a professional evaluation of your child's prospects and capability to earn a living and to manage financial assets. If your son or daughter is already an adult, you should have a fairly clear understanding of his or her capabilities.

But if your child is younger, it may be more difficult to predict the future. In such cases, you should take a conservative view. It is better to anticipate all possibilities, good and bad, in such a way that you do not limit your loved one's potential or set him or her up for unrealistic expectations. Remember, too, that you can change your estate plan as more information about your child becomes available.

Second: Carefully inventory your financial affairs. Estimate the size of your estate (what you own) if you should die within the next year or the next ten years. Keep in mind that the will you write governs your affairs at the time of your death, and so it must be flexible enough to meet a variety of situations. Of course you can always write a new will, but you may never actually write it due to hectic schedules, procrastination, or oversight. Thus, the will you have written must have sufficient flexibility to meet life's ever changing circumstances.

Third: Consider the living arrangements of your son or daughter with a disability. Your child's living arrangements after your death are of paramount importance. Every parent of an individual with a disability should give thought to the questions, "If my spouse and I should die tomorrow, where would our child live? What are the possibilities available to him or her?" The prospective living arrangements of your son or daughter will have a tremendous impact on how your estate should be distributed. Involved in answering the question of living arrangements is whether or not your child will need a guardian or conservator to make decisions for him or her after your death. If you conclude that a guardian or conservator is necessary, you should be prepared to recommend a potential guardian or conservator in your will.

Fourth: Analyze the earning potential of your son or daughter. It is important to determine how much your child can be expected to contribute financially, as a result of employment. If he or she is currently employed, does this employment meet all of his or her living expenses, or only some? If your child is presently too young to be employed, you will have to project into the future. In many cases, even if your son or daughter is employed or expected to be employed at some point in the future, he or she will require additional financial assistance.

Fifth: Consider what government benefits your son or daughter needs and is eligible to receive. Support for a person with a disability will usually come from state and federal benefits. These might be actual case grants, such as social security or supplemental security income, or they might be in-kind support programs, such as subsidized housing or sheltered workshop employment.

In brief, government benefits can be divided into three categories. First are those categories that are unaffected by the financial resources of the beneficiary. For example, social security disability insurance (SSDI) beneficiaries receive their benefits without regard to financial need. Regardless of what the parents leave to a son or daughter with a disability, the social security payments will still be forthcoming once the person has qualified for them.

Second, some government benefits, such as supplemental security income (SSI) and Medicaid, have financial eligibility requirements. If a person with a disability has too many assets or too much income, he or she is not eligible to receive any or all of these benefits. Someone who is eligible due to a lack of financial resources can become ineligible upon inheriting money, property, or other assets. This would lead to a reduction or termination of the SSI benefits for that person. Therefore, if your son or daughter is receiving government benefits that have financial eligibility requirements, it is important to arrange your estate in a manner that will minimize his or her loss of benefits, especially SSI or Medicaid.

Finally, there are government programs available to individuals with disabilities where payment for services is determined according to the person's ability to pay. Many states will charge the individual with a disability for programmatic benefits if he or she has sufficient assets or income. The most striking is the charge that can be levied against residents of state mental institutions. For example, if a resident of a state hospital inherits a substantial sum of money, the state will begin charging the resident for the cost of residency in the state hospital and will continue to charge until all the money is exhausted. Yet the services provided will be no different from the ones that he or she was previously receiving.

Establishing a Will: Four Possible Approaches

Having decided what your son or daughter needs and what you own, you can now consider how best to assist him or her. There are four possible ways to do so.

First, you can disinherit your son or daughter with the disability. No state requires parents to leave money to their children, disabled or not. If your assets are relatively modest and your son or daughter's needs relatively great, the best advice may be to disinherit your child by name and have him or her rely upon federal and state supports after your death. This may be the wisest decision, particularly if you wish to help your other children. Instead of complete disinheritance, you might leave your son or daughter with a disability a gift of modest but sentimental value, such as his or her bedroom furniture. The value of the gift will be small enough not to affect government benefits, but it will indicate your love and concern.

Second, you can leave your son or daughter with a disability an outright gift. For example, suppose your son Tom has a physical disability. You might write a will that states, "I leave one-third of my estate to my son, Tom."

If your child with a disability is not receiving (and is not expected in the future to need) government benefits, this may prove to be a desirable course of action. Your son or daughter, if mentally competent, can hire whatever assistance he or she needs to help with managing the gift. But if your son or daughter has a mental illness or cognitive disability, an outright gift is never a good idea, because this person may not be able to handle the financial responsibilities. If you want to leave a gift to support your child, the use of a trust is far preferable.

Third, you can leave a morally obligated gift to another of your children. Suppose, for example, that the parents have two children: James, who has mental retardation, and Mary, who has no disabilities. The parents leave all of their assets to Mary. Legally, Mary now owns all of the parents' assets and James owns nothing. But prior to their deaths, the parents told Mary that, although they are leaving everything to her, they expect her to use at least half of the money to assist James in whatever way Mary thinks best. They left the money to Mary because they do not wish James to lose his government benefits, and they think that there are ways that Mary could use the money to help her brother. For example, Mary might provide special gifts to James on holidays or pay for special assistance for James that would not be provided by the government benefit programs. The gift is a moral obligation to Mary because legally she can ignore the parents' wishes and do whatever she wants with the money. It is hers. It is only her conscience that guides her. After the parents' death, if Mary chooses to ignore James and use the money for herself, there is nothing James or anyone else can do about it. Morally obligated gifts are often used by parents with modest-sized estates for whom a trust does not seem desirable. The danger of morally obligated gifts is, of course, that the morally obligated recipient—in our example, Mary—may ignore the wishes of the parents. Even if Mary does not deliberately ignore the obligation, she may encounter circumstances that make it impossible for her to carry out her parents' wishes. Suppose, for example, that Mary or her children become ill or are in great financial need. She may feel under pressure to use the money for her own family, even if it means that James goes unassisted. Moreover, if Mary dies before James, it is possible that Mary's family will not carry on the duty to help James. Finally, in case Mary is divorced, the money may be lost to her former spouse in a settlement.

Morally obligated gifts, therefore, are not a complete solution. They can be useful, however, especially when the parents have a modest amount of money, and do not expect a lifetime of care for their son or daughter with a disability. Rather, they merely want their nondisabled sons or daughters to use some of the inherited money to assist their sibling with special needs.

Fourth, you can establish a trust for your son or daughter with a disability. For many parents who have a child with disabilities, the use of a trust is the most effective way to help that individual. The point of a trust is to keep assets in a form that will be available to your son or daughter, but that will not disqualify him or her for government benefits for which he or she might otherwise be eligible.

In A Parent's Words

It had been in the back of my mind for years, soon after I found out my son Samuel had this lifelong disability. What would the future hold for him when I wasn't there anymore to be his advocate, friend, and supporter? It was both a big and little worry. Big, because it gave me a hole in my gut whenever the questions crept in; and little, in the sense that I tried not to think about it. I'd think: I'll worry about that tomorrow, next week, when he's older, when I'm older.

Of course, I've done things to prepare Samuel for that future he's going to have without me, things like teaching him how to wash clothes and shop. But could I write a will? Make an estate plan? No, for years, I dodged that one totally.

Then, when his voice started to change, it suddenly hit me that he was growing up, that he was older now. That future I was always worrying about, and refusing to worry about, was beginning to arrive. I talked with my husband, and I found out he'd been worrying about Sam's future, too. So he and I went to our lawyer. I was so nervous, to bring all the questions out in the open and look at them. No wonder I'd shoved them under the bed for so long!

But you know, it's funny. Now that we're finished setting up our estate and only need periodically to review our plans, I feel like an enormous burden has been lifted up from me. The big, black, scary shadow is gone. Well, not totally gone, I suppose. I still worry about Samuel, what will happen to him in his life. I guess every parent does that. But now I don't worry in the same way. I know I've done all I can do for that part of his future, something that was extremely important to do, and I am very relieved. Now I feel like we can deal fully with the present day and see to the other things that need to be done to prepare Samuel for life as a man. And that's very exciting.

Section 43.2

The Letter of Intent

"The Letter of Intent," by Richard W. Fee, National Institute on Life Planning for Persons with Disabilities, National Dissemination Center for Children with Disabilities (NICHCY). updated 1994, reviewed 2004.

What Is the Letter of Intent?

Simply put, the Letter of Intent is a document written by you (the parents or guardians) or other family members that describes your son or daughter's history, his or her current status, and what you hope for him or her in the future. You would be wise to write this letter today and add to it as the years go by, updating it when information about your son or daughter changes. To the maximum extent possible, it is also a good idea to involve your child in the writing of this Letter, so that the Letter truly presents and represents your child. The Letter is then ready at any moment to be used by all the individuals who will be involved in caring for your son or daughter should you become ill or disabled yourself, or when you should pass away.

Even though the Letter of Intent is not a legal document, the courts and others can rely upon the Letter for guidance in understanding your son or daughter and the wishes of you, the parents. In this way, you can continue to speak out on behalf of your son or daughter, providing insight and knowledge about his or her own best possible care.

Why Is It Important to Write a Letter of Intent?

A Letter of Intent serves many purposes. First, it spells out in black and white your son or daughter's background and history and his or her present situation. It also describes your wishes, hopes, and desires for his or her future care, and where possible, describes your child's feelings about the present and desires for the future. While you are still living, the Letter can be used by your lawyers and financial planners to draft the proper legal documents (wills and/or trusts) to ensure your wishes are carried out. Once you are no longer able to take care of your son or daughter, due to death or illness—and this is the most important reason to write a Letter of Intent—the Letter gives your son or daughter's future caregivers some insight into how to care for him or her. It provides advice on possible alternatives for his or her care. If your child has a severe disability, caregivers will not have to waste precious time learning the most appropriate behavior or medical management techniques to use. If your child is used to doing things independently and only requires occasional assistance, the Letter can spell out exactly what is needed. The Letter of Intent can describe this very concrete information and much, much more, including valuable information about the personality of your son or daughter—his or her likes, dislikes, talents, special problems, and strengths. Thus, the Letter is a crucial part of any life or estate plan, because it speaks both for and about the person with a disability and his or her family.

When Should Parents Write the Letter of Intent?

The answer is a simple one. Start now. Start today. Procrastination is easy, when your health is good, the future looks bright, and there are a hundred other pressing tasks to be done. But none of us can predict the future. What will happen to your son or daughter, if something happens to you? Will your relatives, friends, lawyer, or the police know where to contact your son or daughter—and will that person know enough about your loved one to know what kind of care is needed and how best to provide it?

Writing the Letter of Intent now is a way to protect your son or daughter from unnecessary chaos and turmoil when he or she must depend upon someone other than you for the care and support that is necessary. The Letter of Intent helps pave your son or daughter's transition by giving future caregivers the information about him or her that they so vitally need.

Preparing the Letter is often an emotional experience for parents and their children. You will need self-discipline and motivation to work past the many painful questions and issues that must be addressed when considering your son or daughter's future.

What Information Goes Into the Letter of Intent?

How can you summarize the life of a person you have watched grow and develop over many years? What can you say that will give insight into and perhaps touch the heart of a careprovider who must suddenly assume some measure of responsibility for your son or daughter?

Basically, the procedures for developing a Letter of Intent are fairly simple. You can write the Letter out longhand, or you can use a computer or typewriter. Do not worry about perfect spelling or grammar; your major concern is that anyone who reads the Letter in the future can understand exactly what you meant and what you would like to see happen in your son or daughter's life. Begin by addressing the Letter to "To Whom It May Concern." In the first paragraph list the current names, addresses, and telephone numbers of the people who should be contacted if anything should happen to you (i.e., other children, case manager, your son or daughter's school principal or employer, lawyer, financial planner, priest, etc.). You might then briefly state the family history; include names, birth dates, and addresses of family members.

The Letter will then need to focus in upon seven potentially major areas of your son or daughter's past, present, and future life. Depending upon your child's needs, these areas may be: housing/residential care, education, employment, medical history and care, behavior management, social environment, and religious environment. You might begin by summarizing your son or daughter's background and present status in each of these areas. Then summarize your wishes, hopes, and desires for his or her best future, listing three or four options in each of these areas. Be sure to discuss your ideas with your son or daughter and to take into consideration his or her feelings on the future. The worksheet shown at the end of this section is useful for this future planning step, which may require much thought and planning before you actually begin to write information into the Letter of Intent.

Take a brief look at the example marked "An Example for Writing a Letter of Intent." This example focuses on only one of the major life areas—Housing/Residential Care—and illustrates how a person named Mrs. Sanders went about writing this section of her Letter of Intent for her son named Chris, a 35-year-old man with developmental disabilities.

How Do I Involve My Son or Daughter in Writing the Letter?

How much you involve your son or daughter in writing the Letter of Intent will depend in large part upon his or her age and the nature and severity of the disability. It is only fitting that young adults and adult children be involved in planning their own lives to the maximum extent possible. Many individuals have disabilities that do not prevent their full or partial participation in the Letter-writing process. Before involving your child, however, you, as parents, might want to talk first among yourselves about the content of the Letter and your ideas regarding your child's future. When you have agreed upon the basic information you feel should go in the Letter, discuss each area with your son or daughter. Ask for your child's input about his or her favorite things to do, what type of education has been enjoyable and what might be pursued in the future, what type of employment he or she enjoys or envisions. Equally crucial to discuss are your child's future living arrangements: How does your child feel about the options you are considering listing in the Letter of Intent?

It is important that your child realize that the Letter is not a binding, legal document; it is written to give guidance, not edicts, to all those involved in caregiving in the future. If you fear that your child will be upset by talking about a future that does not involve you as parents, then you may wish to make the discussion simply about the future—what will happen when your child leaves high school or a post-secondary training program, what your child wants to be or do in the next ten years, where he or she wants to live. You may be surprised to find that discussing the future actually relieves your child. He or she may very well be worrying about what will happen when you are no longer there to provide whatever assistance is needed.

Involving your child in discussing and making decisions about the future may be more difficult if the individual has a disability that severely limits his or her ability to communicate or to judge between a variety of options. You, as parents, are probably the best judges of how much—and how—you can involve a son or daughter with a severe cognitive disability. For these children, the Letter is especially critical; it will serve to communicate the vital information about themselves that they cannot.

An Example for Writing a Letter of Intent

Titling a section of her Letter "Housing/Residential Care," Mrs. Sanders writes that Chris has always lived at home and had a room to himself. She briefly describes the family home and the articles in the home that give Chris special pleasure, such as his portable radio.

She then describes his daily and weekly routine, including the fact that Chris finds great joy in going to dances each week at the local Arc. She briefly lists his favorite clothing, food, games, and so on. She also mentions that each year Chris visits his sister for a week in the summer.

Mrs. Sanders then considers what future living arrangements might be suitable for Chris, and she uses the worksheet at the end of this section (Letter of Intent Worksheet) to jot down three options. Before she transfers these options from the worksheet to her Letter of Intent, she discusses each one with Chris. She does so because he needs to be a key member of the team planning his future life.

Following her talk with Chris, Mrs. Sanders lists the agreed upon information in her Letter of Intent. The first option she lists is the possibility that Chris might live with his sister. As a second possibility, he might live with an old family friend. The third option is residence in a group home. Because this last option may indeed be the one that is finally selected for Chris, Mrs. Sanders takes care to describe the type of group home she thinks he would enjoy. As a mother and lifelong friend to Chris, she sees past his limitations to his strengths, and she notes these down in some detail. Lastly, she expresses her desire that the group home will give him room to grow and build upon those strengths.

Residential care is just one important area for Mrs. Sanders to cover in her Letter of Intent. It takes her a week to complete the other sections. She finds that describing the past is not nearly as difficult as considering the future, but she methodically and systematically works her way through each area, using the worksheet when planning is necessary. The end result is a Letter of Intent that is twelve pages long, handwritten. She feels comfortable that anyone picking up this Letter of Intent will have a head start in getting to know and care for Chris.

What Happens Once the Letter of Intent Is Written?

Once you have written the Letter of Intent about your son or daughter, the first, most important thing to do is to let people know that there is a Letter of Intent available to be consulted. This might mean telling your other children (or relatives, neighbors, friends, workshop director, pastor, or case manager) why you have written the Letter, what type of information it contains, and where the Letter can be found. Put the Letter in an easily accessible place, and make it clearly identifiable. Many parents also make copies of the Letter and give it to their other children (or persons such as a neighbor).

Secondly, you should update the Letter on a regular basis. Select one day out of each year (such as the last day of school or perhaps your son or daughter's birthday) where you will review what you have written and add any new information of importance. Talk with your child each time and incorporate his or her ideas. After each addition, sign and date the Letter. Should something change in your son or daughter's life, such as his or her caseworker or the medication he or she is taking, update the Letter immediately.

In Conclusion

Will your Letter of Intent overcome all of the obstacles to your son or daughter's transition into someone else's care? No, of course not. However, the Letter is of immediate usefulness in coping with your son or daughter's changed situation and, in the long term, will certainly help careproviders understand and care for your loved one.

Letter of Intent Worksheet: Considering Your Son or Daughter's Future

For each applicable area listed, consider your son or daughter's future. List 3–4 options to guide future caregivers in decision making and interaction with your child. Draw upon what you know about your son or daughter, through observation and through discussion with your child, and share what you have learned!

Residence: If something should happen to you tomorrow, where will your son or daughter live?

Education: You have a lifelong perspective of your son or daughter's capabilities. Share it.

Employment: What has your son or daughter enjoyed? Consider his or her goals, aspirations, limitations, etc.

Medical Care: What has and has not worked with your son or daughter? What should future caregivers know?

Behavior Management: What consistent approach has worked best in your absence during difficult transition periods in your son or daughter's life?

Social: What activities make life meaningful for your son or daughter?

Religious: Is there a special church or synagogue or person your son or daughter prefers for fellowship?

Additional Considerations

Advocate/Guardian: Who will look after, fight for, and be a friend to your son or daughter? (List 3–4 options.)

Trustee(s): Who do you trust to manage your son or daughter's supplementary funds? (List 3–4 options.)

Section 43.3

The Special Needs Trust

"The Special Needs Trust," by Richard W. Fee, National Institute on
Life Planning for Persons with Disabilities, National Dissemination
Center for Children with Disabilities (NICHCY), updated 1994, re-
viewed 2004.

Imagine for a moment that one evening, on your way home from a
movie or a dinner party, you and your spouse pass away in an automobile accident. While you were always planning to write a will, you
never actually got around to it, so your modest estate, including some
life insurance, is distributed by the laws of your state. You have two
sons, one with a disability and one without. Each of your sons inherits $100,000.

Your older son, Frank—who does not have a disability—uses his
inheritance to pay off some of his mortgage and splurge on a new car.
In contrast, your younger son Johnny gains nothing and loses much.
Johnny, who has multiple disabilities, does not work and relies solely
on government benefits for housing and medical care. The inheritance causes Johnny to lose those benefits. He must now provide
for his own medical care, which includes the considerable cost of
medicine, personal care attendants, physical therapy, and doctor's
visits. The group home in which he lives begins to charge him for
residency and for the services he receives there. Within two years,
all but $2,000 of the inheritance is gone. At this point Johnny again
becomes eligible for government benefits and is re-instated after
a waiting period of several months—a period in which he uses up the
last of his inheritance. Now there are no funds left to pay for whatever supplemental needs Johnny might have: education, over-the-
counter medicines, dental care beyond what is covered by government
benefits, trips to see his brother or other family members, reading
materials, supplies such as razors, soap, and shampoo. Government
benefits do not cover these types of expenses, and Johnny's parents
are no longer here to do so. The irony of the situation is that, while
an inheritance should ordinarily improve a person's lifestyle, this one
has worsened Johnny's.

493

The Question of Relying on Government Benefits Only

The first question that comes to mind when something like this occurs is one of fairness. Should the government continue to subsidize someone who has money? On one hand, the standard government programs such as SSI and Medicaid were established to help persons who are elderly or who are disabled and living at the poverty level. On the other hand, government benefit programs are paid for out of tax dollars, and eligible individuals are entitled to receive these benefits.

When families consider this question, they should be aware that, while the services available through government benefit programs may be substantial (e.g., medical coverage through Medicaid), the actual cash benefits are generally quite small and force the individual to live way below the poverty level. In 1992, the maximum Federal SSI monthly payment was $422 for an individual. This means that, for an individual with a disability to have any type of meaningful lifestyle, the family or local charities have to provide supplemental assistance.

With changes in the Social Security Administration, the primary government benefit programs are recognizing that family contributions to the person's well-being can only improve his or her overall quality of life. As long as the family's contributions are supplementary in nature, as opposed to duplicating government benefit programs, they are permitted. Thus, the current government benefit programs do permit the family to provide some supplementary income and resources to the person with a disability. However, the government regulations are very strict, and they are carefully monitored.

Special Needs Trust

The only reliable method of making sure that the inheritance actually has a chance of reaching a person with a disability when he or she needs it is through the legal device known as a Special Needs Trust (SNT). The SNT is developed to manage resources while maintaining the individual's eligibility for public assistance benefits. How is this done? Simply put, the family leaves whatever resources it deems appropriate to the trust. The trust is managed by a trustee on behalf of the person with the disability.

While government agencies recognize special needs trusts, they have imposed some very stringent rules and regulations upon them. This is why it is vital that any family contemplating using a SNT consult an experienced attorney—not just one who does general estate planning, but one who is very knowledgeable about SNTs and current government benefit programs. One wrong word or phrase can make the difference between an inheritance that really benefits the person with a disability, and one that causes the person to lose access to a wide range of needed services and assistance. As an illustration of this, suppose that the trust instructed the trustee (manager) to pay the person with the disability $100 a month for life. Such a mandatory income might jeopardize government benefit programs which may only allow him or her to have $70 of income each month.

The first thing that may come to mind for most families who have had experience with government benefits is that the government says that a person with a disability cannot have a trust. Correct. However, the special needs trust does not belong to the person with a disability. The trust is established and administered by someone else. The person with the disability does not have a trust. He or she is nominated as a beneficiary of the trust and is usually the only one who receives the benefits. Furthermore, the trustee (manager) is given the absolute discretion to determine when and how much the person should receive.

Given the government's stringent requirements, it is critical that the trust be carefully worded and show clearly that the trust:

- Is established (grantor, settlor) by the family (persons other than the person with the disability).

- Is managed by a trustee (and successor trustees) other than the person with the disability.

- Gives the trustee the absolute discretion to provide whatever assistance is required.

- Should never give the person with the disability more income or resources than permitted by the government.

- Must be used for supplementary purposes only; it should add to the things provided by the government benefit program, not supplant (replace) them.

- Defines what it means by supplementary/special needs in general terms, as well as in specific terms related to the unique needs of the person with the disability.

- Provides instructions for the person's final arrangement (families should assume that when the individual with the disability dies no relatives will be alive who know what the mother and father would have wanted).

- Determines who should receive the remainder (what is left over) of the trust after the individual with the disability dies.

- Provides choices for successor trustees—people or organizations that might be able to take a personal interest in the welfare of the person with the disability.

- Protects the trust against creditors or government agencies trying to obtain funds to pay for debts of the person or the family.

Since the trust is a legal arrangement that is regulated by the laws of your state, there will be other sections that your attorney may need to insert. It is important to know that, while the majority of public assistance funds come from the federal government (which provides guidelines for SNTs), it is the responsibility of each state government to regulate trusts and administer the federal benefits. As long as the federal guidelines are followed to the letter, the state will accept the SNT, and the trust will fulfill its function.

What the Social Security Administration Has to Say about Special Needs Trusts

The Social Security Administration's publication *Understanding SSI* discusses special needs trusts as follows:

How do resources in this type of trust count in the SSI program?

- Money or property in this type of trust for an SSI beneficiary...does not count toward the SSI resource limits of $1,500 for an individual.

How does money from the trust affect the individual's SSI payments?

- Money paid directly to the providers for items other than the person's food, clothing, and shelter does not reduce SSI payments. (Items that are not food, clothing, or shelter include medical care, telephone bills, education, and entertainment.)

- Money paid directly to the providers for food, clothing, and shelter does not reduce the individual's SSI payments—but only up to a limit.

- Money paid directly to the individual from the trust reduces the SSI payment.

Testamentary or Intervivos Trust: That is the Question!

At one time, the average attorney simply advised parents of an individual with a disability to prepare their Last Wills and Testaments and include a Testamentary Special Needs Trust. Upon the death of the parents, the wills would be probated, and the special needs trust would be created. In simpler days, this was pretty good advice.

Today, most attorneys who are experienced in estate planning for persons with disabilities will advise the family to prepare an Intervivos Special Needs Trust. Intervivos simply means that the trust functions now, while the parents are still living. As a living trust, it should not be confused with the modern estate planning tool for the family's main estate, the Family Revocable Living Trust. These are two very separate trusts. The Family Living Trust is designed to avoid probate, reduce estate taxes, and make for a smoother estate distribution. The Intervivos Special Needs Trust's sole function is to look after the future of the person with the disability.

Parents need not wait until their son or daughter is 18 years old to establish the Intervivos Special Needs Trust; they can establish the trust now. The trust is set up as a checking account at a local bank. Families can place funds into the trust every month and use these funds to cover the normal supplementary expenses of the person with the disability, as well as to save for the future. Using the trust funds to pay for the individual's supplementary expenses is also an excellent way of record keeping, for these expenses are tax-deductible.

An Intervivos or Living Special Needs Trust has other very unique features, such as:

- It is a trust that is separate from the family's main estate.

- The trust is managed by the trustees, who are usually the parents.

- By paying for supplementary items from the checkbook, the family shows the future trustees the types of things that are appropriate to the person's needs and that have passed government scrutiny. The typical government challenge to a SNT comes when a trustee pays for nonsupplementary items. (In contrast, a testamentary trust—one that is created after the parents have died—gives guidelines on how to establish the trust; it does not give specific examples of how to administer it.) The simple checkbook with its stubs can help the future trustees use the Living Special Needs Trust properly and avoid expensive challenges.

- Often relatives (e.g., aunts and uncles, grandparents) would like to leave an inheritance to the person with the disability, but are concerned that if they leave it to the person he or she will lose government benefits or will mismanage the funds. Relatives like the concept of a trust, which is a nice legal way to make sure the person actually receives the full gift. With a testamentary trust, the parents of the person with the disability must die, their estate must be probated, and then the trust will be created. After the trust is created, relatives can leave money to the trust. The better option is to create a living special needs trust now. This permits relatives with tax concerns (i.e., those who need to give money each year to avoid large estate taxes upon their death) to give money into the trust now, rather than only upon their deaths.

In today's society, it has been said that 40–60% of the population will go into a nursing home before they die. The average family's total estate will be completely used up in one year to cover nursing home costs. In their wills, the parents may have generously given everything to the testamentary trust. Unfortunately, after nursing home care and Medicaid expenses, there may be no estate left for the testamentary trust. Even if a portion of the estate remains after the parents die, there may be a six month to six year wait while the estate is being probated. A testamentary trust would not be created or funded during this waiting period. What would happen to the supplementary needs of the person during such a wait?

Having a living special needs trust creates a much more secure scenario for the person with the disability. With this type of trust, the parents would have saved money each month for the future and may have purchased life insurance or transferred assets into the trust. Should they suddenly pass away or have to go into a nursing home, the living trust, which is a private matter, continues to function without interruption. The successor trustee designated by the parents would begin to administer the trust funds within a short period of time (one to two hours). Supplementary assistance to the person with the disability would continue without a break.

Revocable or Irrevocable?

Once the basic details of the trust have been agreed upon, you have to decide whether to lock the door and throw away the key, making it impossible to change the trust, or to hold the key just in case you want to make some changes. With a Revocable trust, you retain the right to add and subtract assets as you go along. With this right, there are some potential consequences. The first and major consequence is that the government considers the trust to be part of your estate. Therefore, when you die, everything in the special needs trust is included in your estate for tax purposes and for potential lawsuits. What happens if someone sues your estate after you are gone? The assets in your special needs trust could be lost in such a lawsuit. Even if you only put a life insurance policy in the trust, it now reverts back to where your creditors and the IRS can lay claim.

If you make your trust Irrevocable, it means that any assets you place in it will remain there for the benefit of the person with the disability. If you need some of these assets later on for your own care, you cannot take them out. The advantages of an irrevocable trust may outweigh the disadvantages, as long as you do not place too much in the trust. If it is set up properly, it is completely separate from your estate. The irrevocable trust is considered a separate entity. It has its own tax number. Any assets that you place in the trust cannot be touched by your creditors for debts, taxes, and so on. Neither can the trust be touched by any creditors of the person with the disability.

What should you do? For younger parents, the answer may be a revocable trust. For older parents, the irrevocable trust may be the only option. Your attorney, in consultation with your financial planner, may be the best resource in making this determination. It is important, however, to have a current Letter of Intent (see Section 43.2), which will help your trustee interpret the legalese of either the revocable or irrevocable trust in light of your hopes and desires for the future.

Trustee: The Manager of Resources

It is one thing to leave resources to a trust, and it is quite another to manage them in such a way as to last the lifetime of the person with the disability. Every trust must have a trustee, someone who will manage the trust's assets. As most special needs trusts are established to provide supplementary assistance, they are generally quite small by bank standards. Ideally, it would be nice to have a local bank manage the trust resources, while taking a personal interest in the individual with the disability. Failing the location of a warm and loving trust officer, at least the bank would manage the funds and hire a social worker to look after the individual. Sadly, very few banks are willing to manage cash assets under $150,000 to $200,000 or become as involved in the person's life as you would wish.

In the case of a living trust and where there are sufficient funds and relatives, the family usually nominates future or successor trustees to manage the trust after the parents die or go into a nursing home. Families may even nominate a group of people to serve as joint trustees—several relatives, perhaps—who together administer the trust. It is important to list an advocacy or disability organization as the last successor trustee. This is because the possibility exists that the human successor trustees will die before the person with the disability. In the event that the human successor trustees are unable to serve, then the advocacy or disability organization may take on the responsibility or be able to recommend someone in their group who could do so. Of course, it is important to discuss this with the disability or advocacy group and obtain consent before listing the organization as a future trustee.

Master Trusts

The average family finds that they must rely on relatives or close friends to manage the trust funds. For many older parents with few surviving friends or relatives, the choice of a competent and caring trustee becomes very difficult or even impossible to find. The oldest son may be a fantastic, loving person to his sister with a disability, but may have difficulty managing his own finances, let alone the assets of the trust.

Many disability-related and other not-for-profit organizations have attempted to resolve this very serious problem by establishing Master Trusts. The individual special needs trusts are generally managed under the umbrella of a master or large trust fund. In this way, the family that may have only $50,000 or less to leave will have the assurance that the funds will be managed properly. The organization also promises to serve as an advocate for the person with the disability. Thus, the parents feel comfortable that someone will visit their son or daughter on a regular basis and look after his or her interests.

As the population grows older and develops nursing care needs, with family members living further apart, and with financial institutions becoming more conservative, the Master Trust may be the only real answer to the dilemma of small trust funds managed by people who actually care about persons with disabilities. Today, the average master trust in the United States is established by a local charity or nonprofit agency to serve persons with one or more disabling conditions. Occasionally, a few charities serving different populations will pool their resources to establish a community trust. Usually these organizations have a full-time executive director, along with a secretary, who work with a Board of Directors. The prospective family pays approximately $500 to $2,000 to receive basic life planning counseling and as a set-up charge. The family generally hires an attorney recommended by the charity to do the basic legal work, which may cost from $500 to $3,000. The charity also refers the family to a reputable financial planner to make sure that the trust is funded properly. The master trust staff will usually meet with the family once a year to make sure that everything is in place. This annual check-up may cost between $50 and $100. Should the parent(s) go into a nursing home; the Master Trust can be activated. Assuming there are sufficient cash reserves in the trust, an advocate will look after the person with the disability. And upon the death of the parents, the trust will be fully activated through guaranteed life insurance proceeds or a portion of the family's estate. This is the ideal.

Unfortunately, although the concept of Master Trusts has been around for many years and may indeed represent the only viable answer to the need of many individuals with disabilities for lifelong care, Master Trusts have yet to find a proven formula for success. The track record for many of these types of trusts is very poor. Many are set up, but fail within three to five years. Why do they fail? Although there are many reasons, basically the average master trust signs up only eight to ten individuals over the three-year start-up period, which is often funded by a grant. When the grant runs out, the Master Trust soon ends, in part because of the cost of hiring and keeping staff to manage the trust, but also because the eight to ten families were usually the key leaders of the organization and the strength of its membership. The majority of other members were never properly introduced to the merits of this fine program. Furthermore, the trust was created and managed by individuals who were primarily interested in the care of loved ones with disabilities, not in the business of marketing the trust to others. To work in the long term, the trust has to be sold in a businesslike, even aggressive manner.

Of course, not all Master Trusts fail. There are some that have operated successfully for many years. However, because the concept of a Master Trust has generally not proven successful, it is essential that families take a hard look at any Master Trust they are considering joining. Families should make sure that, if the trust does end, they have an escape clause whereby they can get back their assets.

Funding a Special Needs Trust

As families do their estate planning for their loved ones, they tend to think of it as a legal issue only. However, the lawyer can only establish the trust for them. Someone has to find the funds to put in it and make sure that there are sufficient funds to last the lifetime of the individual with the disability. That person is a financial planner.

The general perception of a financial planner is someone who is going to try to sell you investments and insurance through high pressure techniques. While the financial planner may very well use various financial products to fund the trust, the more reputable planners realize that most families have limited resources. Therefore, the planner's primary job is to help the family see what resources are available and then reallocate them, so that the future funding of the trust will be realistic.

As with attorneys, there are very few financial planners who have any experience with planning for the future of a person with disabilities. Most are trained to look at the overall family estate and try to provide as many dollars as possible, at the same time looking out for potential problems. When they realize that there is a person with a disability involved, they may react in a very human way; assume that the person will need extra help, and direct more dollars to the person with a disability, without understanding the consequences this might have in terms of the person's government benefits.

An experienced financial planner will examine your Letter of Intent (see section 43.2) and do a detailed financial analysis based on the future costs of supplementary items and advocacy. He or she will then look at the many different resources available to fund the trust now and in the future. (*Costing Out Expenses of the Person with the Disability*, at the end of section 43.3, can be used to list the total monthly expenses of the person with a disability.) When you subtract the total amount of government benefits and personal income of the person from the total monthly expenses, you have identified the amount of supplementary funds needed on a monthly basis by the person with a disability.) The only other major expense will be the cost of advocacy services, which may run from $50 to $200 per hour.

Most families are surprised to learn that they do have a variety of resources within their reach that can be directed to the Special Needs Trust. The options open to a family include:

- **Standard government benefits.** These benefits form the foundation for the future.

- **Savings.** No matter how you look at it, the family will have to save for the future. The government benefit programs have never provided enough for even poverty level existence. A regular savings program is essential to meet the person's supplementary needs in the future.

- **Family assistance.** Family members may wish to provide residential care, supervision, and supplemental assistance in the future.

- **Parents' estate.** Parents may leave a portion or all of their estate to the trust. To keep peace in a large family, parents should leave something for the other children as well.

- **Inheritances.** Relatives or friends who have expressed an interest in the person with the disability should be given instructions and assistance on how to leave a gift to the trust.

- **Property.** Some families want their loved one to live in the same house. The house can be placed in the trust and managed by a local nonprofit agency for the benefit of the person, or expanded into a group home setting.

- **Investments.** Certificates of Deposit, IRAs, KEOGHs, and so on can be directed to the trust.

- **Military benefits.** Some families have elected a Survivor Benefit Option (SBO), so the person with the disability will always have some income and medical care. They may still want a special needs trust to manage the other resources which will supplement the military benefits.

- **Insurance.** For the average family, life insurance may be the only way that they can leave a large lump sum for the future by making small monthly payments. It is also one of the few guaranteed methods of funding a trust. While the above items may fizzle out as people change their minds or the economy falters, a paid-up life insurance policy in an irrevocable trust will guarantee future funds.

- **Other resources.** Many families have resources that are unique to them. The financial planner will help you determine which ones are appropriate for funding the trust.

As families examine ways to fund the trust, they need to keep in mind something very important. Do not forget the other brothers and sisters. While the siblings may be pillars of love and understanding when it comes to their brother or sister with a disability, they have probably seen a great deal of your time and energy spent in the disability arena. They should not be left out at the end. Families tend to assume that, while they must pay for the services of a bank trustee and a guardian/advocate, relatives who take on these responsibilities should do so for free, because that is what families do! The trustee should be directed to pay for whatever services are necessary, whether an agency or relative performs the service. This may mean the difference between a brother driving the fifty miles to his sibling's group home once a week or once every three months.

With proper legal and financial planning, the family can guarantee that the person with the disability will enjoy a comfortable lifestyle after the parents are gone.

Worksheet for Costing Out Expenses of the Person with the Disability

Disabled Person's Income

Government Benefits   _____

Employment   _____

Total Monthly Income   _____

Disabled Person's Expenses

Housing

Rental   _____

Utilities   _____

Maintenance   _____

Cleaning items   _____

Laundry costs   _____

Other   _____

Care Assistance

Live-in   _____

Respite   _____

Custodial   _____

Other   _____

Personal Needs:

Haircuts, beauty shop _____

Telephone (basic, TTY) _____

Cigarettes _____

Books, magazines, etc. _____

Allowance _____

Other _____

Clothing _____

Employment

Transportation _____

Workshop fees _____

Attendant _____

Training _____

Other _____

Education

Transportation _____

Fees _____

Books, materials _____

Other _____

Special Equipment

Environment control _____

Elevator _____

Repair of equipment _____

Computer _____

Audio books _____

Ramp _____

Guide dog _____

Technical instruction _____

Hearing Aids/Batteries _____

Wheelchair _____

Other _____

Medical / Dental Care
  Med/Dental visits   _____
  Therapy   _____
  Nursing services   _____
  Meals for attendants   _____
  Drugs, medicine, etc.   _____
  Transportation   _____
  Other   _____

Food
  Meals, snacks-home   _____
  Outside of home   _____
  Special foods   _____
  Other   _____

Social / Recreational
  Sports   _____
  Special Olympics   _____
  Spectator sports   _____
  Vacation   _____
  TV/VCR or rental   _____
  Camps   _____
  Transportation   _____
  Other   _____

Automobile / Van
  Payments   _____
  Gas/Oil/Maintenance   _____
  Other   _____

Insurance
  Medical/Dental   _____
  Burial   _____
  Automobile/Van   _____
  Housing/Rental   _____
  Other   _____

Miscellaneous

    Other   _____

    Other   _____

    Other   _____

Total Expenses   _____

Subtract monthly income plus government benefits – _____

Difference equals supplementary needs   _____

A Parent's Suggestion

Carol and her husband recently completed their estate plan so that their children would be provided for. They have twin sons who do not have disabilities and a son who has Down Syndrome. Here is what Carol has to say about the process of estate planning.

When my husband and I went to talk the lawyer, we had not really talked much among ourselves first. I thought that since we agreed on almost everything about caring for Frank, our son with Down Syndrome, we would be in agreement about how to provide for his future needs, when we were not around anymore to care and advocate for him.

We found out, though, that we had different ideas. And we found out in the lawyer s office! Then we got home and found out our twins were hurt that we had not consulted them at all, had just assumed they would not want to be responsible for helping Frank after we were gone. So then we did what we should have done before going to see the lawyer—we talked as a family.

So my advice to other parents is: Before going to the lawyer for the first time, talk among yourselves about the future and your ideas for how to provide for your son or daughter with a disability. Then talk to the lawyer. Then return home for more discussion within the family. Then continue working with your lawyer and financial planner to create a plan the family can feel comfortable with.

Part Eight

Additional Help
and Information

Chapter 44

Glossary of Important Muscular Dystrophy Terms

Atrophy. From the Greek words *a*, meaning not, and *trophe*, nourishment. A decrease in the size of an organ or tissue (wasting). Common causes of diseases involving muscle atrophy are a lack of nutrients or blood supply or loss of signals from nerve cells. [2]

Becker muscular dystrophy. A hereditary muscle disorder of late onset, usually in the second or third decade, affecting the proximal muscles with characteristic pseudohypertrophy of the calves; clinical features similar to Duchenne muscular dystrophy but much milder and not a genetic lethal; X-linked recessive inheritance, with both Becker and Duchenne dystrophies caused by mutation in the dystrophin gene on Xp.

Biopsy. Process of removing tissue from patients for diagnostic examination.

Brace. An orthosis or orthopedic appliance that supports or holds in correct position a part of the body and can allow motion at adjacent joints, in contrast to a splint, which prevents motion of the part.

Definitions in this chapter are from *Stedman's Medical Dictionary, 27th Edition*, Copyright © 2000, Lippincott Williams & Wilkins. All rights reserved. Additional terms marked [2] are reprinted from "Simply Stated... Neuromuscular Terminology," *QUEST*, Volume 8, Number 4, August 2001. Reprinted with permission from the Muscular Dystrophy Association, www.mdausa.org. © The Muscular Dystrophy Association. For additional information, call the Muscular Dystrophy Association National Headquarters toll-free at (800) 572-1717. To find an MDA office in your area, look in your local telephone book, or click on "Clinics and Services" on the MDA website.

Chromosome. One of the bodies (normally 46 in somatic cells in humans) in the cell nucleus that is the bearer of genes, has the form of a delicate chromatin filament during interphase, contracts to form a compact cylinder segmented into two arms by the centromere during metaphase and anaphase stages of cell division, and is capable of reproducing its physical and chemical structure through successive cell divisions. In bacteria and other prokaryotes, the chromosome is not enclosed within a nuclear membrane and not subject to a mitotic mechanism. Prokaryotes may have more than one chromosome.

Congenital. Existing at birth, referring to certain mental or physical traits, anomalies, malformations, diseases, etc. which may be either hereditary or due to an influence occurring during gestation up to the moment of birth.

Contracture. Static muscle shortening due to tonic spasm or fibrosis, to loss of muscular balance, the antagonists being paralyzed or to a loss of motion of the adjacent joint.

Creatine kinase (CK). An enzyme catalyzing the reversible transfer of phosphate from phosphocreatine to ADP, forming creatine and ATP; of importance in muscle contraction. Certain isozymes are elevated in plasma following myocardial infarctions.

Dehydration.

1. Deprivation of water.

2. Reduction of water content.

Disability.

1. According to the "International Classification of Impairments, Disabilities, and Handicaps" (World Health Organization), any restriction or lack of ability to perform an activity in a manner or within the range considered normal for a human being. The term disability reflects the consequences of impairment in terms of functional performance and activity by the individual; disabilities thus represent disturbances at the level of the person.

2. An impairment or defect of one or more organs or members.

Distal myopathy. Myopathy affecting predominantly the distal portions of the limbs; onset is usually after age 40, with weakness and wasting of small muscles of the hands. The infantile form [MIM*160300][1] and the Swedish later-onset [MIM*160500][1] are autosomal dominant.

There is a Japanese late-onset type [MIM*254130[1]] that is recessive and is caused by mutation in the gene encoding dysferlin on 2p13.

Dominance of traits. An expression of the apparent physiologic relationship existing between two or more genes that may occupy the same chromosomal locus (alleles). At a specific locus there are three possible combinations of two allelic genes, *A* and *a*: two homozygous (*AA* and *aa*) and one heterozygous (*Aa*). If a heterozygous individual presents only the hereditary characteristic determined by gene *A*, but not *a*, *A* is said to be dominant and *a* recessive; in this case, *AA* and *Aa*, although genotypically distinct, should be phenotypically indistinguishable. If *AA*, *Aa*, and *aa* are distinguishable, each from the others, *A* and *a* are codominant.

Duchenne dystrophy. The most common childhood muscular dystrophy, with onset usually before age 6. Characterized by symmetric weakness and wasting of first the pelvic and crural muscles and then the pectoral and proximal upper extremity muscles; pseudohypertrophy of some muscles, especially the calf; heart involvement; sometimes mild mental retardation; progressive course and early death, usually in adolescence. X-linked inheritance (affects males and transmitted by females). Syn: Duchenne disease, childhood muscular dystrophy, pseudohypertrophic muscular dystrophy.

Dystrophin. A protein found in the sarcolemma of normal muscle; it is missing in individuals with pseudohypertrophic muscular dystrophy and in other forms of muscular dystrophy; its role may be in the linkage of the cytoskeleton of the muscle cell to extracellular protein. Syn: distropin, dystropin.

Dystrophy. From the Greek words *dys*, meaning abnormal or faulty, and *trophe*, nourishment. A disorder caused by defective "nutrition" or metabolism. [2]

Electromyography.

1. The recording of electrical activity generated in muscle for diagnostic purposes; both surface and needle recording electrodes can be used, although characteristically the latter is employed, so that the procedure is also called needle electrode examination.

2. Umbrella term for the entire electrodiagnostic study performed in the EMG laboratory, including not only the needle electrode examination, but also the nerve conduction studies.

Emery-Dreifuss muscular dystrophy. A generally benign type of muscular dystrophy, with onset in childhood or early adulthood. Weakness begins with the pectoral girdle and proximal upper extremity muscles and spreads to the pelvic girdle and distal lower extremity muscles. Contractures of the elbow, flexors, neck flexors, and calf muscles often occur; muscle pseudohypertrophy and mental retardation do not occur. A cardiomyopathy is common. An X-linked inherited disorder, nonallelic to Duchenne muscular dystrophy.

Facioscapulohumeral muscular dystrophy. [MIM*158900];[1] a highly variable hereditary disorder with onset in childhood or adolescence, characterized by weakness and wasting, sometimes asymmetrical, mainly of the muscles of the face, shoulder girdle, arms, and later, pelvic girdle, and legs; autosomal dominant inheritance. Syn: facioscapulohumeral atrophy, Landouzy-Dejerine dystrophy.

Gene deletion. Deletion of a segment of a chromosome too small to be detected cytogenetically, inferred from the phenotype at one particular locus.

Genetic testing. Laboratory studies of human blood or other tissue for the purpose of identifying genetic disorders. Relatively large chromosomal abnormalities such as deletion or transposition are identified by microscopic examination of chromosomes from a cell undergoing mitosis (karyotyping). More subtle aberrations can be detected by DNA probes (fabricated lengths of single-stranded DNA that match parts of the known gene). Genetic testing in the broadest sense includes biochemical testing for abnormal substances, or abnormally high or low concentrations of normal substances, that serve as markers of genetic deficiency or abnormality.

Genetic testing has become a standard procedure in a number of settings: screening for genetic diseases such as hemochromatosis, screening of couples planning to have children for the cystic fibrosis carrier state, and screening for genetic mutations known to increase the risk of certain cancers such as retinoblastoma and early-onset breast cancer. In addition, genetic profiling (genetic fingerprinting) can establish or rule out identity of source for 2 specimens of human material, or parent-child relationship between 2 persons, with a probability of 99.9%.

Home health nurse. A nurse who is responsible for a group of clients in the home setting. Visits clients on a routine basis to assist client and family with care as needed and to teach family the care needed so that the client may remain in his/her home. Syn: visiting nurse.

Hydrotherapy. Therapeutic use of water by external application, either for its pressure effect or as a means of applying physical energy to the tissues. Syn: hydrotherapeutics.

Inherited. Derived from a preformed genetic code present in the parents. Contrast with acquired.

Limb-girdle muscular dystrophy. [MIM*253600];[1] a group of muscular dystrophies, probably heterogeneous in nature. Onset usually in childhood or early adulthood and both sexes affected. Characterized by weakness and wasting, usually symmetrical, of the pelvic girdle muscles, the shoulder girdle muscles, or both, but not the facial muscles. Muscle pseudohypertrophy, heart involvement, and mental retardation are absent. Autosomal dominant and recessive inheritance have been described. Syn: Leyden-Möbius muscular dystrophy, pelvofemoral muscular dystrophy, scapulohumeral muscular dystrophy.

Muscular dystrophy. This term is actually a misnomer based on the wrong assumption made many years ago that muscle was being damaged by a lack of nutrients. In modern usage, it refers to a group of genetic myopathies in which a muscle protein is absent, deficient, or abnormal. The disorders classified as muscular dystrophies are myopathies in which a genetic defect results in structural damage to the muscle. Other myopathies involve damage to the muscle's contraction apparatus or energy production system. [2]

Mutation. A change in the chemistry of a gene that is perpetuated in subsequent divisions of the cell in which it occurs; a change in the sequence of base pairs in the chromosomal molecule.

Myasthenia. From *myo*, meaning muscle; *a*, without; and *sthenos*, strength. Muscle weakness or lack of strength. Today, "myasthenia" refers specifically to muscle weakness resulting from faulty communication between nerve and muscle at the place where nerve and muscle meet (the neuromuscular junction). [2]

Myositis. From the Greek word *myo*, meaning muscle, and the Greek suffix *itis*, meaning inflammation of. An inflammation of the muscle, which can result from infection, injury, or attack by the immune system on muscle tissue [2]

Myopathy. From the Greek words *myo*, meaning muscle, and *pathos*, disease or suffering. Any disease or abnormal condition of voluntary muscle. [2]

Myotonia (adjective myotonic). From *myo*, meaning muscle, and *tonos*, tone. Inability to relax muscles after contraction. [2]

Myotonic dystrophy. This genetic disorder involves (but is not limited to) both myotonia and structural damage to muscles (dystrophy). [2]

Neuropathy. From the Greek words *neuron*, meaning nerve or sinew, and *pathos*, disease or suffering. Any disease of the nervous system. Amyotrophic lateral sclerosis and spinal muscular atrophy, in which loss of nerve cells prevents muscles from working, are neuropathies, as are diseases in which nerve fibers malfunction, such as Charcot-Marie-Tooth and Dejerine-Sottas disease. [2]

Occupational therapy (OT). Therapeutic use of self-care, work, and recreational activities to increase independent function, enhance development, and prevent disability; may include adaptation of tasks or environment to achieve maximum independence and optimum quality of life.

Osteoporosis. Reduction in the quantity of bone or atrophy of skeletal tissue; an age-related disorder characterized by decreased bone mass and increased susceptibility to fractures. (In muscular dystrophy, osteoporosis occurs from lack of weight bearing activities.)

Physical therapy (PT).

1. Treatment of pain, disease, or injury by physical means; Syn: physiotherapy.

2. The profession concerned with promotion of health, with prevention of physical disabilities, with evaluation and rehabilitation of persons disabled by pain, disease, or injury, and with treatment by physical therapeutic measures as opposed to medical, surgical, or radiologic measures.

Prenatal screening. Screening for the detection of fetal disease, usually by ultrasound examination or by testing amnionic fluid obtained by amniocentesis. Other screening techniques include testing maternal serum and placental biopsy.

Scoliosis. Abnormal lateral and rotational curvature of the vertebral column. Depending on the etiology, there may be one curve, or primary and secondary compensatory curves; scoliosis may be "fixed" as a result of muscle and/or bone deformity or "mobile" as a result of unequal muscle contraction.

Spinal muscular atrophy. The muscle wasting or atrophy in this genetic disorder results from loss of signals from nerve cells in the spinal cord. [2]

Tracheotomy. The operation of incising the trachea, usually intended to be temporary.

X-linked inheritance. The pattern of inheritance that may result from a mutant gene on an X chromosome.

Note

1. **MIM Numbers.** The catalog assignment for a mendelian trait in the MIM [*Mendelian Inheritance in Man*] system. If the initial digit is 1, the trait is deemed autosomal dominant; if 2, autosomal recessive; if 3, X-linked. Wherever a trait defined in this glossary has a MIM number, the number from the 12th edition of MIM, is given in square brackets with or without an asterisk (asterisks indicate that the mode of inheritance is known; a number symbol (#) before an entry number means that the phenotype can be caused by mutation in any of 2 or more genes) as appropriate; e.g., Pelizaeus-Merzbacher disease [MIM*169500] is a well-established, autosomal, dominant, mendelian disorder.

Chapter 45

Directory of Organizations with Muscular Dystrophy Information

Alliance for Technology Access
1304 Southpoint Blvd., Suite 240
Petaluma, CA 94954
Phone: 707-778-3011
TTY: 707-778-3015
Fax: 707-765-2080
Website: http://www.ataccess.org
E-mail: ATAinfo@ATAccess.org

American Academy of Audiology
11730 Plaza America Drive
Suite 300
Reston, VA 20190
Toll-Free: 800-AAA (222)-2336
Phone: 703-790-8466
Fax: 703-790-8631
Website: http://www.audiology
.org/index.php

American Occupational Therapy Association
4720 Montgomery Lane
P.O. Box 31220
Bethesda, MD 20824-1220
Toll-Free: 800-377-8555 (TTY)
Phone: 301-652-2682
Fax: 301-652-7711
Website: http://www.aota.org

American Physical Therapy Association
1111 N. Fairfax St.
Alexandria, VA 22314-1488
Toll-Free: 800-999-2782
Phone: 703-684-2782
TTY: 703-683-6748
Fax: 703-684-7343
Website: http://www.apta.org
E-mail: practice@apta.org

Resources in this chapter were compiled from several sources deemed reliable; all contact information was verified and updated in February 2004.

American School Counselor Association
1101 King Street
Suite 625
Alexandria, VA 22314
Toll-Free: 800-306-4722
Phone: 703-683-2722
Website: http://www
.schoolcounselor.org
E-mail: asca@schoolcounselor.org

American Speech-Language-Hearing Association
10801 Rockville Pike
Rockville, MD 20852
Toll-Free (Public): 800-638-8255
Toll-Free (Professionals/
Students): 800-498-2071
Phone: 301-571-0457 (V/TTY)
Website: http://www.asha.org
E-mail: actioncenter@asha.org

American Therapeutic Recreation Association
1414 Prince Street, Suite 204
Alexandria, VA 22314
Phone: 703-683-9420
Fax: 703-683-9431
Website: http://www.atra-tr.org/
atra.htm
E-mail: atra@atra-tr.org

Facioscapulohumeral Dystrophy (FSHD) Society
3 Westwood Road
Lexington, MA 02420
Phone: 781-860-0501
Fax: 781-860-0599
Website: http://
www.fshsociety.org
E-mail: info@fshsociety.org

International Myotonic Dystrophy Organization
P.O. Box 1121
Sunland, CA 91041-1121
Toll-Free: 866-679-7954
Phone: 818-951-2311
Website: http://www
.myotonicdystrophy.org
E-mail: info@myotonicdystrophy
.org

Muscular Dystrophy Association
3300 East Sunrise Drive
Tucson, AZ 85718-3208
Toll-Free: 800-572-1717
Phone: 520-529-2000
Fax: 520-529-5300
Website: http://www.mdausa.org
E-mail: mda@mdausa.org

Muscular Dystrophy Australia
GPO Box 9932
Melbourne, 3001 Australia
Phone: 011-61-3-9320-9555
Fax: 011-61-3-9320-9596
Website: http://www.mda.org.au
E-mail: info@mda.org.au

Muscular Dystrophy Campaign
7-11 Prescott Place
London, England
SW4 6BS
Phone: 011-44-020-7720-8055
Fax: 011-44-020-7498-0670
Website: http://www.muscular-dystrophy.org
E-mail: info@muscular-dystrophy.org

Muscular Dystrophy Family Foundation
2330 North Meridian Street
Indianapolis, IN 46208-5730
Toll-Free: 800-544-1213
Phone: 317-923-6333
Fax: 317-923-6334
Website: http://www.mdff.org
E-mail: mdff@mdff.org

National Ability Center
3991 E. Highway 248
P.O. Box 682799
Phone: 435-649-3991 (V/TDD)
Fax: 435-658-3992
Park City, UT 84098
Website: http://codyco.tripod.com/nationalabilitycenter
E-mail: nac1985.org

National Consortium for Physical Education and Recreation for Individuals with Disabilities (NCPERID)
School of Physical Education, Wellness, and Sport Studies
University of South Florida
4202 E. Fowler Ave. PED 214
Tampa, FL 33620-8600
Phone: 813-974-3443
Fax: 813-974-4979
Website: http://ncperid.usf.edu

National Disability Sports Alliance
25 West Independence Way
Kingston, RI 02881
Phone: 401-792-7130
Fax: 401-792-7130
Website: http://ww.ndsaonline.org
E-mail: info@ndsaonline.org

National Dissemination Center for Children with Disabilities (also known as NICHCY)
P.O. Box 1492
Washington, DC 20013
Toll-Free: 800-695-0285 (V/TTY)
Fax: 202-884-8441
Website: http://www.nichcy.org
E-mail: nichcy@aed.org

National Institutes of Health (NIH)
9000 Rockville Pike
Bethesda, MD 20892
Phone: 301-496-4000
Website: http://www.nih.gov
E-mail: nihinfo@od.nih.gov

National Institute of Neurological Disorders and Stroke
P.O. Box 5801
Bethesda, MD 20824
Toll-Free: 800-352-9424
Phone: 301-496-5751
TTY: 301-468-5981
Website: http://www.ninds.nih.gov

National Organization on Disability
910 Sixteenth St., N.W.
Suite 600
Washington, DC, 20006
Phone: 202-293-5960
Fax: 202-293-7999
TTY: 202-293-5968
Website: http://www.nod.org
E-mail: ability@nod.org

National Osteoporosis Foundation
1232 22nd Street N.W.
Washington, DC 20037-1292
Phone: 202-223-2226
Website: http://www.nof.org
E-mail: communications@nof.org

Parent Project Muscular Dystrophy (PPMD)
1012 North University Blvd.
Middletown, OH 45042
Toll-Free: 800-714-KIDS (5437)
Phone: 513-424-0696
Fax: 513-425-9907
Website: http://
www.parentprojectmd.org
E-mail: info@parentprojectmd.org

Pathways Awareness Foundation
150 North Michigan Ave.
Suite 2100
Chicago, IL 60601
Toll-Free: 800-955-2445
Website: http://www
.pathwaysawareness.org
E-mail: friends@
pathwaysawareness.org

RESNA
Rehabilitative Engineering &
Assistive Technology of North
America
1700 N. Moore Street
Suite 1540
Arlington, VA 22209-1903
Phone: 703-524-6686
TTY: 703-524-6639
Fax: 703-524-6630
Website: http://www.resna.org
E-mail: natloffice@resna.org

U.S. Department of Education
Office of Special Education and
Rehabilitative Services
400 Maryland Ave., S.W.
Washington, DC 20202
Toll Free: 800-872-5327
Phone: 202-205-5465
Website: http://www.ed.gov/
about/offices/list/osers/
index.html

Chapter 46

Directory of On-Line Providers of Information and Equipment for People with Muscular Dystrophy

Listed Alphabetically by Company Name

Action Products, Inc.

Website: http://www.actionproducts.com/rehab.html

Wheelchair cushions and seating systems, knee and elbow pads, and full mattress pads.

Advanced Respiratory

Website: http://www.abivest.com

The Vest system is an easy-to-use airway clearance device for both children and adults.

Bruno Independent Living Aids, Inc.

Website: http://www.bruno.com

Stair lifts, power chairs, scooters, vehicle lifts, stair lifts and Turning Automotive Seating™ (TAS).

The information in this chapter is excerpted with permission from the Muscular Dystrophy Family Foundation®, www.mdff.org. The Muscular Dystrophy Family Foundation provides information, emotional support, and financial assistance toward adaptive equipment or individuals and families affected by neuromuscular diseases on a national level. © 2002 Muscular Dystrophy Family Foundation.

Bunni-Steps Design

Website: http://bunnisteps.com/productprofile.asp

Revolutionary assistive technology for exercise, fitness, therapy, and wellness.

Contemporary Products, Inc.

Website: http://www.contemporaryproducts.com

Equipment for respiratory care.

Deming Designs, Inc.

Website: http://www.beachwheelchair.com

Specialized wheelchairs and walkers to use on the beach.

Economic Mobility, Inc.

Website: http://www.toiletlift.com

Lift that aids in standing from the toilet.

E-Z-On Products, Inc. of Florida

Website: http://www.ezonpro.com

Exceptional safety solutions for transporting children and adults.

EZ-Step, Inc.

Website: http://www.ez-step.com

A specialized cane that makes stair climbing easier.

Farley Technologies, Inc.

Website: http://www.vwcdexpo.com/
btemplate.cfm?s_booth=860741&keywords=&show=57&type=5&clk=1

Innovative and unique products for the disabled.

Great Ideas Inc./Solution Comfortseat

Website: http://bidets.us/sol-models.htm

Personal hygiene assistive products.

Guldmann, Inc.

Website: http://www.guldmann.com/index.php?newlang=us

Ceiling lifts, floor lifts, ramps, lifting platforms, and beds.

Kaye Products, Inc.

Website: http://www.kayeproducts.com

Walking aids and durable medical equipment.

Kayjae Manufacturing Co., Inc.

Website: http://www.kayjae.com

Portable table that works well with wheelchairs.

Keybowl™, Inc.

Website: http://www.keybowl.com/kb/index?page=home

OrbiTouch Keyless Keyboard.

Magitek.com, LLC.

Website: http://www.magitek.com

Specializing in human interface drive controls.

Mobility Products & Design

Website: http://www.mobilityproductsdesign.com/products.asp

Customized driving controls.

Muscular Dystrophy Family Foundation®

Website: http://www.vwcdexpo.com/exhibitor_indexmdff.htm

Detailed resource list.

MyMedMart, Inc.

Website: http://www.mymedmart.com/MMM_BASE

Home health care supplies and equipment.

No-Rinse Laboratories, LLC.

Website: http://www.norinse.com

Products that clean without being rinsed for head-to-toe cleanliness.

Rehab Designs, Inc.

Website: http://www.rehabdesigns.com

Rehabilitation equipment specialists.

Ryno Mobility Corporation

Website: http://www.rynomobility.com

Handicapped-accessible pickup truck and 4x4.

Snug Seat
Website: http://www.snugseat.com

Pediatric rehabilitation products and adult aids for daily living.

Surehands Lift & Care Systems
Website: http://www.surehands.com

Lift and care and self-care systems.

Tendercare4kids
Website: http://www.tendercare4kids.com

Products for children with special needs.

Touch Turner
Website: http://www.touchturner.com

Page turning devices.

Voice Factor
Website: http://www.voicefactor.com

Computer program that makes speech into text.

Publications and Magazines

Active Living Magazine
Website: http://www.cripworld.com/themall/activeliving.shtml

Disabled Dealer Magazine
Website: http://www.disableddealer.com

Exceptional Parent Magazine
Website: http://exceptionalparent.com

Flaghouse, Inc.
Website: http://www.activitiesforlife.com

Special populations and rehabilitation catalog.

In Motion Magazine
Website: http://www.inmotionmagazine.com

National Disability Sports Alliance
Website: http://www.eparent.com/resources/associations/ndsa.htm

New Mobility Magazine
Website: http://www.icdri.org/News/NewMobiity.htm

Palaestra
Website: http://www.palaestra.com/

Forum of sport, physical education, and recreation for those with disabilities.

PN/Paraplegia News
Website: http://www.pvamagazines.com/pnnews

News and information magazine for people with mobility impairments.

SATH (Society for Accessible Travel and Hospitality)/Open World
Website: http://www.sath.org

Sports 'n Spokes
Website: http://www.pvamagazines.com/sns

Today's Caregiver Magazine
Website: http://caregiver.com

Index

Index

Page numbers followed by 'n' indicate a footnote. Page numbers in *italics* indicate a table or illustration.

A

accessibility issues, Duchenne muscular dystrophy 423–24

"Accurate and Affordable Diagnosis of Duchenne Muscular Dystrophy" (Zeigler) 159n

ACE inhibitors *see* angiotensin-converting enzyme inhibitors

acetaminophen 65, 270

Achilles tendons
release 289–92
stretching exercices 425–26

acid maltase deficiency 49, 51

Acsadi, Gyula 228

Action Products, Inc., Web site address 523

Active Living Magazine, Web site address 526

activities of daily living
communication 352–53, 408–9
dressing 349–52
eating 358–60
exercising 360–61
grooming 357

activities of daily living, continued
housekeeping 355
mobility 353–54
physical therapy 235
recreation 354–55
sleeping 356, 422, 427
toileting 357–58, 397
transfers 353–54

Actonel (risedronate) 196, *199*

Adapt-Ability, Inc., contact information 345

"Adaptations for Boys with Duchenne Muscular Dystrophy and Adults and Children with Muscular Dystrophy and Allied Neuromuscular Conditions" (Muscular Dystrophy Campaign) 333n

adenosine 5'-triphospate (ATP) 29

adenosine 5-triphospate (ATP) 34, 43

adhalin 126

adolescents
Becker muscular dystrophy 88–89
Duchenne muscular dystrophy 79, 83, 85
Emery-Dreifuss muscular dystrophy 95
facioscapulohumeral muscular dystrophy 5, 115

adolescents, continued
fluid intake 400–401
ventilation support 250–51
Advanced Respiratory
contact information 253
Web site address 523
AFO *see* ankle-foot orthoses
African Americans, osteoporosis 191
age factor
breathing difficulties 246–47
facioscapulohumeral muscular dystrophy 110, 111
mobility stages 429–35
osteoporosis 191
Alberta Children's Hospital, contact information 119
albuterol 306
alcifediol *198*
Aldactone (spironolactone) *210*
alendronate 196, *199*
Alliance for Technology Access, contact information 463, 519
Alora *198*
alpha-beta blockers, congestive heart failure *210*
alpha-sarcoglycan 126
ALS *see* amyotrophic lateral sclerosis
Amalfitano, Andrea 228
Amen *198*
American Academy of Audiology, contact information 463, 519
American Massage Therapy Association (AMTA), contact information 278
American Occupational Therapy Association, contact information 463, 519
American Physical Therapy Association, contact information 242, 463, 519
American School Counselor Association, contact information 463, 520
American Speech-Language-Hearing Association (ASHA), contact information 464, 520
American Therapeutic Recreation Association, contact information 464, 520
aminoglycoside antibiotics 8

AMTA *see* American Massage Therapy Association
amyotrophic lateral sclerosis (ALS)
bone marrow transplantation 231
described 516
gene therapy 228
inflammations 221
physical therapy 236
tracheostomy 257
anabolic steroids 306–7
"Anaesthetics" (Muscular Dystrophy Campaign) 213n
Androderm *199*
anesthesia
congestive heart failure 208–9
inheritable myopathies 17
metabolic disorders 48–49
muscular dystrophy 213–17
myotonic muscular dystrophy 143
angiotensin-converting enzyme inhibitors (ACE inhibitors), congestive heart failure *210*
animal studies
bone marrow transplantation 230
Duchenne muscular dystrophy 7
dysferlin gene 9–10
gene therapy 228
gentamicin 224
gentamycin 307
utrophin 224
ankle-foot orthoses (AFO) *136*, 238, 295
ankles, passive stretches 311, *312*
antibiotic medications
chest infections 250
Duchenne muscular dystrophy 8
scoliosis surgery 286
anxiety, pain management 271
A-Plus Medical, contact information 401
Appel, Stanley 231
Archer, Robert Lee 273
Aristocort (triamcinolone) 192
arrhythmia, described 201, 202–3
arthrogryposis, described 70
artistic programs, described 443–44
art therapy 444
ASHA *see* American Speech-Language-Hearing Association
aspiration, feeding tubes 387, 389

aspirin 65, 270
assisted cough flow 251
assisted ventilation, congestive heart failure 208
assistive devices
limb-girdle muscular dystrophy 125
ptosis *137*, 153
assistive technology devices 444–45
assistive technology services 445–46
Asta, Linda 396
ataxia, mitochondrial encephalomyopathy 32
Athena Diagnostics, Inc., contact information 149, 156, 165
ATP *see* adenosine 5'-triphospate
ATP synthase, described 29
atrophy, defined 511
atropine 270
audiology 447
augmentative communication devices 445
autoimmune diseases
inflammations 220–21
research 225–26
autologous blood donation, described 282
autosomal, described 122–23
autosomal dominant inheritance
central core disease 21
described *153*
Emery-Dreyfuss muscular dystrophy *98*, 98–99
facioscapulohumeral muscular dystrophy 5, 109
hyperkalemic periodic paralysis 20
hypokalemic periodic paralysis 20
limb-girdle muscular dystrophy 122–23, 127–29
myotonic muscular dystrophy 4
myotubular myopathy 23
nemaline myopathy 21, 22
paramyotonia congenita 19
Thomsen's myotonia congenita 18
autosomal recessive inheritance
acid maltase deficiency 51
Becker-type myotonia congenita 18
carnitine deficiency 54
carnitine palmityl transferase deficiency 54

autosomal recessive inheritance, continued
congenital muscular dystrophy 70, *70*
debrancher enzyme deficiency 51
lactate dehydrogenase deficiency 53
limb-girdle muscular dystrophy 122–23, 129–32
myoadenylate deaminase deficiency 54
myotubular myopathy 23
nemaline myopathy 18, 22
phosphofructokinase deficiency 52
phosphorylase deficiency 52
autosomes, described 109
Avonex (beta-interferon-1a) 226
azathioprine 64, 221

B

Bach, John 256, 257–58, 260, 261–62, 265
Barohn, Richard 192, 195
"The Basics of Muscular Dystrophy and Beyond" (PPMD) 77n
Becker, Peter Emil 77
"Becker MD" (Muscular Dystrophy Campaign) 87n
Becker muscular dystrophy (BMD)
cardiac problems 201–11
defined 511
described 6–8
muscle biopsy 174
overview 87–94
"Becker Muscular Dystrophy" (Cleveland Clinic Foundation) 87n
Benditt, Joshua 258
beta blockers, congestive heart failure *210*
beta-interferon-1a 226
beta-sarcoglycan 127
bilevel positive airway pressure devices 255–56
biofeedback, breathing techniques 263
biopsy
Becker muscular dystrophy 92
congenital muscular dystrophy 71
defined 511
Duchenne muscular dystrophy 81

biopsy, continued
  facioscapulohumeral muscular dystrophy 110
  inheritable myopathies 24
  metabolic diseases of muscle 55
  mitochondrial chronic external ophthalmoplegia 155–56
  myositis 64
  overview 171–75
BiPAP 250, 255
bisphosphonates 196–97
Blalock, J. Edwin 226
blood pressure, congestive heart failure 206–7
BMD *see* Becker muscular dystrophy
bone density, osteoporosis 192–93
bone fractures 421
bone marrow transplantation, muscular dystrophy 230
Bowler, M. A. 133n
braces
  defined 511
  Duchenne muscular dystrophy 295–99
breast cancer, hormone supplementation 196
breathing exercises 249
breathing techniques 246–65
breath stacking 251, 261, 262
BromptonPac 250
bronchodilators, chest infections 250
Bruno Independent Living Aids, Inc.
  contact information 346
  Web site address 523
Bunni-Steps Design, Web site address 524
Byrne, Barry 227

C

CalBurst *198*
calcifediol 195
calcinosis 65
calcitonin 196, *199*
calcitriol *198*
calcium
  foods 190–91
  muscle contraction 14
  osteoporosis prevention 194–95

calcium blockers 307
Calcort (deflazacort) 192
Calderol (calcifediol) 195, *198*
calipers 295
Campbell, Kevin 9
cancer
  hormone supplementation 196
  myositis 62–63
carbamazepine 268
carbohydrate-processing disorders, described 51–53
cardiac arrhythmia, described 201–3
cardiac care
  Becker muscular dystrophy 92
  inheritable myopathies 17–18
  metabolic disorders 49
  myopathies 33
cardiac catheterization, described 211
cardiomyopathy, described 201–4, 211
caregivers
  breath stacking 262
  myotonic muscular dystrophy 147–48
  see also home health care
care guidelines 421–23
carnitine 34, 45
carnitine deficiency 49, 54
carnitine palmityl transferase deficiency (CPT) 47, 54, 381
carvedilol *210*
catabolic steroids 304–5
cataracts, myotonic muscular dystrophy 142–43, 145
catheters
  external 396
  Foley catheter, described 284
  infections 395
CAT scan *see* computed tomography
caveolin 125
CEC *see* Council for Exceptional Children
CellCept (mycophenolate mofetil) 226
central core disease
  anesthesia 216
  described 16
  malignant hyperthermia 17
centronuclear myopathy 22–23
certified nursing attendants *see* home health care

Chamberlain, Jeffrey 227, 228
channelopathies
  described 16
  diagnosis 24
Charcot-Marie Tooth disease, described 516
children
  Becker muscular dystrophy 88
  calcium supplements 195
  central core disease 21
  congenital muscular dystrophy 72–
  73
  Duchenne muscular dystrophy 6,
  79, 82–84, 168
  facioscapulohumeral muscular dystrophy 116
  fluid intake 400–401
  Kearns Sayre syndrome 155
  lung capacity 247
  mobility stages 429–35
  muscle biopsy 171–72
  muscular dystrophy diagnosis 405–
  13
  myopathies 16
  myotonic muscular dystrophy 134,
  141
  physical therapy 234, 237–38
  progressive external ophthalmoplegia 33
  ptosis 33
  ventilation support 250–51
  see also infants
Children's Hospital of Eastern
  Ontario, contact information 119, 156
chimeraplasts 8
chlorambucil 64
chloride, muscle contraction 14
cholecalciferol *198*
chorionic villus sampling (CVS)
  congenital muscular dystrophy 74
  embryo screening 182
chromosomes
  defined 512
  distal muscular dystrophies *104*
  facioscapulohumeral muscular dystrophy 108–9
  limb-girdle muscular dystrophy
  125–32
Citracal *198*

CK *see* creatine kinase
Cleveland Clinic Foundation
  Becker muscular dystrophy publication 87n
  contact information 94
clinical trials
  gene replacement therapy 7–8
  muscular dystrophy treatment 225–
  31
clothing, toileting 394–95
coenzyme Q10 34
colchicine 65
CombiPatch *199*
computed tomography (CAT scan; CT
  scan), mitochondrial diseases 37
conduction block, described 33
congenital, defined 512
congenital muscular dystrophy, overview 69–75
congenital myopathies 16
congenital myotubular myopathy, cardiac care 17–18
congestive heart failure, described
  204–11
Contemporary Products, Inc., Web
  site address 524
continuous positive airway pressure
  (CPAP) 250–51
contractions
  described 14
  pain management 269
contractures
  Achilles tendon release 289–90
  defined 512
  Duchenne muscular dystrophy 294,
  309
Cooke, David A. 267n
coping strategies
  disabilities 329–32, 408–13
  family and friends 415–20
Coreg (carvedilol) *210*
Cori's disease *see* debrancher enzyme
  deficiency
coronary artery disease, described 202
corticosteroids
  calcium supplements 195
  Duchenne muscular dystrophy 64–65
  nutritional issues 301
  osteoporosis 192

CoughAssist 251, 252–53, 258, 262–63
Council for Exceptional Children
   (CEC), contact information 470
counseling
   muscular dystrophy diagnosis 409,
      431
   parents 449
   students 447–48, 452
CPAP *see* continuous positive airway
   pressure
CPEO *see* mitochondrial chronic external ophthalmoplegia
CPK *see* phosphocreatine kinase
CPT *see* carnitine palmityl transferase deficiency
cramping, pain management 268–69
creatine 306
creatine kinase (CK)
   anesthesia 215
   Becker muscular dystrophy 92
   congenital muscular dystrophy 71
   defined 512
   Duchenne muscular dystrophy 81,
      306
   limb-girdle muscular dystrophy 123
   myositis 64
   tests 167–70
"Creatine Kinase (Total) Test"
   (McKesson Health Solutions) 167n
creatine phosphate 34
Crinone *198*
CT scan *see* computed tomography
cultural programs, described 443–44
curvature of spine *see* scoliosis
cyclophosphamide 64, 226
cyclosporine 64
Cycrin *198*
cytokines, inflammations 220, 221

D

dance therapy 444
Davies, Kay 224–25
Day, John W. 163–65, 225
debrancher enzyme deficiency
   cardiac care 49
   described 51–52
   pain management 268

Decadron (dexamethasone) 192
deflazacort 192, 305, 424
dehydration
   defined 512
   prevention 397–401
"Dehydration" (Muscular Dystrophy
   Campaign) 393n
Dejerine-Sottas disease, described
   516
DeKleine, Alison 308n, 363n
Del Bene, Maura 398
delta-sarcoglycan 127
Deltasone (prednisone) 192
Deming Designs, Inc., Web site address 524
dermatomyositis
   heart problems 202
   inflammations 221
   muscle biopsy 175
   overview 59–66
   pain management 267–68
   treatment 192
dexamethasone 192
DEXA test *see* dual-energy x-ray
   absorptiometry test
diabetes mellitus, myotonic muscular
   dystrophy 143
diet and nutrition
   Becker muscular dystrophy 92
   breathing problems 248
   congestive heart failure 207
   contraction prevention 269
   coping strategies 422–23, 424–25
   Duchenne muscular dystrophy 299–
      303
   hyperkalemic periodic paralysis 20
   hypokalemic periodic paralysis 20–
      21
   osteoporosis prevention 193, 194–95
digoxin *210*
Dilantin (phenytoin) 268
dilated cardiomyopathy, described 204
diplopia, defined 152
disability
   coping strategies 329–32, 408–13
   defined 512
   estate planning 478–79
   home health care 379–85
   mobility 429–30

Disabled Dealer Magazine, Web site address 526
"Discussing Muscular Dystrophy" (Muscular Dystrophy Association - Australia) 415n
distal muscular dystrophy, overview 103–6
distal myopathy, described 103–6
distal mypoathy with vocal cord and pharyngeal weakness *104*, 106
diuretics, congestive heart failure *210*
DMD *see* Duchenne muscular dystrophy
DNA (deoxyribonucleic acid)
  Duchenne muscular dystrophy 160
  facioscapulohumeral muscular dystrophy 108–9, 111–12, 116–18
  genetic tests 182
  myotonic muscular dystrophy 165
DNA probes, genetic testing 514
DOE *see* US Department of Education
dominance of traits, defined 513
dowager's hump 190
DP90 250
DS Medica, contact information 401
dual-energy x-ray absorptiometry test (DEXA test) 193
Duchenne, buillaume Benjamin Amand 77
Duchenne dystrophy, defined 513
Duchenne-like muscular dystrophy 130–31
Duchenne muscular dystrophy (DMD)
  cardiac problems 201–11
  coping strategies 415–20
  described 6–8
  gentamicin 224
  home health care 383
  inflammations 220–21
  muscle biopsy 174
  overview 77–85
  prednisone 223–24
  respiratory muscle weakness 246–47
  treatment 192, 294–325
  utrophin 224–25
Duke University Medical Center, limb-girdle muscular dystrophy publication 121n
Dyrenium (triamterene) *210*

dysferlin 9–10, 104, 105, 126
dysphagia
  defined 152
  described 62
dyspnea, described 205
dystal myopathy, defined 512–13
dystrophin
  Becker muscular dystrophy 6, 79, *80*, 87–88
  cardiomyopathy 203
  defined 513
  Duchenne muscular dystrophy 8, 79, *80*, 160, 174, 299–300
  gentamicin 224
  immune system 228

E

ECG *see* electrocardiogram
echocardiogram
  congestive heart failure 211
  pregnancy 209–10
Economic Mobility, Inc., Web site address 524
edema, described 205–6, 211
Education of All Handicapped Children Act 438
"Effects of Facioscapulohumeral Muscular Dystrophy" (MDA) 107n
EHA *see* Education of All Handicapped Children Act
EKG *see* electrocardiogram
elbows, passive stretches 315, *315*
electrocardiogram (ECG; EKG)
  congestive heart failure 209
  heart problems 139
  mitochondrial chronic external ophthalmoplegia 155
  mitochondrial diseases 39
electroencephalogram (EEG)
  mitochondrial diseases 37
  scoliosis 282
electromyography (EMG)
  Becker muscular dystrophy 92
  congenital muscular dystrophy 71
  defined 513
  facioscapulohumeral muscular dystrophy 110

electromyography (EMG), continued
metabolic diseases of muscle 55
muscle activity 24
myositis 63–64
myotonic muscular dystrophy 146
overview 177–80
emerin 99
Emery-Dreifuss muscular dystrophy
defined 514
heart problems 202, 203
overview 95–99
EMG *see* electromyography
emotional concerns
diet and nutrition 302–3
muscular dystrophy diagnosis 405–
8, 417–18
encephalomyopathy, described 32–34
endocrine myopathies, described 25–
26
endometrial cancer, hormone supplementation 196
endoscope 388
enzymes, metabolic diseases 45–46
ergocalciferol *198*
ERIC Clearinghouse on Disabilites
and Gifted Education, children with
disabilities publication 465n
estate planning, overview 478–86
Estrace *198*
Estraderm *198*
Estratest *199*
Estrig *198*
estrogens, osteoporosis prevention
195–96, *198*
Eulenburg's disease, described 18–19
Evista (raloxifene) 196, *199*
Exceptional Parent Magazine, Web
site address 526
"Excessive Daytime Sleeping and
Myotonic Dystrophy" (Bowler) 133n
exercise
Becker muscular dystrophy 88
congestive heart failure 205, 207–8,
211
Duchenne muscular dystrophy 294,
426–27
metabolic diseases of muscle 49–51,
55
osteoporosis 191–92, 197–98

exercise intolerance
metabolic diseases 47
myopathy 31
exercises
breathing 249
Duchenne muscular dystrophy 308–
25, 318–25
limb-girdle muscular dystrophy 125
range of motion 235
exertional fatigue *see* exercise intolerance
exons, Duchenne muscular dystrophy
160
expiration, described 247
exsufflation belt, described 260–61
external ophthalmoplegia, defined 151
E-Z-On Products, Inc. of Florida, Web
site address 524
EZ-Step, Inc., Web site address 524

F

"Facioscapulohumeral Disease" (FSH
Society) 107n
Facioscapulohumeral Dystrophy
(FSHD) Society, contact information
113, 520
facioscapulohumeral muscular dys-
trophy (FSHD)
defined 514
described 5–6
inflammations 220
overview 107–19
treatment 225
FacioScapuloHumeral Society (FSH
Society), facioscapulohumeral dis-
ease publication 107n
"Facts about Duchenne and Becker
Muscular Dystrophies" (MDA) 77n
"Facts about Metabolic Diseases of
Muscle" (MDA) 43n
"Facts about Mitochondrial Myopa-
thies" (MDA) 26n
"Facts about Myopathies" (MDA) 12n
"Facts about Myotonic Dystrophy"
(MDA) 133n
"Facts about Polymyositis and Der-
matomyositis" (MDA) 59n

"Facts About Rare Muscular Dystrophies" (MDA) 103n
FAPE *see* free appropriate public education
Farley Technologies, Inc., Web site address 524
Farrell, Kathleen 397
fat-processing disorders, described 54
"Faulty Gene is Key to Understanding Myotonic Dystrophy" (Lai) 133n
"Faulty Muscle Repair Implicated in Muscular Dystrophies" (Zeigler) 3n
Fee, Richard W. 486n, 493n
feeding tubes
  described 153
  overview 387–92
FemHRT *199*
FemPatch *198*
financial considerations
  electromyography 180
  individualized education programs 443
  massage therapy 272
  special needs trusts 502–7
Finnish distal myopathy *104*, 104–5
Flaghouse, Inc., Web site address 526
Flanigan, Kevin 159–61
flu *see* influenza
fluid intake 399–400
Forbes' disease *see* debrancher enzyme deficiency
Fosamax (alendronate) 196, 197, *199*
fosinopril *210*
free appropriate public education (FAPE) 438, 441, 443
Friedreich's ataxia
  heart problems 202
  toileting difficulties 395
Frolik, Lawrence A. 478n
"From Steroids to Stem Cells" (Stimson) 223n
"From Where I Sit" (Shipley) 329n
FSHD *see* Facioscapulohumeral Dystrophy Society; facioscapulohumeral muscular dystrophy
FSH Society *see* FacioScapuloHumeral Society
Fukuyama congenital muscular dystrophy 74
furosemide *210*

G

gamma-sarcoglycan 126
"Gastrostomy" (Muscular Dystrophy Campaign) 387n
gastrostomy tubes *see* feeding tubes
gender factor
  Becker muscular dystrophy 90
  calcium supplements 194
  Duchenne muscular dystrophy 6, 77–79
  myotubular myopathy 23
  osteoporosis 190–91
gene deletion, defined 514
general anesthetic *see* anesthesia
gene replacement therapy, Duchenne muscular dystrophy 7–8
genes
  Becker muscular dystrophy 6–7
  Duchenne muscular dystrophy 6–7
  facioscapulohumeral muscular dystrophy 5, 108–9, 116–18
  limb-girdle muscular dystrophy 121
  metabolic diseases 45–46
  mitochondrial diseases 39–40
  mitochondrial myopathies 29–30
  muscular dystrophy 14, 223
  myositis 62, 63
  myotonic muscular dystrophy 5, 148–49
  see also heredity
Gene Tests, contact information 186
gene therapy
  limb-girdle muscular dystrophy 226–27
  muscle diseases 228–29
  vector delivery 227
genetic counseling, Duchenne muscular dystrophy 81
genetic defects
  facioscapulohumeral muscular dystrophy 116–18
  metabolic diseases of muscle 43
"Genetics and LGMD" (Duke University Medical Center) 121n
genetic tests
  Becker muscular dystrophy 92
  congenital muscular dystrophy 74

genetic tests, continued
  defined 514
  inheritable myopathies 24
  metabolic diseases of muscle 55
  mitochondrial diseases 39
  myotonic muscular dystrophy 163
  overview 181–86
gentamicin 8, 224, 307
glucocorticoids 304
glycogenosis type 2 *see* acid maltase
  deficiency
glycogenosis type 3 *see* debrancher
  enzyme deficiency
glycogenosis type 5 *see* phosphorylase
  deficiency
glycogenosis type 7 *see* phosphofructokinase deficiency
glycogenosis type 9 *see* phosphoglycerate kinase deficiency
glycogenosis type 10 *see* phosphoglycerate mutase deficiency
glycogenosis type 11 *see* lactate
  dehydrogenase deficiency
government benefits
  described 482–83
  special needs trusts 493–94
Gower's distal myopathy *104*, 105
Great Ideas Inc./Solution
  Comfortseat, Web site address 524
"The Great Trach Escape" (Wahl)
  254n
g-tubes (gastrostomy tubes) *see* feeding tubes
"A Guide for Parents: Section 3 - General Care" (Muscular Dystrophy Association - Australia) 421n
"A Guide for Parents: Section 5 -
  Everyday Living" (Muscular Dystrophy Association - Australia) 429n
Guldmann, Inc., Web site address 524
Gussoni, Emmanuela 230
Gwinn-Hardy, Katrina 117

H

Hayek Oscillator 251
Hayes, Sheila 234, 236–37, 238–39
headaches, pain management 270

heart disease
  anesthesia 214–15
  Emery-Dreyfuss muscular dystro-
    phy 96
  myotonic muscular dystrophy 139
  neuromuscular disorders 201–11
heart failure
  described 204–11
  metabolic disorders 49
"The Heart is a Muscle, Too - Frequently Asked Questions about
  Cardiac Problems" (Wahl) 201n
heart transplantation, congestive
  heart failure 209
Hemovac, described 284
Henderson, Richard 192–93
Hepp, P. 59
Herediary inclusion-body myositis
  (HIBM) 105–6
hereditary inclusion-body myositis
  (HIBM) *104*
heredity
  Becker muscular dystrophy 90–91
  congenital muscular dystrophy 73
  distal muscular dystrophies 103–6
  Duchenne muscular dystrophy 6,
    81–82
  Emery-Dreyfuss muscular dystro-
    phy 97–99, *98*
  facioscapulohumeral muscular dys-
    trophy 107, 109
  limb-girdle muscular dystrophy
    122–23
  metabolic diseases of muscle 55–56
  mitochondrial chronic external oph-
    thalmoplegia 155
  mitochondrial diseases 39–40
  myopathies 14–24
  myositis 60–61
  myotonic muscular dystrophy 4–5
  oculopharyngeal muscular dystro-
    phy 153
  see also genes
Hernandez-Reif, Maria 272, 274–75
HIBM *see* Herediary inclusion-body
  myositis
hips, passive stretches *313*, 313–14,
  314
histamine, inflammations 220

home health care, overview 379–85
"Home Health Care: Home Is Where
the Help Is" (Ivory) 379n
home health nurse, defined 514–15
hormones, osteoporosis prevention
195–96
horseback riding 426
Huang, Leaf 228
Huard, Johnny 230
huffing, described 249
Hutterite dystrophy 132
hydrocortisone 304
hydrotherapy, defined 515
hydroxychloroquine 65
hyperkalemic periodic paralysis 17–
18, 19–20
hyperthermia, anesthesia 216
hyperthyroid myopathy, described 25
hypertrophic cardiomyopathy, described 204
hypokalemic periodic paralysis 19,
20–21
hypothyroid myopathy, described 25–
26
hypoventilation, nocturnal 246–48

I

ibuprofen 65
IDEA *see* Individuals with Disabilities Act
ideal body weight, Duchenne muscular
dystrophy 301
IFSP *see* individualized family service
plan
immune system
inflammation 220, 267–68
myositis 60, 63
immunosuppressants, inflammations
221
incentive spirometer, described 283
Inderal (propranolol) *210*
individualized education programs
(IEP)
assistive technology services 446
described 441–43
mitochondrial diseases 33
special education process rights 467

individualized family service plan
(IFSP) 467, 468–69
Individuals with Disabilities Education Act (IDEA) 233, 243–44, 438–
65
special education process rights
465–67
infants
central core disease 21
congenital muscular dystrophy 69–
70
facioscapulohumeral muscular dystrophy 110
myotonic muscular dystrophy 133,
144
myotubular myopathy 23
Pompe's disease 51
see also children
inflammatory myopathies *see* dermatomyositis; polymyositis
influenza vaccine 249
inherited, defined 515
In Motion Magazine, Web site address 526
inotropes, congestive heart failure
210
inspiratory muscles, described 247
insurance coverage
airway clearing devices 251
genetic testing 185
physical therapy 239–40
International Myotonic Dystrophy
Organization, contact information
149, 520
International Ventilator Users Network (IVUN), contact information
265
interstitial lung disease 66
intervivos trusts 497–98
intravenous immunoglobulin (IVIg)
65
ion channel defects 14–15, 17, 19
ion channels, muscle contraction 14–
15
iron lungs, described 256
irrevocable trusts 499
isoforms 204
isosorbide dinitrate *210*
IVIG 221

IVIg *see* intravenous immunoglobulin
Ivory, Phil 379n
IVUN *see* International Ventilator
   Users Network

J

Jabre, Joe F. 177n
J.H. Emerson, contact information
   253
joint flexibility 289–90

K

KAFO *see* knee-ankle-foot orthoses
Kaplan, Marla 273, 278
karyotyping, described 514
Kaye Products, Inc., Web site address
   525
Kayjae Manufacturing Co., Inc., Web
   site address 525
Kearns Sayre syndrome (KSS) 35,
   155
Keybowl, Inc., Web site address 525
kinase 5
King, Wendy M. 273
"Kitchen Adaptations" (Muscular
   Dystrophy Campaign) 333n
knee-ankle-foot orthoses (KAFO) 238,
   295–99
knees, passive stretches 311–13, *312*
KSS *see* Kearns-Sayre syndrome
Kunkel, Louis 229, 230

L

lactate dehydrogenase deficiency 53
lactic acidosis 30
Lai, Katie 133n
Lambert-Eaton syndrome
   inflammations 221
   treatment 192
laminA/C 125
laminin-m *see* merosin
Landouzy-Déjérine disease *see*
   facioscapulohumeral muscular dystrophy

Lanoxicaps (digoxin) *210*
Lanoxin (digoxin) *210*
Lasix (furosemide) *210*
L-carnitine 34
learning disabilities, Duchenne muscular dystrophy 424
Lee, Mike 396
Leigh's syndrome 35
"The Letter of Intent" (Fee) 486n
letter of intent, described 486–92
leukotrienes, inflammations 220
life expectancy
   Duchenne muscular dystrophy 418–
      19
   facioscapulohumeral muscular dys-
      trophy 110
limb-girdle muscular dystrophy
   (LGMD)
   clinical trials 8
   defined 515
   gene therapy 226–27
   heredity 104, 106
   home health care 383
   muscle biopsy 174
   overview 121–32
"Limb-Girdle Muscular Dystrophy"
   (Muscular Dystrophy Canada) 121n
lisinopril *210*
local anesthetic *see* anesthesia
logrolling, described 283
long leg braces 295
Lopressor (metoprolol) *210*
LTV950 261
Luque rod, described 281
lysosomal storage disease *see* acid
   maltase deficiency

M

macrophages, inflammations 220
Maddak, Inc., contact information
   346
Magitek.com, LLC, Web site address
   525
magnetic resonance imaging (MRI)
   Duchenne muscular dystrophy 81
   mitochondrial diseases 37
   myositis 64

"Making Breathing Easier" (Muscular Dystrophy Campaign) 246n
malignant hyperthermia 17, 21
Manitoba Hutterite dystrophy 132
Markesbery distal myopathy *104*, 104–5
Marulic, Carol 198–99
"Marvelous Massage" (Sowell) 267n
massage therapy, pain management 271–78
master trusts 500–502
maternally inherited Leigh's syndrome (MILS) 35
Maxi-Aids, Inc., contact information 346
McCardle's disease *see* phosphorylase deficiency
McKesson Health Solutions, LLC, creatine kinase test publication 167n
McMichael, Robert 197
MDA *see* Muscular Dystrophy Association
MDS *see* mitochondrial DNA depletion syndrome
MedicAlert bracelets
congestive heart failure 209
metabolic disorders 48
MedicAlert Foundation International, contact information 211
medical services, described 448
Medicare, airway clearing devices 251
Mendell, Jerry 226–27
menopause
osteoporosis 191
osteoporosis prevention 194–96
merosin 69, 71, 73–75, 99, 174
MERRF *see* myoclonus epilepsy with ragged red fibers
Mestinon 269, 272
metabolic diseases of muscle, overview 43–57
methotrexate 64, 221
methylphenidate 141
methylprednisolone 64
metoclopramide 139
metoprolol *210*
Miacalcin (calcitonin) 196, *199*
microdystrophins 228

microglia 221
milk
osteoporosis 190
osteoporosis prevention 194–95
MILS *see* maternally inherited Leigh's syndrome
mitochondria
central core disease 21
described 26–27, 39–40
metabolic diseases of muscle 43
mitochondrial DNA depletion syndrome (MDS) 35
mitochondrial encephalomyopathy
described 32
lactic acidosis, and strokelike episodes (MELAS) 35–36
mitochondrial myopathies, overview 26–42
mitochondrial myopathy, pain management 268
mitochondrial neurogastrointestinal encephalomyopathy (MNGIE) 36
mitosis, genetic testing 514
Miyoshi distal myopathy *104*, 105, 130
MMD *see* myotonic muscular dystrophy
MNGIE *see* mitochondrial neurogastrointestinal encephalomyopathy
mobility
age factor 429–35
Duchenne muscular dystrophy 425
Mobility Products and Design, Web site address 525
Mobility Transfer Systems, contact information 402
modafinil 142
Moeschen, Pat 272
Molecular Genetics Testing Laboratory, contact information 119
Monopril (fosinopril) *210*
motor neurons, physical therapy 236–37
movement therapy 444
MRI *see* magnetic resonance imaging
Muir, David 260
"Muscle Biopsies" (Muscular Dystrophy Campaign) 171n

muscle biopsy, described 171–75
muscle contraction, described 14–15, *15*
muscle contractures, described 95
muscle relaxants, anesthesia 215
muscles, described 308–9
muscle tone, described 14
muscle weakness, metabolic diseases 48
muscular dystrophy
  defined 515
  described 134, 279
  home adaptations 333–47
  overview 3–10
  treatment 3–4, 223–31
  see also Becker muscular dystrophy; congenital muscular dystrophy; distal muscular dystrophy; Duchenne muscular dystrophy; Emery-Dreifuss muscular dystrophy; facioscapulohumeral muscular dystrophy; limb-girdle muscular dystrophy; myotonic muscular dystrophy; spinal muscular dystrophy
Muscular Dystrophy Association (MDA)
  contact information 41, 56, 93, 149, 211, 520
  publications
    Becker muscular dystrophy 77n
    cardiac problems 201n
    coping strategies 349n
    cratine kinase test 167n
    dermatomyositis 59n
    disability coping strategies 329n
    Duchenne muscular dystrophy 77n
    facioscapulohumeral muscular dystrophy 107n
    home health care 379n
    inflammation 219n
    massage 267n
    mitochondrial myopathies 26n
    muscle metabolic diseases 43n
    muscular dystrophy treatment 223n
    myopathies 12n
    myotonic muscular dystrophy 133n

Muscular Dystrophy Association (MDA), continued
  publications, continued
    noninvasive ventilation 254n
    osteoporosis 189n
    pain management 267n
    physical therapy 233n
    polymyositis 59n
    rare muscular dystrophies 103n
    terminology 511n
    toileting management 393n
Muscular Dystrophy Association - Australia
  publications
    facioscapulohumeral muscular dystrophy 107n
    muscular dystrophy daily life 421n
    muscular dystrophy discussions 415n
    muscular dystrophy everyday living 429n
    school physical programs 471n
Muscular Dystrophy Australia, contact information 520
Muscular Dystrophy Campaign
  contact information 217, 520
  publications
    adaptations 333n
    anesthesia 213n
    Becker muscular dystrophy 87n
    breathing difficulty 246n
    Duchenne muscular dystrophy 77n
    Duchenne muscular dystrophy treatment 308n
    feeding tubes 387n
    hydration management 393n
    muscle biopsies 171n
    ocular myopathies 151n
    wheelchairs 363n
Muscular Dystrophy Canada,limb-girdle muscular dystrophy publication 121n
Muscular Dystrophy Family Foundation
  contact information 94, 521
  Web site address 525
music therapy 444

mutation, defined 515
myasthenia, defined 515
myasthenia gravis
  contractions 269
  cramping 268
  inflammations 221
  treatment 192
  vaccine 226
mycophenolate mofetil 226
MyMedMart, Inc.
  contact information 346
  Web site address 525
myoadenylate deaminase deficiency
  54
myocardium, described 206–7
myoclonus epilepsy with ragged red
  fibers (MERRF) 36
myofascial release, described 276
myoglobinuria, described 48
myopathy
  defined 516
  described 31–34
  overview 12–26
myophosphorylase deficiency *see*
  phosphorylase deficiency
myositis
  defined 59, 515
  inflammations 221
  overview 59–66
  pain management 267–68
  see also dermatomyositis; heredi-
    tary inclusion-body myositis;
    polymyositis
myotolin 125
myotonia
  defined 516
  described 4, 133–34, 138
myotonia congenita, described 18
myotonic muscular dystrophy
  (MMD)
  defined 516
  described 4–5
  heart problems 202, 203
  inflammations 220, 269
  overview 133–49
  treatment 225
myotubular myopathy, described 22–
  23

N

naproxen 65
NARP *see* neuropathy, ataxia, and re-
  tinitis pigmentosa
nasal pillows, described 255
nasal ventilation, described 250
National Ability Center, contact infor-
  mation 521
National Consortium for Physical
  Education and Recreation for Indi-
  viduals with Disabilities
  (NCPERID), contact information
  464, 521
National Disability Sports Alliance
  contact information 521
  Web site address 526
National Dissemination Center for
  Children with Disabilities
  (NICHCY)
  contact information 243, 413, 465,
    470, 521
  publications
    children with disabilities 438n
    estate planning 478n
    letters of intent 486n
    special needs trusts 493n
National Institute of Art and Dis-
  abilities (NIAD), contact informa-
  tion 464
National Institute of Neurological
  Disorders and Stroke (NINDS)
  contact information 521
  facioscapulohumeral muscular dys-
    trophy publication 107n
National Institutes of Health (NIH),
  contact information 521
National Organization on Disability,
  contact information 521
National Osteoporosis Foundation,
  contact information 200, 522
National Registry of Myotonic Dystrophy and FSHD Patients and
  Family Members, contact information 118
NCPERID *see* National Consortium for
  Physical Education and Recreation
  for Individuals with Disabilities

nemaline myopathy
  biopsy 173
  cardiac care 17–18
  described 16, 21–22
neuromuscular disorders
  anesthesia risks 213–17
  breathing difficulties 246–51
  cardiac problems 201–11
  inflammations 219–21
  osteoporosis 189
  see also Becker muscular dystrophy;
    Duchenne muscular dystrophy;
    Emery-Dreifuss muscular dys-
    trophy; facioscapulohumeral
    muscular dystrophy; limb-girdle
    muscular dystrophy; muscular
    dystrophy; myotonic muscular
    dystrophy; spinal muscular dys-
    trophy
neuropathy, ataxia, and retinitis
  pigmentosa (NARP) 36
neuropathy, defined 516
New Angle Products, contact information 401
New Mobility Magazine, Web site address 527
"A New Test for Myotonic Dystrophy:
  Exposing an Enemy That's Too Big
  to See" (Zeigler) 163n
NIAD see National Institute of Art
  and Disabilities
NICHCY see National Dissemination
  Center for Children with Disabilities
Nichols, Yvonne 240
night splints 295, 316–17
NIH see National Institutes of Health
NINDS see National Institute of Neu-
  rological Disorders and Stroke
Nippy 250
Nissen's fundoplication 392
Nonaka distal myopathy 104, 105
noninvasive ventilation techniques
  254–65
nonsteroidal anti-inflammatory drugs
  (NSAID) 65, 269
No-Rinse Laboratories, LLC, Web site
  address 525
NSAID see nonsteroidal anti-inflam-
  matory drugs

"Nutritional Issues for Duchenne
  Muscular Dystrophy" (PPMD) 299n

O

obesity
  breathing problems 248
  Duchenne muscular dystrophy 302,
    425
obstructive sleep apnea 248, 251
occupational therapy (OT)
  Becker muscular dystrophy 92
  defined 516
  Duchenne muscular dystrophy 294–
    95
  facioscapulohumeral muscular dys-
    trophy 112
  limb-girdle muscular dystrophy 125
  mobility 429–30
  versus physical therapy 234
  students 448–49
"Ocular Myopathies" (Muscular Dystrophy Campaign) 151n
oculopharyngeal muscular dystrophy
  (OPMD) 151–54, 156
Oddis, Chester 197
"The Older Child with Duchenne
  Muscular Dystrophy" (Muscular
  Dystrophy Campaign) 77n
"101 Hints to 'Help-with-Ease' for Patients with Neuromuscular Disease"
  (MDA) 349n
OnTheGo
  contact information 402
  described 397
ophthalmoplegic muscular dystrophy,
  overview 151–56
OPMD see oculopharyngeal muscular
  dystrophy
Oppenheimer, Edward 258–59, 262–
  63
Orasone (prednisone) 192
orthoses
  ankle-foot 136, 238
  distal muscular dystropies 106
  knee-ankle-foot 238
orthotists, splints 295
Os-Cal 198

oscillation vest 262–63
osteoblasts, described 190, 196
osteoclasts, described 190
osteoporosis
defined 516
Duchenne muscular dystrophy 301–2
overview 189–200
OT *see* occupational therapy
"Overview of Estate Planning Issues"
(Frolik) 478n
oximeters, breathing techniques 263
oxygen, congestive heart failure 204–5
oxygen therapy, congestive heart failure 208

P

"Pain, Pain, Go Away" (Robinson)
267n
pain management
neuromuscular disease 267–78
patient controlled analgesia 283
Palaestra, Web site address 527
Pandya, Shree 234, 235–36, 238–39,
240, 241–42
paramyotonia congenita
described 18–19
diagnosis 24
parental concerns
family and friends 415–20
muscular dystrophy diagnosis 405–
13
Parent Project Muscular Dystrophy
(PPMD)
contact information 427, 522
publications
Duchenne muscular dystrophy
treatment 294n
muscular dystrophy basics 77n
muscular dystrophy daily life
421n
physical therapy 294n
respiratory difficulty 246n
splints and braces 294n
wheelchairs 363n
"Parents and Family: Daily Life"
(PPMD) 421n
Parent to Parent programs 408

passive stretching, Duchenne muscular dystrophy 310–17
Passy-Muir speaking valve 260
Pathways Awareness Foundation,
contact information 522
patient-controlled analgesia (PCA)
283, 285
PCA *see* patient controlled analgesia
PCR test *see* polymerase chain reaction
peak cough flow 251
Pearson syndrome 36
PEG *see* percutaneous endoscopic
gastrostomy
Penn, Audrey S. 3n
PEO *see* progressive external
ophthalmoplegia
percutaneous endoscopic gastrostomy
(PEG) 388
percutaneous tenotomy 291
periodic paralysis
described 19
diagnosis 24
personal assistants *see* home health
care
personal care attendants *see* home
health care
PGD *see* preimplantation genetic diagnosis
phenytoin 268
PHI *see* Post-Polio Health International
phosphocreatine kinase (CPK) 167
phosphofructokinase deficiency 52–53
phosphoglycerate kinase deficiency 53
phosphoglycerate mutase deficiency 53
phosphorylase deficiency
described 52
pain management 268
physical education, muscular dystrophy students 471–76
physical therapy (PT)
Becker muscular dystrophy 92
defined 516
Duchenne muscular dystrophy 294–
95
limb-girdle muscular dystrophy 125
mobility 425
overview 233–44
students 449–50

"Physical Therapy - Flexibility, Fitness, and Fun" (Wahl) 233n
physiotherapy
  Achilles tendon release 289
  breathing difficulties 249
  Duchenne muscular dystrophy 310
  mobility 429–30
pigmentary retinopathy 155
Pinczewski, Steve 272
Pittman, Gregory L. 273, 276
plasmapheresis, described 65
PLV-100 volume ventilator 257, 261
pneumobelt, described 260–61
pneumococcal vaccine 249
pneumonia, tracheostomy 258
PN/Paraplegia News, Web site address 527
polymerase chain reaction (PCR test) 164
polymyositis
  heart problems 202
  inflammations 220–21
  muscle biopsy 175
  overview 59–66
  pain management 267–68
  treatment 192
Pompe's disease 228
Pompe's disease (infantile form) *see* acid maltase deficiency
Post-Polio Health International (PHI), contact information 265
posture
  breathing difficulties 249
  Duchenne muscular dystrophy 317–18
  wheelchairs 364–68
potassium
  anesthesia 215
  muscle contraction 14
  periodic paralyses 19
PPMD *see* Parent Project Muscular Dystrophy
prednisolone 192, 224
prednisone 64, 192, 195, 221, 223–24, 225–26, 268, 270, 304–5, 424
pregnancy
  echocardiogram 209–10
  myotonic muscular dystrophy 141
preimplantation genetic diagnosis (PGD) 182

Prelone (prednisolone) 192
prenatal screening
  defined 516
  facioscapulohumeral muscular dystrophy 112
Prinivil (lisinopril) *210*
progestin, osteoporosis prevention 196, *198*, *199*
progressive external ophthalmoplegia (PEO) 31, 33, 36–37
Prometrium *198*
propranolol *210*
prostaglandins, inflammations 220, 221
protein deficiencies, heart problems 203–4
proteins
  metabolic diseases 45
  mitochondrial myopathies 29
  muscular dystrophy 9–10
  myotonic muscular dystrophy 5
Provera *198*
Provigil (modafinil) 142
psychological services, students 450–51
PT *see* physical therapy
ptosis
  defined 151
  described 31, 33, 137
Public Law 94-142 *see* Education of All Handicapped Children Act
Public Law 101-476 *see* Individuals with Disabilities Education Act
pulmonary edema, described 205–6, 211
Pulmonetic Systems, Inc., contact information 265

Q

Quackwatch, Web site address 186
quinine 268

R

raloxifene 196, *199*
"Range of Specifications and Wheelchair Features" (Muscular Dystrophy Campaign) 363n

Ranum, Laura 163–65, 225
rashes, dermatomyositis 59, 60, 62
R.D. Equipment, contact information 402
reactive oxygen species 30
recreation, students 451–52
"Recreation Options" (Muscular Dystrophy - Australia) 471n
reduction surgery, described 209
Reglan (metoclopramide) 139
Rehab Designs, Inc.
    contact information 347
    Web site address 525
related services, overview 439–60
"Related Services for School-Aged Children with Disabilities" (NICHCY) 438n
RESNA, contact information 464, 522
respiratory care
    Becker muscular dystrophy 92
    easier breathing techniques 246–65
    inheritable myopathies 17
    metabolic disorders 49
    myopathies 32
    myotonic muscular dystrophy 138
respiratory infections
    noninvasive ventilation 264
    tracheostomy 258
respite care 430
revocable trusts 499
Reye's syndrome 270
rhabdomyolysis
    creatine kinase levels 168
    exercise intolerance 47
    myopathy 31
"Rights and Responsibilities of Parents of Children with Disabilities: Update 1999" (ERIC Clearinghouse) 465n
risedronate 196, *199*
Ritalin (methylphenidate) 141
Robinson, Richard 267n
Robison, Jenny 236, 239, 240
Rocaltrol (calcitriol) *198*
Rochester Medical Corporation, contact information 402
rod body disease 21–22
Rothstein, Jeffrey 231
Ryno Mobility Corporation, Web site address 525

S

safety issues, physical education 475
salbutamol 250
sarcoglycan 203
SATH (Society for Accessible Travel and Hospitality)/Open World, Web site address 527
SCAIP sequencing *see* single condition amplification/internal primer sequencing
SCARMD *see* severe childhood autosomal recessive muscular dystrophy
school health services, students 453
sciatica 421
scoliosis
    breathing difficulties 249
    defined 516–17
    respiratory muscles 247
    treatment 279–87
scopolamine 270
see mitochondrial chronic external ophthalmoplegia (CPEO) 151, 154–56
selective estrogen receptor modulators (SERMs) 196
septal myotomy, described 209
SERMs *see* selective estrogen receptor modulators
serotonin 275
severe childhood autosomal recessive muscular dystrophy (SCARMD) 131
sexuality, muscular dystrophy diagnosis 432
Shiatsu, described 276
Shipley, Sandy 329n
shoulders, passive stretches 316, *316*
side effects, prednisone 305
"Simply Stated ... Inflammation" (MDA) 511n
"Simply Stated ... Neuromuscular Terminology" (MDA) 511n
"Simply Stated ... The Creatine Kinase Test" (MDA) 167n
single condition amplification/internal primer (SCAIP sequencing) 160
skeletal pain management 269–70

sleep disorders
  myotonic muscular dystrophy 141–42, 146–48
  nocturnal hypoventilation 246–48
  obstructive sleep apnea 248
  prevention 422
Smith, Patricia McGill 405n
Snug Seat, Web site address 526
social work services 454
sodium
  muscle contraction 14
  paramyotonia congenita 18
Sowell, Carol 267n
special education concerns
  muscular dystrophy 433–34
  parental rights 465–70
"The Special Needs Trust" (Fee) 493n
special needs trusts 493–507
speech therapy
  Duchenne muscular dystrophy 424
  facioscapulohumeral muscular dystrophy 112
  myopathy 31
  myotonic muscular dystrophy 145
  students 454
  swallowing difficulties 66
spinal fusion, described 281
spinal muscular atrophy, described 516
spinal muscular dystrophy
  defined 517
  physical therapy 236
spironolactone *210*
splints, Duchenne muscular dystrophy 295–99
sports, muscular dystrophy students 471–76
Sports 'n Spokes, Web site address 527
Stack, Jennie Borodko 393n
stair step phenomenon, described 122
Stedman, Hansell 228
Stedman's Medical Dictionary (Lippincott Williams and Wilkins) 511n
stem cell therapy
  muscular dystrophy 223
  neuromuscular diseases 229
"Sticks and Stones Break Fragile Bones" (Wahl) 189n
Stimson, Dan 223n

stoma, described 388
strabismus, described 145
stretching exercises
  Achilles tendon 425–26
  ankles 311, *312*
  elbows 315, *315*
  hips *313*, 313–14, *314*
  knees 311–13, *312*
  passive stretching 310–17
  shoulders 316, *316*
  wrists 315, *315*
subacute necrotizing encephalomyopathy 35
supplements
  creatine 306
  osteoporosis prevention 194–95
support systems, muscular dystrophy diagnosis 408–9, 413
Surehands Lift and Care Systems
  contact information 347
  Web site address 526
surgery
  Becker muscular dystrophy 92
  Emery-Dreyfuss muscular dystrophy 97
  scoliosis treatment 280–87
  skeletal pain management 270
surgical procedures
  Achilles tendons 291–92
  cataracts 142–43
  congestive heart failure 209
  facioscapulohumeral muscular dystrophy 112–13
  feeding tubes 388
  Nissen's fundoplication 392
  tracheostomy 255
swallowing difficulty
  feeding tubes 387–88, 389
  myotonic muscular dystrophy 138
Swedish massage, described 275–76
swimming 426

T

Tarui's disease *see* phosphofructokinase deficiency
teachers, muscular dystrophy students 475–76

Tegretol (carbamazepine) 268
"TeleEMG.com Patient's Guide to EMG and Nerve Conduction Studies" (Jabre) 177n
telethonin 127
Tendercare4kids, Web site address 526
terminology, understanding 409–10
testamentary trusts 497–98
"Testimony on Muscular Dystrophy" (Penn) 3n
Testoderm *199*
testosterone 196, *199*
tests
  Becker muscular dystrophy 92
  congenital muscular dystrophy 71
  creatine kinase 167–70
  Duchenne muscular dystrophy 81, 159–61
  facioscapulohumeral muscular dystrophy 110
  heart problems 139
  inheritable myopathies 23–24
  limb-girdle muscular dystrophy 123–24
  metabolic diseases of muscle 55
  mitochondrial diseases 37–39, *38*
  myositis 63–64
  myotonia 145–46
  myotonic muscular dystrophy 163–65
  oculopharyngeal muscular dystrophy 156
  osteoporosis 193
  sleep studies 248
  see also electromyography; genetic tests
thryoxine 25–26
thyroid-stimulating hormones (THS), inheritable myopathy diagnosis 24
thyrotoxic myopathy 25
tibial muscular dystrophy 104
Today's Caregiver Magazine, Web site address 527
toileting
  activities of daily living 357–58
  bowel management 421–22
  overview 393–402
Toprol XL (metoprolol) *210*

Touch Research Institutes, contact information 278
touch therapy 274–75
Touch Turner, Web site address 526
tracheostomy
  defined 517
  described 255, 257
transportation issues, students 455–56
Trautlein, Judith 194–95
"Treating Scoliosis in Muscular Dystrophy" (University of Iowa) 279n
"Treatment for DMD: Respiratory News" (PPMD) 246n
"Treatment for DMD: Wheelchairs FAQ" (PPMD) 363n
"Treatment for Duchenne MD: Physical Therapy" (PPMD) 294n
"Treatment for Duchenne MD: Steroids/Nutritional Supplements/Antibiotics" (PPMD) 299n
triamcinolone 192
triamterene *210*
trigger points, massage therapy 276
triplet repeat disorders 5
trustees, described 499–500
trusts, special needs 493–507
Tums 195, *198*
Tupler, Rossella 117–18, 225

U

ultrasound, osteoporosis diagnosis 193
University of Iowa, scoliosis treatment publication 279n
University of Tennessee Medical Center, contact information 156
Unverricht, H. 59
urinals 396
urinary tract infections, women 398
US Department of Education (DOE), contact information 244, 522
"Use of Physiotherapy in Duchenne MD" (Muscular Dystrophy Campaign) 308n
utrophin 224–25

V

vaccines
  influenza 249
  myasthenia gravis 226
  pneumonia 249
vacuoles, described 106
vasodilation, inflammations 220
vasodilators, congestive heart failure *210*
ventilation devices, breathing assistance 250–53
Ventolin (salbutamol) 250
Vest 262–63
Viroslav, Joseph 260
vitamin D 194–95, *198*
Vogel, Steven 9–10
Voice Factor, Web site address 526
volume ventilators 256–57

W

Wagner, Janis 397
Wahl, Margaret 189n, 201n, 233n, 254n
walkers, Achilles tendon release 291
Welander's distal myopathy, described *104*
"What Is a Good Seating Position?" (Muscular Dystrophy Campaign) 363n
wheelchairs
  accessibility issues 423
  Achilles tendon release 289, 291
  golf 472–73
  home adaptations 333–45
  mobility 430, 431, 432
  orienteering 473

wheelchairs, continued
  overview 363–77
  soccer 472
  softball 472
  toileting 394
"When You've Gotta Go, You've Gotta Go" (Stack) 393n
Whizzy 397
Williams, Tracy 277
wills, estate planning 480–81, 483–85
wrists, passive stretches 315, *315*
wrist supports *136*

X

Xiao, Xiao 227
X-linked inheritance
  Becker muscular dystrophy 90, 91
  defined 517
  Emery-Dreyfuss muscular dystrophy 97–98, *98*
  myotubular myopathy 22–23, *23*
X-linked recessive inheritance, phosphoglycerate kinase deficiency 53
x-rays, osteoporosis 193

Y

yogurt 195
"You Are Not Alone" (Smith) 405n

Z

Z-discs, described 14
Zeigler, Tania 3n, 159n, 163n
Zestril (lisinopril) *210*

Health Reference Series
COMPLETE CATALOG

Adolescent Health Sourcebook

Basic Consumer Health Information about Common Medical, Mental, and Emotional Concerns in Adolescents, Including Facts about Acne, Body Piercing, Mononucleosis, Nutrition, Eating Disorders, Stress, Depression, Behavior Problems, Peer Pressure, Violence, Gangs, Drug Use, Puberty, Sexuality, Pregnancy, Learning Disabilities, and More

Along with a Glossary of Terms and Other Resources for Further Help and Information

Edited by Chad T. Kimball. 658 pages. 2002. 0-7808-0248-9. $78.

"It is written in clear, nontechnical language aimed at general readers. . . . Recommended for public libraries, community colleges, and other agencies serving health care consumers."
—*American Reference Books Annual, 2003*

"Recommended for school and public libraries. Parents and professionals dealing with teens will appreciate the easy-to-follow format and the clearly written text. This could become a 'must have' for every high school teacher." —*E-Streams, Jan '03*

"A good starting point for information related to common medical, mental, and emotional concerns of adolescents." —*School Library Journal, Nov '02*

"This book provides accurate information in an easy to access format. It addresses topics that parents and caregivers might not be aware of and provides practical, useable information." —*Doody's Health Sciences Book Review Journal, Sep-Oct '02*

"Recommended reference source."
—*Booklist, American Library Association, Sep '02*

■

AIDS Sourcebook, 3rd Edition

Basic Consumer Health Information about Acquired Immune Deficiency Syndrome (AIDS) and Human Immunodeficiency Virus (HIV) Infection, Including Facts about Transmission, Prevention, Diagnosis, Treatment, Opportunistic Infections, and Other Complications, with a Section for Women and Children, Including Details about Associated Gynecological Concerns, Pregnancy, and Pediatric Care

Along with Updated Statistical Information, Reports on Current Research Initiatives, a Glossary, and Directories of Internet, Hotline, and Other Resources

Edited by Dawn D. Matthews. 664 pages. 2003. 0-7808-0631-X. $78.

ALSO AVAILABLE: *AIDS Sourcebook, 1st Edition.* Edited by Karen Bellenir and Peter D. Dresser. 831 pages. 1995. 0-7808-0031-1. $78.

AIDS Sourcebook, 2nd Edition. Edited by Karen Bellenir. 751 pages. 1999. 0-7808-0225-X. $78.

"The 3rd edition of the *AIDS Sourcebook*, part of Omnigraphics' *Health Reference Series*, is a welcome update. . . . This resource is highly recommended for academic and public libraries."
—*American Reference Books Annual, 2004*

"Excellent sourcebook. This continues to be a highly recommended book. There is no other book that provides as much information as this book provides."
—*AIDS Book Review Journal, Dec-Jan 2000*

"Recommended reference source."
—*Booklist, American Library Association, Dec '99*

"A solid text for college-level health libraries."
—*The Bookwatch, Aug '99*

Cited in *Reference Sources for Small and Medium-Sized Libraries, American Library Association, 1999*

■

Alcoholism Sourcebook

Basic Consumer Health Information about the Physical and Mental Consequences of Alcohol Abuse, Including Liver Disease, Pancreatitis, Wernicke-Korsakoff Syndrome (Alcoholic Dementia), Fetal Alcohol Syndrome, Heart Disease, Kidney Disorders, Gastrointestinal Problems, and Immune System Compromise and Featuring Facts about Addiction, Detoxification, Alcohol Withdrawal, Recovery, and the Maintenance of Sobriety

Along with a Glossary and Directories of Resources for Further Help and Information

Edited by Karen Bellenir. 613 pages. 2000. 0-7808-0325-6. $78.

"This title is one of the few reference works on alcoholism for general readers. For some readers this will be a welcome complement to the many self-help books on the market. Recommended for collections serving general readers and consumer health collections."
—*E-Streams, Mar '01*

"This book is an excellent choice for public and academic libraries."
—*American Reference Books Annual, 2001*

"Recommended reference source."
—*Booklist, American Library Association, Dec '00*

"Presents a wealth of information on alcohol use and abuse and its effects on the body and mind, treatment, and prevention." —*SciTech Book News, Dec '00*

"Important new health guide which packs in the latest consumer information about the problems of alcoholism." —*Reviewer's Bookwatch, Nov '00*

SEE ALSO *Drug Abuse Sourcebook, Substance Abuse Sourcebook*

Allergies Sourcebook, 2nd Edition

Basic Consumer Health Information about Allergic Disorders, Triggers, Reactions, and Related Symptoms, Including Anaphylaxis, Rhinitis, Sinusitis, Asthma, Dermatitis, Conjunctivitis, and Multiple Chemical Sensitivity

Along with Tips on Diagnosis, Prevention, and Treatment, Statistical Data, a Glossary, and a Directory of Sources for Further Help and Information

Edited by Annemarie S. Muth. 598 pages. 2002. 0-7808-0376-0. $78.

ALSO AVAILABLE: *Allergies Sourcebook, 1st Edition.* Edited by Allan R. Cook. 611 pages. 1997. 0-7808-0036-2. $78.

"This book brings a great deal of useful material together. . . . This is an excellent addition to public and consumer health library collections."
— *American Reference Books Annual, 2003*

"This second edition would be useful to laypersons with little or advanced knowledge of the subject matter. This book would also serve as a resource for nursing and other health care professions students. It would be useful in public, academic, and hospital libraries with consumer health collections." — *E-Streams, Jul '02*

■

Alternative Medicine Sourcebook, 2nd Edition

Basic Consumer Health Information about Alternative and Complementary Medical Practices, Including Acupuncture, Chiropractic, Herbal Medicine, Homeopathy, Naturopathic Medicine, Mind-Body Interventions, Ayurveda, and Other Non-Western Medical Traditions

Along with Facts about such Specific Therapies as Massage Therapy, Aromatherapy, Qigong, Hypnosis, Prayer, Dance, and Art Therapies, a Glossary, and Resources for Further Information

Edited by Dawn D. Matthews. 618 pages. 2002. 0-7808-0605-0. $78.

ALSO AVAILABLE: *Alternative Medicine Sourcebook, 1st Edition.* Edited by Allan R. Cook. 737 pages. 1999. 0-7808-0200-4. $78.

"Recommended for public, high school, and academic libraries that have consumer health collections. Hospital libraries that also serve the public will find this to be a useful resource." — *E-Streams, Feb '03*

"Recommended reference source."
— *Booklist, American Library Association, Jan '03*

"An important alternate health reference."
— *MBR Bookwatch, Oct '02*

"A great addition to the reference collection of every type of library." — *American Reference Books Annual, 2000*

Alzheimer's Disease Sourcebook, 3rd Edition

Basic Consumer Health Information about Alzheimer's Disease, Other Dementias, and Related Disorders, Including Multi-Infarct Dementia, AIDS Dementia Complex, Dementia with Lewy Bodies, Huntington's Disease, Wernicke-Korsakoff Syndrome (Alcohol-Reated Dementia), Delirium, and Confusional States

Along with Information for People Newly Diagnosed with Alzheimer's Disease and Caregivers, Reports Detailing Current Research Efforts in Prevention, Diagnosis, and Treatment, Facts about Long-Term Care Issues, and Listings of Sources for Additional Information

Edited by Karen Bellenir. 645 pages. 2003. 0-7808-0666-2. $78.

ALSO AVAILABLE: *Alzheimer's, Stroke & 29 Other Neurological Disorders Sourcebook, 1st Edition.* Edited by Frank E. Bair. 579 pages. 1993. 1-55888-748-2. $78.

ALSO AVAILABLE: *Alzheimer's Disease Sourcebook, 2nd Edition.* Edited by Karen Bellenir. 524 pages. 1999. 0-7808-0223-3. $78.

"This very informative and valuable tool will be a great addition to any library serving consumers, students and health care workers."
— *American Reference Books Annual, 2004*

"This is a valuable resource for people affected by dementias such as Alzheimer's. It is easy to navigate and includes important information and resources."
— *Doody's Review Service, Feb. 2004*

"Recommended reference source."
— *Booklist, American Library Association, Oct '99*

SEE ALSO *Brain Disorders Sourcebook*

■

Arthritis Sourcebook, 2nd Edition

Basic Consumer Health Information about Osteoarthritis, Rheumatoid Arthritis, Other Rheumatic Disorders, Infectious Forms of Arthritis, and Diseases with Symptoms Linked to Arthritis, Featuring Facts about Diagnosis, Pain Management, and Surgical Therapies

Along with Coping Strategies, Research Updates, a Glossary, and Resources for Additional Help and Information

Edited by Amy L. Sutton. 600 pages. 2004. 0-7808-0667-0. $78.

ALSO AVAILABLE: *Arthritis Sourcebook, 1st Edition.* Edited by Allan R. Cook. 550 pages. 1998. 0-7808-0201-2. $78.

". . . accessible to the layperson."
— *Reference and Research Book News, Feb '99*

Asthma Sourcebook

Basic Consumer Health Information about Asthma, Including Symptoms, Traditional and Nontraditional Remedies, Treatment Advances, Quality-of-Life Aids, Medical Research Updates, and the Role of Allergies, Exercise, Age, the Environment, and Genetics in the Development of Asthma

Along with Statistical Data, a Glossary, and Directories of Support Groups, and Other Resources for Further Information

Edited by Annemarie S. Muth. 628 pages. 2000. 0-7808-0381-7. $78.

"A worthwhile reference acquisition for public libraries and academic medical libraries whose readers desire a quick introduction to the wide range of asthma information." *— Choice, Association of College & Research Libraries, Jun '01*

"Recommended reference source."
— Booklist, American Library Association, Feb '01

"Highly recommended." *— The Bookwatch, Jan '01*

"There is much good information for patients and their families who deal with asthma daily."
— American Medical Writers Association Journal, Winter '01

"This informative text is recommended for consumer health collections in public, secondary school, and community college libraries and the libraries of universities with a large undergraduate population."
— American Reference Books Annual, 2001

■

Attention Deficit Disorder Sourcebook

Basic Consumer Health Information about Attention Deficit/Hyperactivity Disorder in Children and Adults, Including Facts about Causes, Symptoms, Diagnostic Criteria, and Treatment Options Such as Medications, Behavior Therapy, Coaching, and Homeopathy

Along with Reports on Current Research Initiatives, Legal Issues, and Government Regulations, and Featuring a Glossary of Related Terms, Internet Resources, and a List of Additional Reading Material

Edited by Dawn D. Matthews. 470 pages. 2002. 0-7808-0624-7. $78.

"Recommended reference source."
— Booklist, American Library Association, Jan '03

"This book is recommended for all school libraries and the reference or consumer health sections of public libraries." *— American Reference Books Annual, 2003*

■

Back & Neck Disorders Sourcebook

Basic Information about Disorders and Injuries of the Spinal Cord and Vertebrae, Including Facts on Chiropractic Treatment, Surgical Interventions, Paralysis, and Rehabilitation

Along with Advice for Preventing Back Trouble

Edited by Karen Bellenir. 548 pages. 1997. 0-7808-0202-0. $78.

"The strength of this work is its basic, easy-to-read format. Recommended."
— Reference and User Services Quarterly, American Library Association, Winter '97

■

Blood & Circulatory Disorders Sourcebook

Basic Information about Blood and Its Components, Anemias, Leukemias, Bleeding Disorders, and Circulatory Disorders, Including Aplastic Anemia, Thalassemia, Sickle-Cell Disease, Hemochromatosis, Hemophilia, Von Willebrand Disease, and Vascular Diseases

Along with a Special Section on Blood Transfusions and Blood Supply Safety, a Glossary, and Source Listings for Further Help and Information

Edited by Karen Bellenir and Linda M. Shin. 554 pages. 1998. 0-7808-0203-9. $78.

"Recommended reference source."
— Booklist, American Library Association, Feb '99

"An important reference sourcebook written in simple language for everyday, non-technical users."
— Reviewer's Bookwatch, Jan '99

■

Brain Disorders Sourcebook

Basic Consumer Health Information about Strokes, Epilepsy, Amyotrophic Lateral Sclerosis (ALS/Lou Gehrig's Disease), Parkinson's Disease, Brain Tumors, Cerebral Palsy, Headache, Tourette Syndrome, and More

Along with Statistical Data, Treatment and Rehabilitation Options, Coping Strategies, Reports on Current Research Initiatives, a Glossary, and Resource Listings for Additional Help and Information

Edited by Karen Bellenir. 481 pages. 1999. 0-7808-0229-2. $78.

"Belongs on the shelves of any library with a consumer health collection." *— E-Streams, Mar '00*

"Recommended reference source."
— Booklist, American Library Association, Oct '99

***SEE ALSO** Alzheimer's Disease Sourcebook*

■

Breast Cancer Sourcebook, 2nd Edition

Basic Consumer Health Information about Breast Cancer, Including Facts about Risk Factors, Prevention, Screening and Diagnostic Methods, Treatment Options, Complementary and Alternative Therapies, Post-Treatment Concerns, Clinical Trials, Special Risk Populations, and New Developments in Breast Cancer Research

Along with Breast Cancer Statistics, a Glossary of Related Terms, and a Directory of Resources for Additional Help and Information

Edited by Sandra J. Judd. 600 pages. 2004. 0-7808-0668-9. $78.

ALSO AVAILABLE: Breast Cancer Sourcebook, 1st Edition. Edited by Edward J. Prucha and Karen Bellenir. 580 pages. 2001. 0-7808-0244-6. $78.

"It would be a useful reference book in a library or on loan to women in a support group."
— *Cancer Forum, Mar '03*

"Recommended reference source."
— *Booklist, American Library Association, Jan '02*

"This reference source is highly recommended. It is quite informative, comprehensive and detailed in nature, and yet it offers practical advice in easy-to-read language. It could be thought of as the 'bible' of breast cancer for the consumer." — *E-Streams, Jan '02*

"The broad range of topics covered in lay language make the *Breast Cancer Sourcebook* an excellent addition to public and consumer health library collections."
— *American Reference Books Annual 2002*

"From the pros and cons of different screening methods and results to treatment options, *Breast Cancer Sourcebook* provides the latest information on the subject."
— *Library Bookwatch, Dec '01*

"This thoroughgoing, very readable reference covers all aspects of breast health and cancer. . . . Readers will find much to consider here. Recommended for all public and patient health collections."
— *Library Journal, Sep '01*

SEE ALSO Cancer Sourcebook for Women, Women's Health Concerns Sourcebook

▪

Breastfeeding Sourcebook

Basic Consumer Health Information about the Benefits of Breastmilk, Preparing to Breastfeed, Breastfeeding as a Baby Grows, Nutrition, and More, Including Information on Special Situations and Concerns Such as Mastitis, Illness, Medications, Allergies, Multiple Births, Prematurity, Special Needs, and Adoption

Along with a Glossary and Resources for Additional Help and Information

Edited by Jenni Lynn Colson. 388 pages. 2002. 0-7808-0332-9. $78.

SEE ALSO Pregnancy & Birth Sourcebook

"Particularly useful is the information about professional lactation services and chapters on breastfeeding when returning to work. . . . *Breastfeeding Sourcebook* will be useful for public libraries, consumer health libraries, and technical schools offering nurse assistant training, especially in areas where Internet access is problematic."
— *American Reference Books Annual, 2003*

Burns Sourcebook

Basic Consumer Health Information about Various Types of Burns and Scalds, Including Flame, Heat, Cold, Electrical, Chemical, and Sun Burns

Along with Information on Short-Term and Long-Term Treatments, Tissue Reconstruction, Plastic Surgery, Prevention Suggestions, and First Aid

Edited by Allan R. Cook. 604 pages. 1999. 0-7808-0204-7. $78.

"This is an exceptional addition to the series and is highly recommended for all consumer health collections, hospital libraries, and academic medical centers."
— *E-Streams, Mar '00*

"This key reference guide is an invaluable addition to all health care and public libraries in confronting this ongoing health issue."
— *American Reference Books Annual, 2000*

"Recommended reference source."
— *Booklist, American Library Association, Dec '99*

SEE ALSO Skin Disorders Sourcebook

▪

Cancer Sourcebook, 4th Edition

Basic Consumer Health Information about Major Forms and Stages of Cancer, Featuring Facts about Head and Neck Cancers, Lung Cancers, Gastrointestinal Cancers, Genitourinary Cancers, Lymphomas, Blood Cell Cancers, Endocrine Cancers, Skin Cancers, Bone Cancers, Sarcomas, and Others, and Including Information about Cancer Treatments and Therapies, Identifying and Reducing Cancer Risks, and Strategies for Coping with Cancer and the Side Effects of Treatment

Along with a Cancer Glossary, Statistical and Demographic Data, and a Directory of Sources for Additional Help and Information

Edited by Karen Bellenir. 1,119 pages. 2003. 0-7808-0633-6. $78.

ALSO AVAILABLE: Cancer Sourcebook, 1st Edition. Edited by Frank E. Bair. 932 pages. 1990. 1-55888-888-8. $78.

New Cancer Sourcebook, 2nd Edition. Edited by Allan R. Cook. 1,313 pages. 1996. 0-7808-0041-9. $78.

Cancer Sourcebook, 3rd Edition. Edited by Edward J. Prucha. 1,069 pages. 2000. 0-7808-0227-6. $78.

"With cancer being the second leading cause of death for Americans, a prodigious work such as this one, which locates centrally so much cancer-related information, is clearly an asset to this nation's citizens and others." — *Journal of the National Medical Association, 2004*

"This title is recommended for health sciences and public libraries with consumer health collections."
— *E-Streams, Feb '01*

". . . can be effectively used by cancer patients and their families who are looking for answers in a language they can understand. Public and hospital libraries should have it on their shelves."
— *American Reference Books Annual, 2001*

Cancer Sourcebook for Women, 2nd Edition

Basic Consumer Health Information about Gynecologic Cancers and Related Concerns, Including Cervical Cancer, Endometrial Cancer, Gestational Trophoblastic Tumor, Ovarian Cancer, Uterine Cancer, Vaginal Cancer, Vulvar Cancer, Breast Cancer, and Common Non-Cancerous Uterine Conditions, with Facts about Cancer Risk Factors, Screening and Prevention, Treatment Options, and Reports on Current Research Initiatives

Along with a Glossary of Cancer Terms and a Directory of Resources for Additional Help and Information

Edited by Karen Bellenir. 604 pages. 2002. 0-7808-0226-8. $78.

ALSO AVAILABLE: Cancer Sourcebook for Women, 1st Edition. Edited by Allan R. Cook and Peter D. Dresser. 524 pages. 1996. 0-7808-0076-1. $78.

Cardiovascular Diseases & Disorders Sourcebook, 1st Edition

SEE Heart Diseases & Disorders Sourcebook, 2nd Edition

Caregiving Sourcebook

Basic Consumer Health Information for Caregivers, Including a Profile of Caregivers, Caregiving Responsibilities and Concerns, Tips for Specific Conditions, Care Environments, and the Effects of Caregiving

Along with Facts about Legal Issues, Financial Information, and Future Planning, a Glossary, and a Listing of Additional Resources

Edited by Joyce Brennfleck Shannon. 600 pages. 2001. 0-7808-0331-0. $78.

Child Abuse Sourcebook

Basic Consumer Health Information about the Physical, Sexual, and Emotional Abuse of Children, with Additional Facts about Neglect, Munchausen Syndrome by Proxy (MSBP), Shaken Baby Syndrome, and Controversial Issues Related to Child Abuse, Such as Withholding Medical Care, Corporal Punishment, and Child Maltreatment in Youth Sports, and Featuring Facts about Child Protective Services, Foster Care, Adoption, Parenting Challenges, and Other Abuse Prevention Efforts

Along with a Glossary of Related Terms and Resources for Additional Help and Information

Edited by Dawn D. Matthews. 620 pages. 2004. 0-7808-0705-7. $78.

Childhood Diseases & Disorders Sourcebook

Basic Consumer Health Information about Medical Problems Often Encountered in Pre-Adolescent Children, Including Respiratory Tract Ailments, Ear Infections, Sore Throats, Disorders of the Skin and Scalp, Digestive and Genitourinary Diseases, Infectious Diseases, Inflammatory Disorders, Chronic Physical and Developmental Disorders, Allergies, and More

Along with Information about Diagnostic Tests, Common Childhood Surgeries, and Frequently Used Medications, with a Glossary of Important Terms and Resource Directory

Edited by Chad T. Kimball. 662 pages. 2003. 0-7808-0458-9. $78.

Colds, Flu & Other Common Ailments Sourcebook

Basic Consumer Health Information about Common Ailments and Injuries, Including Colds, Coughs, the Flu, Sinus Problems, Headaches, Fever, Nausea and Vomiting, Menstrual Cramps, Diarrhea, Constipation, Hemorrhoids, Back Pain, Dandruff, Dry and Itchy Skin, Cuts, Scrapes, Sprains, Bruises, and More

Along with Information about Prevention, Self-Care, Choosing a Doctor, Over-the-Counter Medications, Folk Remedies, and Alternative Therapies, and Including a Glossary of Important Terms and a Directory of Resources for Further Help and Information

Edited by Chad T. Kimball. 638 pages. 2001. 0-7808-0435-X. $78.

"A good starting point for research on common illnesses. It will be a useful addition to public and consumer health library collections."
— American Reference Books Annual 2002

"Will prove valuable to any library seeking to maintain a current, comprehensive reference collection of health resources. . . . Excellent reference."
— The Bookwatch, Aug '01

"Recommended reference source."
— Booklist, American Library Association, July '01

■

Communication Disorders Sourcebook

Basic Information about Deafness and Hearing Loss, Speech and Language Disorders, Voice Disorders, Balance and Vestibular Disorders, and Disorders of Smell, Taste, and Touch

Edited by Linda M. Ross. 533 pages. 1996. 0-7808-0077-X. $78.

"This is skillfully edited and is a welcome resource for the layperson. It should be found in every public and medical library." *— Booklist Health Sciences Supplement, American Library Association, Oct '97*

■

Congenital Disorders Sourcebook

Basic Information about Disorders Acquired during Gestation, Including Spina Bifida, Hydrocephalus, Cerebral Palsy, Heart Defects, Craniofacial Abnormalities, Fetal Alcohol Syndrome, and More

Along with Current Treatment Options and Statistical Data

Edited by Karen Bellenir. 607 pages. 1997. 0-7808-0205-5. $78.

"Recommended reference source."
— Booklist, American Library Association, Oct '97

SEE ALSO *Pregnancy & Birth Sourcebook*

Consumer Issues in Health Care Sourcebook

Basic Information about Health Care Fundamentals and Related Consumer Issues, Including Exams and Screening Tests, Physician Specialties, Choosing a Doctor, Using Prescription and Over-the-Counter Medications Safely, Avoiding Health Scams, Managing Common Health Risks in the Home, Care Options for Chronically or Terminally Ill Patients, and a List of Resources for Obtaining Help and Further Information

Edited by Karen Bellenir. 618 pages. 1998. 0-7808-0221-7. $78.

"Both public and academic libraries will want to have a copy in their collection for readers who are interested in self-education on health issues."
— American Reference Books Annual, 2000

"The editor has researched the literature from government agencies and others, saving readers the time and effort of having to do the research themselves. Recommended for public libraries."
— Reference and User Services Quarterly, American Library Association, Spring '99

"Recommended reference source."
— Booklist, American Library Association, Dec '98

■

Contagious Diseases Sourcebook

Basic Consumer Health Information about Infectious Diseases Spread by Person-to-Person Contact through Direct Touch, Airborne Transmission, Sexual Contact, or Contact with Blood or Other Body Fluids, Including Hepatitis, Herpes, Influenza, Lice, Measles, Mumps, Pinworm, Ringworm, Severe Acute Respiratory Syndrome (SARS), Streptococcal Infections, Tuberculosis, and Others

Along with Facts about Disease Transmission, Antimicrobial Resistance, and Vaccines, with a Glossary and Directories of Resources for More Information

Edited by Karen Bellenir. 625 pages. 2004. 0-7808-0736-7. $78.

■

Contagious & Non-Contagious Infectious Diseases Sourcebook

Basic Information about Contagious Diseases like Measles, Polio, Hepatitis B, and Infectious Mononucleosis, and Non-Contagious Infectious Diseases like Tetanus and Toxic Shock Syndrome, and Diseases Occurring as Secondary Infections Such as Shingles and Reye Syndrome

Along with Vaccination, Prevention, and Treatment Information, and a Section Describing Emerging Infectious Disease Threats

Edited by Karen Bellenir and Peter D. Dresser. 566 pages. 1996. 0-7808-0075-3. $78.

Death & Dying Sourcebook

Basic Consumer Health Information for the Layperson about End-of-Life Care and Related Ethical and Legal Issues, Including Chief Causes of Death, Autopsies, Pain Management for the Terminally Ill, Life Support Systems, Insurance, Euthanasia, Assisted Suicide, Hospice Programs, Living Wills, Funeral Planning, Counseling, Mourning, Organ Donation, and Physician Training

Along with Statistical Data, a Glossary, and Listings of Sources for Further Help and Information

Edited by Annemarie S. Muth. 641 pages. 1999. 0-7808-0230-6. $78.

"Public libraries, medical libraries, and academic libraries will all find this sourcebook a useful addition to their collections."
— American Reference Books Annual, 2001

"An extremely useful resource for those concerned with death and dying in the United States."
— Respiratory Care, Nov '00

"Recommended reference source."
— Booklist, American Library Association, Aug '00

"This book is a definite must for all those involved in end-of-life care." — Doody's Review Service, 2000

Dental Care & Oral Health Sourcebook, 2nd Edition

Basic Consumer Health Information about Dental Care, Including Oral Hygiene, Dental Visits, Pain Management, Cavities, Crowns, Bridges, Dental Implants, and Fillings, and Other Oral Health Concerns, Such as Gum Disease, Bad Breath, Dry Mouth, Genetic and Developmental Abnormalities, Oral Cancers, Orthodontics, and Temporomandibular Disorders

Along with Updates on Current Research in Oral Health, a Glossary, a Directory of Dental and Oral Health Organizations, and Resources for People with Dental and Oral Health Disorders

Edited by Amy L. Sutton. 609 pages. 2003. 0-7808-0634-4. $78.

ALSO AVAILABLE: Oral Health Sourcebook, 1st Edition. Edited by Allan R. Cook. 558 pages. 1997. 0-7808-0082-6. $78.

"This book could serve as a turning point in the battle to educate consumers in issues concerning oral health."
— American Reference Books Annual, 2004

"Unique source which will fill a gap in dental sources for patients and the lay public. A valuable reference tool even in a library with thousands of books on dentistry. Comprehensive, clear, inexpensive, and easy to read and use. It fills an enormous gap in the health care literature." — Reference and User Services Quarterly, American Library Association, Summer '98

"Recommended reference source."
— Booklist, American Library Association, Dec '97

Depression Sourcebook

Basic Consumer Health Information about Unipolar Depression, Bipolar Disorder, Postpartum Depression, Seasonal Affective Disorder, and Other Types of Depression in Children, Adolescents, Women, Men, the Elderly, and Other Selected Populations

Along with Facts about Causes, Risk Factors, Diagnostic Criteria, Treatment Options, Coping Strategies, Suicide Prevention, a Glossary, and a Directory of Sources for Additional Help and Information

Edited by Karen Belleni. 602 pages. 2002. 0-7808-0611-5. $78.

"Depression Sourcebook is of a very high standard. Its purpose, which is to serve as a reference source to the lay reader, is very well served."
— Journal of the National Medical Association, 2004

"Invaluable reference for public and school library collections alike." — Library Bookwatch, Apr '03

"Recommended for purchase."
— American Reference Books Annual, 2003

Diabetes Sourcebook, 3rd Edition

Basic Consumer Health Information about Type 1 Diabetes (Insulin-Dependent or Juvenile-Onset Diabetes), Type 2 Diabetes (Noninsulin-Dependent or Adult-Onset Diabetes), Gestational Diabetes, Impaired Glucose Tolerance (IGT), and Related Complications, Such as Amputation, Eye Disease, Gum Disease, Nerve Damage, and End-Stage Renal Disease, Including Facts about Insulin, Oral Diabetes Medications, Blood Sugar Testing, and the Role of Exercise and Nutrition in the Control of Diabetes

Along with a Glossary and Resources for Further Help and Information

Edited by Dawn D. Matthews. 622 pages. 2003. 0-7808-0629-8. $78.

ALSO AVAILABLE: Diabetes Sourcebook, 1st Edition. Edited by Karen Bellenir and Peter D. Dresser. 827 pages. 1994. 1-55888-751-2. $78.

Diabetes Sourcebook, 2nd Edition. Edited by Karen Bellenir. 688 pages. 1998. 0-7808-0224-1. $78.

"This edition is even more helpful than earlier versions. . . . It is a truly valuable tool for anyone seeking readable and authoritative information on diabetes."
— American Reference Books Annual, 2004

"An invaluable reference." — Library Journal, May '00

Selected as one of the 250 "Best Health Sciences Books of 1999." — Doody's Rating Service, Mar-Apr 2000

"Provides useful information for the general public."
— Healthlines, University of Michigan Health Management Research Center, Sep/Oct '99

". . . provides reliable mainstream medical information . . . belongs on the shelves of any library with a consumer health collection." — E-Streams, Sep '99

"Recommended reference source."
— Booklist, American Library Association, Feb '99

Diet & Nutrition Sourcebook, 2nd Edition

Basic Consumer Health Information about Dietary Guidelines, Recommended Daily Intake Values, Vitamins, Minerals, Fiber, Fat, Weight Control, Dietary Supplements, and Food Additives

Along with Special Sections on Nutrition Needs throughout Life and Nutrition for People with Such Specific Medical Concerns as Allergies, High Blood Cholesterol, Hypertension, Diabetes, Celiac Disease, Seizure Disorders, Phenylketonuria (PKU), Cancer, and Eating Disorders, and Including Reports on Current Nutrition Research and Source Listings for Additional Help and Information

Edited by Karen Bellenir. 650 pages. 1999. 0-7808-0228-4. $78.

ALSO AVAILABLE: *Diet & Nutrition Sourcebook, 1st Edition.* Edited by Dan R. Harris. 662 pages. 1996. 0-7808-0084-2. $78.

"This book is an excellent source of basic diet and nutrition information." *— Booklist Health Sciences Supplement, American Library Association, Dec '00*

"This reference document should be in any public library, but it would be a very good guide for beginning students in the health sciences. If the other books in this publisher's series are as good as this, they should all be in the health sciences collections."
—American Reference Books Annual, 2000

"This book is an excellent general nutrition reference for consumers who desire to take an active role in their health care for prevention. Consumers of all ages who select this book can feel confident they are receiving current and accurate information." *— Journal of Nutrition for the Elderly, Vol. 19, No. 4, '00*

"Recommended reference source."
—Booklist, American Library Association, Dec '99

SEE ALSO *Digestive Diseases & Disorders Sourcebook, Eating Disorders Sourcebook, Gastrointestinal Diseases & Disorders Sourcebook, Vegetarian Sourcebook*

Digestive Diseases & Disorders Sourcebook

Basic Consumer Health Information about Diseases and Disorders that Impact the Upper and Lower Digestive System, Including Celiac Disease, Constipation, Crohn's Disease, Cyclic Vomiting Syndrome, Diarrhea, Diverticulosis and Diverticulitis, Gallstones, Heartburn, Hemorrhoids, Hernias, Indigestion (Dyspepsia), Irritable Bowel Syndrome, Lactose Intolerance, Ulcers, and More

Along with Information about Medications and Other Treatments, Tips for Maintaining a Healthy Digestive Tract, a Glossary, and Directory of Digestive Diseases Organizations

Edited by Karen Bellenir. 335 pages. 2000. 0-7808-0327-2. $78.

"This title would be an excellent addition to all public or patient-research libraries."
—American Reference Books Annual, 2001

"This title is recommended for public, hospital, and health sciences libraries with consumer health collections." *— E-Streams, Jul-Aug '00*

"Recommended reference source."
—Booklist, American Library Association, May '00

SEE ALSO *Diet & Nutrition Sourcebook, Eating Disorders Sourcebook, Gastrointestinal Diseases & Disorders Sourcebook*

Disabilities Sourcebook

Basic Consumer Health Information about Physical and Psychiatric Disabilities, Including Descriptions of Major Causes of Disability, Assistive and Adaptive Aids, Workplace Issues, and Accessibility Concerns

Along with Information about the Americans with Disabilities Act, a Glossary, and Resources for Additional Help and Information

Edited by Dawn D. Matthews. 616 pages. 2000. 0-7808-0389-2. $78.

"It is a must for libraries with a consumer health section." *— American Reference Books Annual 2002*

"A much needed addition to the Omnigraphics *Health Reference Series*. A current reference work to provide people with disabilities, their families, caregivers or those who work with them, a broad range of information in one volume, has not been available until now. . . . It is recommended for all public and academic library reference collections." *— E-Streams, May '01*

"An excellent source book in easy-to-read format covering many current topics; highly recommended for all libraries." *— Choice, Association of College and Research Libraries, Jan '01*

"Recommended reference source."
—Booklist, American Library Association, Jul '00

Domestic Violence Sourcebook, 2nd Edition

Basic Consumer Health Information about the Causes and Consequences of Abusive Relationships, Including Physical Violence, Sexual Assault, Battery, Stalking, and Emotional Abuse, and Facts about the Effects of Violence on Women, Men, Young Adults, and the Elderly, with Reports about Domestic Violence in Selected Populations, and Featuring Facts about Medical Care, Victim Assistance and Protection, Prevention Strategies, Mental Health Services, and Legal Issues

Along with a Glossary of Related Terms and Resources for Additional Help and Information

Edited by Dawn D. Matthews. 628 pages. 2004. 0-7808-0669-7. $78.

ALSO AVAILABLE: *Domestic Violence & Child Abuse Sourcebook, 1st Edition.* Edited by Helene Henderson. 1,064 pages. 2001. 0-7808-0235-7. $78.

"Interested lay persons should find the book extremely beneficial. . . . A copy of *Domestic Violence and Child Abuse Sourcebook* should be in every public library in the United States."

— *Social Science & Medicine, No. 56, 2003*

"This is important information. The Web has many resources but this sourcebook fills an important societal need. I am not aware of any other resources of this type." — *Doody's Review Service, Sep '01*

"Recommended for all libraries, scholars, and practitioners." — *Choice,*
Association of College & Research Libraries, Jul '01

"Recommended reference source."
— *Booklist, American Library Association, Apr '01*

"Important pick for college-level health reference libraries." — *The Bookwatch, Mar '01*

"Because this problem is so widespread and because this book includes a lot of issues within one volume, this work is recommended for all public libraries."
— *American Reference Books Annual, 2001*

■

Drug Abuse Sourcebook, 2nd Edition

Basic Consumer Health Information about Illicit Substances of Abuse and the Misuse of Prescription and Over-the-Counter Medications, Including Depressants, Hallucinogens, Inhalants, Marijuana, Stimulants, and Anabolic Steroids

Along with Facts about Related Health Risks, Treatment Programs, Prevention Programs, a Glossary of Abuse and Addiction Terms, a Glossary of Drug-Related Street Terms, and a Directory Resources for More Information

Edited by Catherine Ginther. 600 pages. 2004. 0-7808-0740-5. $78.

ALSO AVAILABLE: Drug Abuse Sourcebook, 1st Edition. Edited by Karen Bellenir. 629 pages. 2000. 0-7808-0242-X. $78.

"Containing a wealth of information . . . . This resource belongs in libraries that serve a lower-division undergraduate or community college clientele as well as the general public." — *Choice, Association of College and Research Libraries, Jun '01*

"Recommended reference source."
— *Booklist, American Library Association, Feb '01*

"Highly recommended." — *The Bookwatch, Jan '01*

"Even though there is a plethora of books on drug abuse, this volume is recommended for school, public, and college libraries."
— *American Reference Books Annual, 2001*

SEE ALSO *Alcoholism Sourcebook, Substance Abuse Sourcebook*

Ear, Nose & Throat Disorders Sourcebook

Basic Information about Disorders of the Ears, Nose, Sinus Cavities, Pharynx, and Larynx, Including Ear Infections, Tinnitus, Vestibular Disorders, Allergic and Non-Allergic Rhinitis, Sore Throats, Tonsillitis, and Cancers That Affect the Ears, Nose, Sinuses, and Throat

Along with Reports on Current Research Initiatives, a Glossary of Related Medical Terms, and a Directory of Sources for Further Help and Information

Edited by Karen Bellenir and Linda M. Shin. 576 pages. 1998. 0-7808-0206-3. $78.

"Overall, this sourcebook is helpful for the consumer seeking information on ENT issues. It is recommended for public libraries."
— *American Reference Books Annual, 1999*

"Recommended reference source."
— *Booklist, American Library Association, Dec '98*

■

Eating Disorders Sourcebook

Basic Consumer Health Information about Eating Disorders, Including Information about Anorexia Nervosa, Bulimia Nervosa, Binge Eating, Body Dysmorphic Disorder, Pica, Laxative Abuse, and Night Eating Syndrome

Along with Information about Causes, Adverse Effects, and Treatment and Prevention Issues, and Featuring a Section on Concerns Specific to Children and Adolescents, a Glossary, and Resources for Further Help and Information

Edited by Dawn D. Matthews. 322 pages. 2001. 0-7808-0335-3. $78.

"Recommended for health science libraries that are open to the public, as well as hospital libraries. This book is a good resource for the consumer who is concerned about eating disorders." — *E-Streams, Mar '02*

"This volume is another convenient collection of excerpted articles. Recommended for school and public library patrons; lower-division undergraduates; and two-year technical program students." — *Choice, Association of College & Research Libraries, Jan '02*

"Recommended reference source." — *Booklist, American Library Association, Oct '01*

SEE ALSO *Diet & Nutrition Sourcebook, Digestive Diseases & Disorders Sourcebook, Gastrointestinal Diseases & Disorders Sourcebook*

■

Emergency Medical Services Sourcebook

Basic Consumer Health Information about Preventing, Preparing for, and Managing Emergency Situations, When and Who to Call for Help, What to Expect in the Emergency Room, the Emergency Medical Team, Patient Issues, and Current Topics in Emergency Medicine

Along with Statistical Data, a Glossary, and Sources of Additional Help and Information

Edited by Jenni Lynn Colson. 494 pages. 2002. 0-7808-0420-1. $78.

"Handy and convenient for home, public, school, and college libraries. Recommended."
— *Choice, Association of College and Research Libraries, Apr '03*

"This reference can provide the consumer with answers to most questions about emergency care in the United States, or it will direct them to a resource where the answer can be found."
— *American Reference Books Annual, 2003*

"Recommended reference source."
— *Booklist, American Library Association, Feb '03*

■

Endocrine & Metabolic Disorders Sourcebook

Basic Information for the Layperson about Pancreatic and Insulin-Related Disorders Such as Pancreatitis, Diabetes, and Hypoglycemia; Adrenal Gland Disorders Such as Cushing's Syndrome, Addison's Disease, and Congenital Adrenal Hyperplasia; Pituitary Gland Disorders Such as Growth Hormone Deficiency, Acromegaly, and Pituitary Tumors; Thyroid Disorders Such as Hypothyroidism, Graves' Disease, Hashimoto's Disease, and Goiter; Hyperparathyroidism; and Other Diseases and Syndromes of Hormone Imbalance or Metabolic Dysfunction

Along with Reports on Current Research Initiatives

Edited by Linda M. Shin. 574 pages. 1998. 0-7808-0207-1. $78.

"Omnigraphics has produced another needed resource for health information consumers."
— *American Reference Books Annual, 2000*

"Recommended reference source."
— *Booklist, American Library Association, Dec '98*

■

Environmental Health Sourcebook, 2nd Edition

Basic Consumer Health Information about the Environment and Its Effect on Human Health, Including the Effects of Air Pollution, Water Pollution, Hazardous Chemicals, Food Hazards, Radiation Hazards, Biological Agents, Household Hazards, Such as Radon, Asbestos, Carbon Monoxide, and Mold, and Information about Associated Diseases and Disorders, Including Cancer, Allergies, Respiratory Problems, and Skin Disorders

Along with Information about Environmental Concerns for Specific Populations, a Glossary of Related Terms, and Resources for Further Help and Information

Edited by Dawn D. Matthews. 673 pages. 2003. 0-7808-0632-8. $78.

ALSO AVAILABLE: *Environmentally Induced Disorders Sourcebook, 1st Edition.* Edited by Allan R. Cook. 620 pages. 1997. 0-7808-0083-4. $78.

"This recently updated edition continues the level of quality and the reputation of the numerous other volumes in Omnigraphics' *Health Reference Series.***"**
— *American Reference Books Annual, 2004*

"Recommended reference source."
— *Booklist, American Library Association, Sep '98*

"This book will be a useful addition to anyone's library." — *Choice Health Sciences Supplement, Association of College and Research Libraries, May '98*

". . . a good survey of numerous environmentally induced physical disorders . . . a useful addition to anyone's library."
— *Doody's Health Sciences Book Reviews, Jan '98*

". . . provide[s] introductory information from the best authorities around. Since this volume covers topics that potentially affect everyone, it will surely be one of the most frequently consulted volumes in the *Health Reference Series.***"** — *Rettig on Reference, Nov '97*

■

Environmentally Induced Disorders Sourcebook, 1st Edition

SEE Environmental Health Sourcebook, 2nd Edition

■

Ethnic Diseases Sourcebook

Basic Consumer Health Information for Ethnic and Racial Minority Groups in the United States, Including General Health Indicators and Behaviors, Ethnic Diseases, Genetic Testing, the Impact of Chronic Diseases, Women's Health, Mental Health Issues, and Preventive Health Care Services

Along with a Glossary and a Listing of Additional Resources

Edited by Joyce Brennfleck Shannon. 664 pages. 2001. 0-7808-0336-1. $78.

"Recommended for health sciences libraries where public health programs are a priority."
— *E-Streams, Jan '02*

"Not many books have been written on this topic to date, and the *Ethnic Diseases Sourcebook* **is a strong addition to the list. It will be an important introductory resource for health consumers, students, health care personnel, and social scientists. It is recommended for public, academic, and large hospital libraries."**
— *American Reference Books Annual 2002*

"Recommended reference source."
— *Booklist, American Library Association, Oct '01*

"Will prove valuable to any library seeking to maintain a current, comprehensive reference collection of health resources. . . . An excellent source of health information about genetic disorders which affect particular ethnic and racial minorities in the U.S."
— *The Bookwatch, Aug '01*

Eye Care Sourcebook, 2nd Edition

Basic Consumer Health Information about Eye Care and Eye Disorders, Including Facts about the Diagnosis, Prevention, and Treatment of Common Refractive Problems Such as Myopia, Hyperopia, Astigmatism, and Presbyopia, and Eye Diseases, Including Glaucoma, Cataract, Age-Related Macular Degeneration, and Diabetic Retinopathy

Along with a Section on Vision Correction and Refractive Surgeries, Including LASIK and LASEK, a Glossary, and Directories of Resources for Additional Help and Information

Edited by Amy L. Sutton. 543 pages. 2003. 0-7808-0635-2. $78.

ALSO AVAILABLE: Ophthalmic Disorders Sourcebook, 1st Edition. Edited by Linda M. Ross. 631 pages. 1996. 0-7808-0081-8. $78.

". . . a solid reference tool for eye care and a valuable addition to a collection."
— American Reference Books Annual, 2004

Family Planning Sourcebook

Basic Consumer Health Information about Planning for Pregnancy and Contraception, Including Traditional Methods, Barrier Methods, Hormonal Methods, Permanent Methods, Future Methods, Emergency Contraception, and Birth Control Choices for Women at Each Stage of Life

Along with Statistics, a Glossary, and Sources of Additional Information

Edited by Amy Marcaccio Keyzer. 520 pages. 2001. 0-7808-0379-5. $78.

"Recommended for public, health, and undergraduate libraries as part of the circulating collection."
— E-Streams, Mar '02

"Information is presented in an unbiased, readable manner, and the sourcebook will certainly be a necessary addition to those public and high school libraries where Internet access is restricted or otherwise problematic." — American Reference Books Annual 2002

"Recommended reference source."
— Booklist, American Library Association, Oct '01

"Will prove valuable to any library seeking to maintain a current, comprehensive reference collection of health resources. . . . Excellent reference."
— The Bookwatch, Aug '01

SEE ALSO Pregnancy & Birth Sourcebook

Fitness & Exercise Sourcebook, 2nd Edition

Basic Consumer Health Information about the Fundamentals of Fitness and Exercise, Including How to Begin and Maintain a Fitness Program, Fitness as a Lifestyle, the Link between Fitness and Diet, Advice for Specific Groups of People, Exercise as It Relates to Specific Medical Conditions, and Recent Research in Fitness and Exercise

Along with a Glossary of Important Terms and Resources for Additional Help and Information

Edited by Kristen M. Gledhill. 646 pages. 2001. 0-7808-0334-5. $78.

ALSO AVAILABLE: Fitness & Exercise Sourcebook, 1st Edition. Edited by Dan R. Harris. 663 pages. 1996. 0-7808-0186-5. $78.

"This work is recommended for all general reference collections."
— American Reference Books Annual 2002

"Highly recommended for public, consumer, and school grades fourth through college."
— E-Streams, Nov '01

"Recommended reference source." — Booklist, American Library Association, Oct '01

"The information appears quite comprehensive and is considered reliable. . . . This second edition is a welcomed addition to the series."
— Doody's Review Service, Sep '01

"This reference is a valuable choice for those who desire a broad source of information on exercise, fitness, and chronic-disease prevention through a healthy lifestyle." — American Medical Writers Association Journal, Fall '01

"Will prove valuable to any library seeking to maintain a current, comprehensive reference collection of health resources. . . . Excellent reference."
— The Bookwatch, Aug '01

Food & Animal Borne Diseases Sourcebook

Basic Information about Diseases That Can Be Spread to Humans through the Ingestion of Contaminated Food or Water or by Contact with Infected Animals and Insects, Such as Botulism, E. Coli, Hepatitis A, Trichinosis, Lyme Disease, and Rabies

Along with Information Regarding Prevention and Treatment Methods, and Including a Special Section for International Travelers Describing Diseases Such as Cholera, Malaria, Travelers' Diarrhea, and Yellow Fever, and Offering Recommendations for Avoiding Illness

Edited by Karen Bellenir and Peter D. Dresser. 535 pages. 1995. 0-7808-0033-8. $78.

"Targeting general readers and providing them with a single, comprehensive source of information on selected topics, this book continues, with the excellent caliber of its predecessors, to catalog topical information on health matters of general interest. Readable and thorough, this valuable resource is highly recommended for all libraries."
— Academic Library Book Review, Summer '96

"A comprehensive collection of authoritative information." — Emergency Medical Services, Oct '95

Food Safety Sourcebook

Basic Consumer Health Information about the Safe Handling of Meat, Poultry, Seafood, Eggs, Fruit Juices, and Other Food Items, and Facts about Pesticides, Drinking Water, Food Safety Overseas, and the Onset, Duration, and Symptoms of Foodborne Illnesses, Including Types of Pathogenic Bacteria, Parasitic Protozoa, Worms, Viruses, and Natural Toxins

Along with the Role of the Consumer, the Food Handler, and the Government in Food Safety; a Glossary, and Resources for Additional Help and Information

Edited by Dawn D. Matthews. 339 pages. 1999. 0-7808-0326-4. $78.

"This book is recommended for public libraries and universities with home economic and food science programs." — *E-Streams, Nov '00*

"Recommended reference source."
—*Booklist, American Library Association, May '00*

"This book takes the complex issues of food safety and foodborne pathogens and presents them in an easily understood manner. [It does] an excellent job of covering a large and often confusing topic."
—*American Reference Books Annual, 2000*

■

Forensic Medicine Sourcebook

Basic Consumer Information for the Layperson about Forensic Medicine, Including Crime Scene Investigation, Evidence Collection and Analysis, Expert Testimony, Computer-Aided Criminal Identification, Digital Imaging in the Courtroom, DNA Profiling, Accident Reconstruction, Autopsies, Ballistics, Drugs and Explosives Detection, Latent Fingerprints, Product Tampering, and Questioned Document Examination

Along with Statistical Data, a Glossary of Forensics Terminology, and Listings of Sources for Further Help and Information

Edited by Annemarie S. Muth. 574 pages. 1999. 0-7808-0232-2. $78.

"Given the expected widespread interest in its content and its easy to read style, this book is recommended for most public and all college and university libraries."
— *E-Streams, Feb '01*

"Recommended for public libraries."
—*Reference & User Services Quarterly, American Library Association, Spring 2000*

"Recommended reference source."
—*Booklist, American Library Association, Feb '00*

"A wealth of information, useful statistics, references are up-to-date and extremely complete. This wonderful collection of data will help students who are interested in a career in any type of forensic field. It is a great resource for attorneys who need information about types of expert witnesses needed in a particular case. It also offers useful information for fiction and nonfiction writers whose work involves a crime. A fascinating compilation. All levels." — *Choice, Association of College and Research Libraries, Jan 2000*

"There are several items that make this book attractive to consumers who are seeking certain forensic data.... This is a useful current source for those seeking general forensic medical answers."
—*American Reference Books Annual, 2000*

■

Gastrointestinal Diseases & Disorders Sourcebook

Basic Information about Gastroesophageal Reflux Disease (Heartburn), Ulcers, Diverticulosis, Irritable Bowel Syndrome, Crohn's Disease, Ulcerative Colitis, Diarrhea, Constipation, Lactose Intolerance, Hemorrhoids, Hepatitis, Cirrhosis, and Other Digestive Problems, Featuring Statistics, Descriptions of Symptoms, and Current Treatment Methods of Interest for Persons Living with Upper and Lower Gastrointestinal Maladies

Edited by Linda M. Ross. 413 pages. 1996. 0-7808-0078-8. $78.

"... very readable form. The successful editorial work that brought this material together into a useful and understandable reference makes accessible to all readers information that can help them more effectively understand and obtain help for digestive tract problems."
— *Choice, Association of College & Research Libraries, Feb '97*

SEE ALSO *Diet & Nutrition Sourcebook, Digestive Diseases & Disorders, Eating Disorders Sourcebook*

■

Genetic Disorders Sourcebook, 2nd Edition

Basic Consumer Health Information about Hereditary Diseases and Disorders, Including Cystic Fibrosis, Down Syndrome, Hemophilia, Huntington's Disease, Sickle Cell Anemia, and More; Facts about Genes, Gene Research and Therapy, Genetic Screening, Ethics of Gene Testing, Genetic Counseling, and Advice on Coping and Caring

Along with a Glossary of Genetic Terminology and a Resource List for Help, Support, and Further Information

Edited by Kathy Massimini. 768 pages. 2001. 0-7808-0241-1. $78.

ALSO AVAILABLE: *Genetic Disorders Sourcebook, 1st Edition.* Edited by Karen Bellenir. 642 pages. 1996. 0-7808-0034-6. $78.

"Recommended for public libraries and medical and hospital libraries with consumer health collections."
— *E-Streams, May '01*

"Recommended reference source."
— *Booklist, American Library Association, Apr '01*

"Important pick for college-level health reference libraries." — *The Bookwatch, Mar '01*

"Provides essential medical information to both the general public and those diagnosed with a serious or fatal genetic disease or disorder." —*Choice, Association of College and Research Libraries, Jan '97*

Head Trauma Sourcebook

Basic Information for the Layperson about Open-Head and Closed-Head Injuries, Treatment Advances, Recovery, and Rehabilitation

Along with Reports on Current Research Initiatives

Edited by Karen Bellenir. 414 pages. 1997. 0-7808-0208-X. $78.

Headache Sourcebook

Basic Consumer Health Information about Migraine, Tension, Cluster, Rebound and Other Types of Headaches, with Facts about the Cause and Prevention of Headaches, the Effects of Stress and the Environment, Headaches during Pregnancy and Menopause, and Childhood Headaches

Along with a Glossary and Other Resources for Additional Help and Information

Edited by Dawn D. Matthews. 362 pages. 2002. 0-7808-0337-X. $78.

"Highly recommended for academic and medical reference collections." — *Library Bookwatch, Sep '02*

Health Insurance Sourcebook

Basic Information about Managed Care Organizations, Traditional Fee-for-Service Insurance, Insurance Portability and Pre-Existing Conditions Clauses, Medicare, Medicaid, Social Security, and Military Health Care

Along with Information about Insurance Fraud

Edited by Wendy Wilcox. 530 pages. 1997. 0-7808-0222-5. $78.

"Particularly useful because it brings much of this information together in one volume. This book will be a handy reference source in the health sciences library, hospital library, college and university library, and medium to large public library."
— *Medical Reference Services Quarterly, Fall '98*

Awarded "Books of the Year Award"
— *American Journal of Nursing, 1997*

"The layout of the book is particularly helpful as it provides easy access to reference material. A most useful addition to the vast amount of information about health insurance. The use of data from U.S. government agencies is most commendable. Useful in a library or learning center for healthcare professional students."
— *Doody's Health Sciences Book Reviews, Nov '97*

Health Reference Series Cumulative Index 1999

A Comprehensive Index to the Individual Volumes of the Health Reference Series, Including a Subject Index, Name Index, Organization Index, and Publication Index

Along with a Master List of Acronyms and Abbreviations

Edited by Edward J. Prucha, Anne Holmes, and Robert Rudnick. 990 pages. 2000. 0-7808-0382-5. $78.

"This volume will be most helpful in libraries that have a relatively complete collection of the Health Reference Series." — *American Reference Books Annual, 2001*

"Essential for collections that hold any of the numerous Health Reference Series titles."
— *Choice, Association of College and Research Libraries, Nov '00*

Healthy Aging Sourcebook

Basic Consumer Health Information about Maintaining Health through the Aging Process, Including Advice on Nutrition, Exercise, and Sleep, Help in Making Decisions about Midlife Issues and Retirement, and Guidance Concerning Practical and Informed Choices in Health Consumerism

Along with Data Concerning the Theories of Aging, Different Experiences in Aging by Minority Groups, and Facts about Aging Now and Aging in the Future; and Featuring a Glossary, a Guide to Consumer Help, Additional Suggested Reading, and Practical Resource Directory

Edited by Jenifer Swanson. 536 pages. 1999. 0-7808-0390-6. $78.

"Recommended reference source."
— *Booklist, American Library Association, Feb '00*

SEE ALSO *Physical & Mental Issues in Aging Sourcebook*

Healthy Children Sourcebook

Basic Consumer Health Information about the Physical and Mental Development of Children between the Ages of 3 and 12, Including Routine Health Care, Preventative Health Services, Safety and First Aid, Healthy Sleep, Dental Care, Nutrition, and Fitness, and Featuring Parenting Tips on Such Topics as Bedwetting, Choosing Day Care, Monitoring TV and Other Media, and Establishing a Foundation for Substance Abuse Prevention

Along with a Glossary of Commonly Used Pediatric Terms and Resources for Additional Help and Information.

Edited by Chad T. Kimball. 647 pages. 2003. 0-7808-0247-0. $78.

"It is hard to imagine that any other single resource exists that would provide such a comprehensive guide of timely information on health promotion and disease prevention for children aged 3 to 12."
— *American Reference Books Annual, 2004*

"The strengths of this book are many. It is clearly written, presented and structured."
— *Journal of the National Medical Association, 2004*

Healthy Heart Sourcebook for Women

Basic Consumer Health Information about Cardiac Issues Specific to Women, Including Facts about Major Risk Factors and Prevention, Treatment and Control Strategies, and Important Dietary Issues

Along with a Special Section Regarding the Pros and Cons of Hormone Replacement Therapy and Its Impact on Heart Health, and Additional Help, Including Recipes, a Glossary, and a Directory of Resources

Edited by Dawn D. Matthews. 336 pages. 2000. 0-7808-0329-9. $78.

"A good reference source and recommended for all public, academic, medical, and hospital libraries."
— Medical Reference Services Quarterly, Summer '01

"Because of the lack of information specific to women on this topic, this book is recommended for public libraries and consumer libraries."
— American Reference Books Annual, 2001

"Contains very important information about coronary artery disease that all women should know. The information is current and presented in an easy-to-read format. The book will make a good addition to any library." *— American Medical Writers Association Journal, Summer '00*

"Important, basic reference."
— Reviewer's Bookwatch, Jul '00

SEE ALSO *Heart Diseases & Disorders Sourcebook, Women's Health Concerns Sourcebook*

Heart Diseases & Disorders Sourcebook, 2nd Edition

Basic Consumer Health Information about Heart Attacks, Angina, Rhythm Disorders, Heart Failure, Valve Disease, Congenital Heart Disorders, and More, Including Descriptions of Surgical Procedures and Other Interventions, Medications, Cardiac Rehabilitation, Risk Identification, and Prevention Tips

Along with Statistical Data, Reports on Current Research Initiatives, a Glossary of Cardiovascular Terms, and Resource Directory

Edited by Karen Bellenir. 612 pages. 2000. 0-7808-0238-1. $78.

ALSO AVAILABLE: *Cardiovascular Diseases & Disorders Sourcebook, 1st Edition.* Edited by Karen Bellenir and Peter D. Dresser. 683 pages. 1995. 0-7808-0032-X. $78.

"This work stands out as an imminently accessible resource for the general public. It is recommended for the reference and circulating shelves of school, public, and academic libraries."
— American Reference Books Annual, 2001

"Recommended reference source."
— Booklist, American Library Association, Dec '00

"Provides comprehensive coverage of matters related to the heart. This title is recommended for health sciences and public libraries with consumer health collections."
— E-Streams, Oct '00

SEE ALSO *Healthy Heart Sourcebook for Women*

Household Safety Sourcebook

Basic Consumer Health Information about Household Safety, Including Information about Poisons, Chemicals, Fire, and Water Hazards in the Home

Along with Advice about the Safe Use of Home Maintenance Equipment, Choosing Toys and Nursery Furniture, Holiday and Recreation Safety, a Glossary, and Resources for Further Help and Information

Edited by Dawn D. Matthews. 606 pages. 2002. 0-7808-0338-8. $78.

"This work will be useful in public libraries with large consumer health and wellness departments."
— American Reference Books Annual, 2003

"As a sourcebook on household safety this book meets its mark. It is encyclopedic in scope and covers a wide range of safety issues that are commonly seen in the home." *— E-Streams, Jul '02*

Hypertension Sourcebook

Basic Consumer Health Information about the Causes, Diagnosis, and Treatment of High Blood Pressure, with Facts about Consequences, Complications, and Co-Occurring Disorders, Such as Coronary Heart Disease, Diabetes, Stroke, Kidney Disease, and Hypertensive Retinopathy, and Issues in Blood Pressure Control, Including Dietary Choices, Stress Management, and Medications

Along with Reports on Current Research Initiatives and Clinical Trials, a Glossary, and Resources for Additional Help and Information

Edited by Dawn D. Matthews and Karen Bellenir. 600 pages. 2004. 0-7808-0674-3. $78.

Immune System Disorders Sourcebook

Basic Information about Lupus, Multiple Sclerosis, Guillain-Barré Syndrome, Chronic Granulomatous Disease, and More

Along with Statistical and Demographic Data and Reports on Current Research Initiatives

Edited by Allan R. Cook. 608 pages. 1997. 0-7808-0209-8. $78.

Infant & Toddler Health Sourcebook

Basic Consumer Health Information about the Physical and Mental Development of Newborns, Infants, and Toddlers, Including Neonatal Concerns, Nutrition Recommendations, Immunization Schedules, Common Pediatric Disorders, Assessments and Milestones, Safety Tips, and Advice for Parents and Other Caregivers

Along with a Glossary of Terms and Resource Listings for Additional Help

Edited by Jenifer Swanson. 585 pages. 2000. 0-7808-0246-2. $78.

"As a reference for the general public, this would be useful in any library." — *E-Streams, May '01*

"Recommended reference source."
— *Booklist, American Library Association, Feb '01*

"This is a good source for general use."
— *American Reference Books Annual, 2001*

■

Infectious Diseases Sourcebook

Basic Consumer Health Information about Non-Contagious Bacterial, Viral, Prion, Fungal, and Parasitic Diseases Spread by Food and Water, Insects and Animals, or Environmental Contact, Including Botulism, E. Coli, Encephalitis, Legionnaires' Disease, Lyme Disease, Malaria, Plague, Rabies, Salmonella, Tetanus, and Others, and Facts about Newly Emerging Diseases, Such as Hantavirus, Mad Cow Disease, Monkeypox, and West Nile Virus

Along with Information about Preventing Disease Transmission, the Threat of Bioterrorism, and Current Research Initiatives, with a Glossary and Directory of Resources for More Information

Edited by Karen Bellenir. 634 pages. 2004. 0-7808-0675-1. $78.

■

Injury & Trauma Sourcebook

Basic Consumer Health Information about the Impact of Injury, the Diagnosis and Treatment of Common and Traumatic Injuries, Emergency Care, and Specific Injuries Related to Home, Community, Workplace, Transportation, and Recreation

Along with Guidelines for Injury Prevention, a Glossary, and a Directory of Additional Resources

Edited by Joyce Brennfleck Shannon. 696 pages. 2002. 0-7808-0421-X. $78.

"This publication is the most comprehensive work of its kind about injury and trauma."
— *American Reference Books Annual, 2003*

"This sourcebook provides concise, easily readable, basic health information about injuries. . . . This book is well organized and an easy to use reference resource suitable for hospital, health sciences and public libraries with consumer health collections."
— *E-Streams, Nov '02*

"Practitioners should be aware of guides such as this in order to facilitate their use by patients and their families."
— *Doody's Health Sciences Book Review Journal, Sep-Oct '02*

"Recommended reference source."
— *Booklist, American Library Association, Sep '02*

"Highly recommended for academic and medical reference collections."
— *Library Bookwatch, Sep '02*

Kidney & Urinary Tract Diseases & Disorders Sourcebook

Basic Information about Kidney Stones, Urinary Incontinence, Bladder Disease, End Stage Renal Disease, Dialysis, and More

Along with Statistical and Demographic Data and Reports on Current Research Initiatives

Edited by Linda M. Ross. 602 pages. 1997. 0-7808-0079-6. $78.

■

Learning Disabilities Sourcebook, 2nd Edition

Basic Consumer Health Information about Learning Disabilities, Including Dyslexia, Developmental Speech and Language Disabilities, Non-Verbal Learning Disorders, Developmental Arithmetic Disorder, Developmental Writing Disorder, and Other Conditions That Impede Learning Such as Attention Deficit/ Hyperactivity Disorder, Brain Injury, Hearing Impairment, Klinefelter Syndrome, Dyspraxia, and Tourette Syndrome

Along with Facts about Educational Issues and Assistive Technology, Coping Strategies, a Glossary of Related Terms, and Resources for Further Help and Information

Edited by Dawn D. Matthews. 621 pages. 2003. 0-7808-0626-3. $78.

ALSO AVAILABLE: Learning Disabilities Sourcebook, 1st Edition. Edited by Linda M. Shin. 579 pages. 1998. 0-7808-0210-1. $78.

"The second edition of *Learning Disabilities Sourcebook* far surpasses the earlier edition in that it is more focused on information that will be useful as a consumer health resource."
— *American Reference Books Annual, 2004*

"Teachers as well as consumers will find this an essential guide to understanding various syndromes and their latest treatments. [An] invaluable reference for public and school library collections alike."
— *Library Bookwatch, Apr '03*

Named "Outstanding Reference Book of 1999."
— *New York Public Library, Feb 2000*

"An excellent candidate for inclusion in a public library reference section. It's a great source of information. Teachers will also find the book useful. Definitely worth reading."
— *Journal of Adolescent & Adult Literacy, Feb 2000*

"Readable . . . provides a solid base of information regarding successful techniques used with individuals who have learning disabilities, as well as practical suggestions for educators and family members. Clear language, concise descriptions, and pertinent information for contacting multiple resources add to the strength of this book as a useful tool." — *Choice, Association of College and Research Libraries, Feb '99*

"Recommended reference source."
— *Booklist, American Library Association, Sep '98*

"A useful resource for libraries and for those who don't have the time to identify and locate the individual publications." — *Disability Resources Monthly, Sep '98*

Leukemia Sourcebook

Basic Consumer Health Information about Adult and Childhood Leukemias, Including Acute Lymphocytic Leukemia (ALL), Chronic Lymphocytic Leukemia (CLL), Acute Myelogenous Leukemia (AML), Chronic Myelogenous Leukemia (CML), and Hairy Cell Leukemia, and Treatments Such as Chemotherapy, Radiation Therapy, Peripheral Blood Stem Cell and Marrow Transplantation, and Immunotherapy

Along with Tips for Life During and After Treatment, a Glossary, and Directories of Additional Resources

Edited by Joyce Brennfleck Shannon. 587 pages. 2003. 0-7808-0627-1. $78.

"Unlike other medical books for the layperson, . . . the language does not talk down to the reader. . . . This volume is highly recommended for all libraries."
—American Reference Books Annual, 2004

■

Liver Disorders Sourcebook

Basic Consumer Health Information about the Liver and How It Works; Liver Diseases, Including Cancer, Cirrhosis, Hepatitis, and Toxic and Drug Related Diseases; Tips for Maintaining a Healthy Liver; Laboratory Tests, Radiology Tests, and Facts about Liver Transplantation

Along with a Section on Support Groups, a Glossary, and Resource Listings

Edited by Joyce Brennfleck Shannon. 591 pages. 2000. 0-7808-0383-3. $78.

"A valuable resource."
—American Reference Books Annual, 2001

"This title is recommended for health sciences and public libraries with consumer health collections."
—E-Streams, Oct '00

"Recommended reference source."
—Booklist, American Library Association, Jun '00

■

Lung Disorders Sourcebook

Basic Consumer Health Information about Emphysema, Pneumonia, Tuberculosis, Asthma, Cystic Fibrosis, and Other Lung Disorders, Including Facts about Diagnostic Procedures, Treatment Strategies, Disease Prevention Efforts, and Such Risk Factors as Smoking, Air Pollution, and Exposure to Asbestos, Radon, and Other Agents

Along with a Glossary and Resources for Additional Help and Information

Edited by Dawn D. Matthews. 678 pages. 2002. 0-7808-0339-6. $78.

"This title is a great addition for public and school libraries because it provides concise health information on the lungs."
—American Reference Books Annual, 2003

"Highly recommended for academic and medical reference collections." *—Library Bookwatch, Sep '02*

Medical Tests Sourcebook, 2nd Edition

Basic Consumer Health Information about Medical Tests, Including Age-Specific Health Tests, Important Health Screenings and Exams, Home-Use Tests, Blood and Specimen Tests, Electrical Tests, Scope Tests, Genetic Testing, and Imaging Tests, Such as X-Rays, Ultrasound, Computed Tomography, Magnetic Resonance Imaging, Angiography, and Nuclear Medicine

Along with a Glossary and Directory of Additional Resources

Edited by Joyce Brennfleck Shannon. 654 pages. 2004. 0-7808-0670-0. $78.

ALSO AVAILABLE: *Medical Tests, 1st Edition.* Edited by Joyce Brennfleck Shannon. 691 pages. 1999. 0-7808-0243-8. $78.

"Recommended for hospital and health sciences libraries with consumer health collections."
—E-Streams, Mar '00

"This is an overall excellent reference with a wealth of general knowledge that may aid those who are reluctant to get vital tests performed."
—Today's Librarian, Jan 2000

"A valuable reference guide."
—American Reference Books Annual, 2000

■

Men's Health Concerns Sourcebook, 2nd Edition

Basic Consumer Health Information about the Medical and Mental Concerns of Men, Including Theories about the Shorter Male Lifespan, the Leading Causes of Death and Disability, Physical Concerns of Special Significance to Men, Reproductive and Sexual Concerns, Sexually Transmitted Diseases, Men's Mental and Emotional Health, and Lifestyle Choices That Affect Wellness, Such as Nutrition, Fitness, and Substance Use

Along with a Glossary of Related Terms and a Directory of Organizational Resources in Men's Health

Edited by Robert Aquinas McNally. 644 pages. 2004. 0-7808-0671-9. $78.

ALSO AVAILABLE: *Men's Health Concerns Sourcebook, 1st Edition.* Edited by Allan R. Cook. 738 pages. 1998. 0-7808-0212-8. $78.

"This comprehensive resource and the series are highly recommended."
—American Reference Books Annual, 2000

"Recommended reference source."
—Booklist, American Library Association, Dec '98

■

Mental Health Disorders Sourcebook, 2nd Edition

Basic Consumer Health Information about Anxiety Disorders, Depression and Other Mood Disorders, Eating Disorders, Personality Disorders, Schizophrenia, and More, Including Disease Descriptions, Treatment Options, and Reports on Current Research Initiatives

Along with Statistical Data, Tips for Maintaining Mental Health, a Glossary, and Directory of Sources for Additional Help and Information

Edited by Karen Bellenir. 605 pages. 2000. 0-7808-0240-3. $78.

ALSO AVAILABLE: Mental Health Disorders Sourcebook, 1st Edition. Edited by Karen Bellenir. 548 pages. 1995. 0-7808-0040-0. $78.

"Well organized and well written."
—American Reference Books Annual, 2001

"Recommended reference source."
—Booklist, American Library Association, Jun '00

■

Mental Retardation Sourcebook

Basic Consumer Health Information about Mental Retardation and Its Causes, Including Down Syndrome, Fetal Alcohol Syndrome, Fragile X Syndrome, Genetic Conditions, Injury, and Environmental Sources

Along with Preventive Strategies, Parenting Issues, Educational Implications, Health Care Needs, Employment and Economic Matters, Legal Issues, a Glossary, and a Resource Listing for Additional Help and Information

Edited by Joyce Brennfleck Shannon. 642 pages. 2000. 0-7808-0377-9. $78.

"Public libraries will find the book useful for reference and as a beginning research point for students, parents, and caregivers."
—American Reference Books Annual, 2001

"The strength of this work is that it compiles many basic fact sheets and addresses for further information in one volume. It is intended and suitable for the general public. This sourcebook is relevant to any collection providing health information to the general public."
—E-Streams, Nov '00

"From preventing retardation to parenting and family challenges, this covers health, social and legal issues and will prove an invaluable overview."
—Reviewer's Bookwatch, Jul '00

■

Movement Disorders Sourcebook

Basic Consumer Health Information about Neurological Movement Disorders, Including Essential Tremor, Parkinson's Disease, Dystonia, Cerebral Palsy, Huntington's Disease, Myasthenia Gravis, Multiple Sclerosis, and Other Early-Onset and Adult-Onset Movement Disorders, Their Symptoms and Causes, Diagnostic Tests, and Treatments

Along with Mobility and Assistive Technology Information, a Glossary, and a Directory of Additional Resources

Edited by Joyce Brennfleck Shannon. 655 pages. 2003. 0-7808-0628-X. $78.

". . . a good resource for consumers and recommended for public, community college and undergraduate libraries."
—American Reference Books Annual, 2004

■

Muscular Dystrophy Sourcebook

Basic Consumer Health Information about Congenital, Childhood-Onset, and Adult-Onset Forms of Muscular Dystrophy, Such as Duchenne, Becker, Emery-Dreifuss, Distal, Limb-Girdle, Facioscapulohumeral (FSHD), Myotonic, and Ophthalmoplegic Muscular Dystrophies, Including Facts about Diagnostic Tests, Medical and Physical Therapies, Management of Co-Occurring Conditions, and Parenting Guidelines

Along with Practical Tips for Home Care, a Glossary, and Directories of Additional Resources

Edited by Joyce Brennfleck Shannon. 577 pages. 2004. 0-7808-0676-X. $78.

■

Obesity Sourcebook

Basic Consumer Health Information about Diseases and Other Problems Associated with Obesity, and Including Facts about Risk Factors, Prevention Issues, and Management Approaches

Along with Statistical and Demographic Data, Information about Special Populations, Research Updates, a Glossary, and Source Listings for Further Help and Information

Edited by Wilma Caldwell and Chad T. Kimball. 376 pages. 2001. 0-7808-0333-7. $78.

"The book synthesizes the reliable medical literature on obesity into one easy-to-read and useful resource for the general public."
—American Reference Books Annual 2002

"This is a very useful resource book for the lay public."
—Doody's Review Service, Nov '01

"Well suited for the health reference collection of a public library or an academic health science library that serves the general population." *—E-Streams, Sep '01*

"Recommended reference source."
—Booklist, American Library Association, Apr '01

" Recommended pick both for specialty health library collections and any general consumer health reference collection." *— The Bookwatch, Apr '01*

■

Ophthalmic Disorders Sourcebook, 1st Edition

SEE Eye Care Sourcebook, 2nd Edition

■

Oral Health Sourcebook

SEE Dental Care & Oral Health Sourcebook, 2nd Ed.

Osteoporosis Sourcebook

Basic Consumer Health Information about Primary and Secondary Osteoporosis and Juvenile Osteoporosis and Related Conditions, Including Fibrous Dysplasia, Gaucher Disease, Hyperthyroidism, Hypophosphatasia, Myeloma, Osteopetrosis, Osteogenesis Imperfecta, and Paget's Disease

Along with Information about Risk Factors, Treatments, Traditional and Non-Traditional Pain Management, a Glossary of Related Terms, and a Directory of Resources

Edited by Allan R. Cook. 584 pages. 2001. 0-7808-0239-X. $78.

"This would be a book to be kept in a staff or patient library. The targeted audience is the layperson, but the therapist who needs a quick bit of information on a particular topic will also find the book useful."
— *Physical Therapy, Jan '02*

"This resource is recommended as a great reference source for public, health, and academic libraries, and is another triumph for the editors of Omnigraphics."
— *American Reference Books Annual 2002*

"Recommended for all public libraries and general health collections, especially those supporting patient education or consumer health programs."
— *E-Streams, Nov '01*

"Will prove valuable to any library seeking to maintain a current, comprehensive reference collection of health resources. . . . From prevention to treatment and associated conditions, this provides an excellent survey."
— *The Bookwatch, Aug '01*

"Recommended reference source."
— *Booklist, American Library Association, July '01*

SEE ALSO *Women's Health Concerns Sourcebook*

◼

Pain Sourcebook, 2nd Edition

Basic Consumer Health Information about Specific Forms of Acute and Chronic Pain, Including Muscle and Skeletal Pain, Nerve Pain, Cancer Pain, and Disorders Characterized by Pain, Such as Fibromyalgia, Shingles, Angina, Arthritis, and Headaches

Along with Information about Pain Medications and Management Techniques, Complementary and Alternative Pain Relief Options, Tips for People Living with Chronic Pain, a Glossary, and a Directory of Sources for Further Information

Edited by Karen Bellenir. 670 pages. 2002. 0-7808-0612-3. $78.

ALSO AVAILABLE: *Pain Sourcebook, 1st Edition.* Edited by Allan R. Cook. 667 pages. 1997. 0-7808-0213-6. $78.

"A source of valuable information. . . . This book offers help to nonmedical people who need information about pain and pain management. It is also an excellent reference for those who participate in patient education."
— *Doody's Review Service, Sep '02*

"The text is readable, easily understood, and well indexed. This excellent volume belongs in all patient

education libraries, consumer health sections of public libraries, and many personal collections."
— *American Reference Books Annual, 1999*

"A beneficial reference." — *Booklist Health Sciences Supplement, American Library Association, Oct '98*

"The information is basic in terms of scholarship and is appropriate for general readers. Written in journalistic style . . . intended for non-professionals. Quite thorough in its coverage of different pain conditions and summarizes the latest clinical information regarding pain treatment." — *Choice, Association of College and Research Libraries, Jun '98*

"Recommended reference source."
— *Booklist, American Library Association, Mar '98*

◼

Pediatric Cancer Sourcebook

Basic Consumer Health Information about Leukemias, Brain Tumors, Sarcomas, Lymphomas, and Other Cancers in Infants, Children, and Adolescents, Including Descriptions of Cancers, Treatments, and Coping Strategies

Along with Suggestions for Parents, Caregivers, and Concerned Relatives, a Glossary of Cancer Terms, and Resource Listings

Edited by Edward J. Prucha. 587 pages. 1999. 0-7808-0245-4. $78.

"An excellent source of information. Recommended for public, hospital, and health science libraries with consumer health collections." — *E-Streams, Jun '00*

"Recommended reference source."
— *Booklist, American Library Association, Feb '00*

"A valuable addition to all libraries specializing in health services and many public libraries."
— *American Reference Books Annual, 2000*

◼

Physical & Mental Issues in Aging Sourcebook

Basic Consumer Health Information on Physical and Mental Disorders Associated with the Aging Process, Including Concerns about Cardiovascular Disease, Pulmonary Disease, Oral Health, Digestive Disorders, Musculoskeletal and Skin Disorders, Metabolic Changes, Sexual and Reproductive Issues, and Changes in Vision, Hearing, and Other Senses

Along with Data about Longevity and Causes of Death, Information on Acute and Chronic Pain, Descriptions of Mental Concerns, a Glossary of Terms, and Resource Listings for Additional Help

Edited by Jenifer Swanson. 660 pages. 1999. 0-7808-0233-0. $78.

"This is a treasure of health information for the layperson." — *Choice Health Sciences Supplement, Association of College & Research Libraries, May 2000*

"Recommended for public libraries."
— *American Reference Books Annual, 2000*

"Recommended reference source."
— *Booklist, American Library Association, Oct '99*

SEE ALSO *Healthy Aging Sourcebook*

Podiatry Sourcebook

Basic Consumer Health Information about Foot Conditions, Diseases, and Injuries, Including Bunions, Corns, Calluses, Athlete's Foot, Plantar Warts, Hammertoes and Clawtoes, Clubfoot, Heel Pain, Gout, and More

Along with Facts about Foot Care, Disease Prevention, Foot Safety, Choosing a Foot Care Specialist, a Glossary of Terms, and Resource Listings for Additional Information

Edited by M. Lisa Weatherford. 380 pages. 2001. 0-7808-0215-2. $78.

"Recommended reference source."
— *Booklist, American Library Association, Feb '02*

"There is a lot of information presented here on a topic that is usually only covered sparingly in most larger comprehensive medical encyclopedias."
— *American Reference Books Annual 2002*

■

Pregnancy & Birth Sourcebook, 2nd Edition

Basic Consumer Health Information about Conception and Pregnancy, Including Facts about Fertility, Infertility, Pregnancy Symptoms and Complications, Fetal Growth and Development, Labor, Delivery, and the Postpartum Period, as Well as Information about Maintaining Health and Wellness during Pregnancy and Caring for a Newborn

Along with Information about Public Health Assistance for Low-Income Pregnant Women, a Glossary, and Directories of Agencies and Organizations Providing Help and Support

Edited by Amy L. Sutton. 626 pages. 2004. 0-7808-0672-7. $78.

ALSO AVAILABLE: Pregnancy & Birth Sourcebook, 1st Edition. Edited by Heather E. Aldred. 737 pages. 1997. 0-7808-0216-0. $78.

"A well-organized handbook. Recommended."
— *Choice, Association of College and Research Libraries, Apr '98*

"Recommended reference source."
— *Booklist, American Library Association, Mar '98*

"Recommended for public libraries."
— *American Reference Books Annual, 1998*

SEE ALSO Congenital Disorders Sourcebook, Family Planning Sourcebook

■

Prostate Cancer Sourcebook

Basic Consumer Health Information about Prostate Cancer, Including Information about the Associated Risk Factors, Detection, Diagnosis, and Treatment of Prostate Cancer

Along with Information on Non-Malignant Prostate Conditions, and Featuring a Section Listing Support and Treatment Centers and a Glossary of Related Terms

Edited by Dawn D. Matthews. 358 pages. 2001. 0-7808-0324-8. $78.

"Recommended reference source."
— *Booklist, American Library Association, Jan '02*

"A valuable resource for health care consumers seeking information on the subject. . . . All text is written in a clear, easy-to-understand language that avoids technical jargon. Any library that collects consumer health resources would strengthen their collection with the addition of the *Prostate Cancer Sourcebook*."
— *American Reference Books Annual 2002*

■

Public Health Sourcebook

Basic Information about Government Health Agencies, Including National Health Statistics and Trends, Healthy People 2000 Program Goals and Objectives, the Centers for Disease Control and Prevention, the Food and Drug Administration, and the National Institutes of Health

Along with Full Contact Information for Each Agency

Edited by Wendy Wilcox. 698 pages. 1998. 0-7808-0220-9. $78.

"Recommended reference source."
— *Booklist, American Library Association, Sep '98*

"This consumer guide provides welcome assistance in navigating the maze of federal health agencies and their data on public health concerns."
— *SciTech Book News, Sep '98*

■

Reconstructive & Cosmetic Surgery Sourcebook

Basic Consumer Health Information on Cosmetic and Reconstructive Plastic Surgery, Including Statistical Information about Different Surgical Procedures, Things to Consider Prior to Surgery, Plastic Surgery Techniques and Tools, Emotional and Psychological Considerations, and Procedure-Specific Information

Along with a Glossary of Terms and a Listing of Resources for Additional Help and Information

Edited by M. Lisa Weatherford. 374 pages. 2001. 0-7808-0214-4. $78.

"An excellent reference that addresses cosmetic and medically necessary reconstructive surgeries. . . . The style of the prose is calm and reassuring, discussing the many positive outcomes now available due to advances in surgical techniques."
— *American Reference Books Annual 2002*

"Recommended for health science libraries that are open to the public, as well as hospital libraries that are open to the patients. This book is a good resource for the consumer interested in plastic surgery."
— *E-Streams, Dec '01*

"Recommended reference source."
— *Booklist, American Library Association, July '01*

Rehabilitation Sourcebook

Basic Consumer Health Information about Rehabilitation for People Recovering from Heart Surgery, Spinal Cord Injury, Stroke, Orthopedic Impairments, Amputation, Pulmonary Impairments, Traumatic Injury, and More, Including Physical Therapy, Occupational Therapy, Speech/ Language Therapy, Massage Therapy, Dance Therapy, Art Therapy, and Recreational Therapy

Along with Information on Assistive and Adaptive Devices, a Glossary, and Resources for Additional Help and Information

Edited by Dawn D. Matthews. 531 pages. 1999. 0-7808-0236-5. $78.

"This is an excellent resource for public library reference and health collections."
— *American Reference Books Annual, 2001*

"Recommended reference source."
— *Booklist, American Library Association, May '00*

∎

Respiratory Diseases & Disorders Sourcebook

Basic Information about Respiratory Diseases and Disorders, Including Asthma, Cystic Fibrosis, Pneumonia, the Common Cold, Influenza, and Others, Featuring Facts about the Respiratory System, Statistical and Demographic Data, Treatments, Self-Help Management Suggestions, and Current Research Initiatives

Edited by Allan R. Cook and Peter D. Dresser. 771 pages. 1995. 0-7808-0037-0. $78.

"Designed for the layperson and for patients and their families coping with respiratory illness. . . . an extensive array of information on diagnosis, treatment, management, and prevention of respiratory illnesses for the general reader." — *Choice, Association of College and Research Libraries, Jun '96*

"A highly recommended text for all collections. It is a comforting reminder of the power of knowledge that good books carry between their covers."
— *Academic Library Book Review, Spring '96*

"A comprehensive collection of authoritative information presented in a nontechnical, humanitarian style for patients, families, and caregivers."
— *Association of Operating Room Nurses, Sep/Oct '95*

SEE ALSO Lung Disorders Sourcebook

∎

Sexually Transmitted Diseases Sourcebook, 2nd Edition

Basic Consumer Health Information about Sexually Transmitted Diseases, Including Information on the Diagnosis and Treatment of Chlamydia, Gonorrhea, Hepatitis, Herpes, HIV, Mononucleosis, Syphilis, and Others

Along with Information on Prevention, Such as Condom Use, Vaccines, and STD Education; And Featuring a Section on Issues Related to Youth and Adolescents, a Glossary, and Resources for Additional Help and Information

Edited by Dawn D. Matthews. 538 pages. 2001. 0-7808-0249-7. $78.

ALSO AVAILABLE: Sexually Transmitted Diseases Sourcebook, 1st Edition. Edited by Linda M. Ross. 550 pages. 1997. 0-7808-0217-9. $78.

"Recommended for consumer health collections in public libraries, and secondary school and community college libraries."
— *American Reference Books Annual 2002*

"Every school and public library should have a copy of this comprehensive and user-friendly reference book."
— *Choice, Association of College & Research Libraries, Sep '01*

"This is a highly recommended book. This is an especially important book for all school and public libraries." — *AIDS Book Review Journal, Jul-Aug '01*

"Recommended reference source."
— *Booklist, American Library Association, Apr '01*

"Recommended pick both for specialty health library collections and any general consumer health reference collection." — *The Bookwatch, Apr '01*

∎

Skin Disorders Sourcebook

Basic Information about Common Skin and Scalp Conditions Caused by Aging, Allergies, Immune Reactions, Sun Exposure, Infectious Organisms, Parasites, Cosmetics, and Skin Traumas, Including Abrasions, Cuts, and Pressure Sores

Along with Information on Prevention and Treatment

Edited by Allan R. Cook. 647 pages. 1997. 0-7808-0080-X. $78.

". . . comprehensive, easily read reference book."
— *Doody's Health Sciences Book Reviews, Oct '97*

SEE ALSO Burns Sourcebook

∎

Sleep Disorders Sourcebook

Basic Consumer Health Information about Sleep and Its Disorders, Including Insomnia, Sleepwalking, Sleep Apnea, Restless Leg Syndrome, and Narcolepsy

Along with Data about Shiftwork and Its Effects, Information on the Societal Costs of Sleep Deprivation, Descriptions of Treatment Options, a Glossary of Terms, and Resource Listings for Additional Help

Edited by Jenifer Swanson. 439 pages. 1998. 0-7808-0234-9. $78.

"This text will complement any home or medical library. It is user-friendly and ideal for the adult reader."
— *American Reference Books Annual, 2000*

"A useful resource that provides accurate, relevant, and accessible information on sleep to the general public. Health care providers who deal with sleep disorders patients may also find it helpful in being prepared to answer some of the questions patients ask."
— *Respiratory Care, Jul '99*

"Recommended reference source."
— *Booklist, American Library Association, Feb '99*

■

Smoking Concerns Sourcebook

Basic Consumer Health Information about Nicotine Addiction and Smoking Cessation, Featuring Facts about the Health Effects of Tobacco Use, Including Lung and Other Cancers, Heart Disease, Stroke, and Respiratory Disorders, Such as Emphysema and Chronic Bronchitis

Along with Information about Smoking Prevention Programs, Suggestions for Achieving and Maintaining a Smoke-Free Lifestyle, Statistics about Tobacco Use, Reports on Current Research Initiatives, a Glossary of Related Terms, and Directories of Resources for Additional Help and Information

Edited by Karen Bellenir. 625 pages. 2004. 0-7808-0323-X. $78.

■

Sports Injuries Sourcebook, 2nd Edition

Basic Consumer Health Information about the Diagnosis, Treatment, and Rehabilitation of Common Sports-Related Injuries in Children and Adults

Along with Suggestions for Conditioning and Training, Information and Prevention Tips for Injuries Frequently Associated with Specific Sports and Special Populations, a Glossary, and a Directory of Additional Resources

Edited by Joyce Brennfleck Shannon. 614 pages. 2002. 0-7808-0604-2. $78.

ALSO AVAILABLE: Sports Injuries Sourcebook, 1st Edition. Edited by Heather E. Aldred. 624 pages. 1999. 0-7808-0218-7. $78.

"This is an excellent reference for consumers and it is recommended for public, community college, and undergraduate libraries."
— *American Reference Books Annual, 2003*

"Recommended reference source."
— *Booklist, American Library Association, Feb '03*

■

Stress-Related Disorders Sourcebook

Basic Consumer Health Information about Stress and Stress-Related Disorders, Including Stress Origins and Signals, Environmental Stress at Work and Home, Mental and Emotional Stress Associated with Depression, Post-Traumatic Stress Disorder, Panic Disorder, Suicide, and the Physical Effects of Stress on the Cardiovascular, Immune, and Nervous Systems

Along with Stress Management Techniques, a Glossary, and a Listing of Additional Resources

Edited by Joyce Brennfleck Shannon. 610 pages. 2002. 0-7808-0560-7. $78.

"Well written for a general readership, the *Stress-Related Disorders Sourcebook* is a useful addition to the health reference literature."
— *American Reference Books Annual, 2003*

"I am impressed by the amount of information. It offers a thorough overview of the causes and consequences of stress for the layperson. . . . A well-done and thorough reference guide for professionals and nonprofessionals alike."
— *Doody's Review Service, Dec '02*

■

Stroke Sourcebook

Basic Consumer Health Information about Stroke, Including Ischemic, Hemorrhagic, Transient Ischemic Attack (TIA), and Pediatric Stroke, Stroke Triggers and Risks, Diagnostic Tests, Treatments, and Rehabilitation Information

Along with Stroke Prevention Guidelines, Legal and Financial Information, a Glossary, and a Directory of Additional Resources

Edited by Joyce Brennfleck Shannon. 606 pages. 2003. 0-7808-0630-1. $78.

"This volume is highly recommended and should be in every medical, hospital, and public library."
— *American Reference Books Annual, 2004*

■

Substance Abuse Sourcebook

Basic Health-Related Information about the Abuse of Legal and Illegal Substances Such as Alcohol, Tobacco, Prescription Drugs, Marijuana, Cocaine, and Heroin; and Including Facts about Substance Abuse Prevention Strategies, Intervention Methods, Treatment and Recovery Programs, and a Section Addressing the Special Problems Related to Substance Abuse during Pregnancy

Edited by Karen Bellenir. 573 pages. 1996. 0-7808-0038-9. $78.

"A valuable addition to any health reference section. Highly recommended."
— *The Book Report, Mar/Apr '97*

". . . a comprehensive collection of substance abuse information that's both highly readable and compact. Families and caregivers of substance abusers will find the information enlightening and helpful, while teachers, social workers and journalists should benefit from the concise format. Recommended."
— *Drug Abuse Update, Winter '96/'97*

SEE ALSO Alcoholism Sourcebook, Drug Abuse Sourcebook

Surgery Sourcebook

Basic Consumer Health Information about Inpatient and Outpatient Surgeries, Including Cardiac, Vascular, Orthopedic, Ocular, Reconstructive, Cosmetic, Gynecologic, and Ear, Nose, and Throat Procedures and More

Along with Information about Operating Room Policies and Instruments, Laser Surgery Techniques, Hospital Errors, Statistical Data, a Glossary, and Listings of Sources for Further Help and Information

Edited by Annemarie S. Muth and Karen Bellenir. 596 pages. 2002. 0-7808-0380-9. $78.

"Large public libraries and medical libraries would benefit from this material in their reference collections."
— *American Reference Books Annual, 2004*

"Invaluable reference for public and school library collections alike." — *Library Bookwatch, Apr '03*

◼

Transplantation Sourcebook

Basic Consumer Health Information about Organ and Tissue Transplantation, Including Physical and Financial Preparations, Procedures and Issues Relating to Specific Solid Organ and Tissue Transplants, Rehabilitation, Pediatric Transplant Information, the Future of Transplantation, and Organ and Tissue Donation

Along with a Glossary and Listings of Additional Resources

Edited by Joyce Brennfleck Shannon. 628 pages. 2002. 0-7808-0322-1. $78.

"Along with these advances [in transplantation technology] have come a number of daunting questions for potential transplant patients, their families, and their health care providers. This reference text is the best single tool to address many of these questions. . . . It will be a much-needed addition to the reference collections in health care, academic, and large public libraries."
— *American Reference Books Annual, 2003*

"Recommended for libraries with an interest in offering consumer health information." — *E-Streams, Jul '02*

"This is a unique and valuable resource for patients facing transplantation and their families."
— *Doody's Review Service, Jun '02*

◼

Traveler's Health Sourcebook

Basic Consumer Health Information for Travelers, Including Physical and Medical Preparations, Transportation Health and Safety, Essential Information about Food and Water, Sun Exposure, Insect and Snake Bites, Camping and Wilderness Medicine, and Travel with Physical or Medical Disabilities

Along with International Travel Tips, Vaccination Recommendations, Geographical Health Issues, Disease Risks, a Glossary, and a Listing of Additional Resources

Edited by Joyce Brennfleck Shannon. 613 pages. 2000. 0-7808-0384-1. $78.

"Recommended reference source."
— *Booklist, American Library Association, Feb '01*

"This book is recommended for any public library, any travel collection, and especially any collection for the physically disabled."
— *American Reference Books Annual, 2001*

◼

Vegetarian Sourcebook

Basic Consumer Health Information about Vegetarian Diets, Lifestyle, and Philosophy, Including Definitions of Vegetarianism and Veganism, Tips about Adopting Vegetarianism, Creating a Vegetarian Pantry, and Meeting Nutritional Needs of Vegetarians, with Facts Regarding Vegetarianism's Effect on Pregnant and Lactating Women, Children, Athletes, and Senior Citizens

Along with a Glossary of Commonly Used Vegetarian Terms and Resources for Additional Help and Information

Edited by Chad T. Kimball. 360 pages. 2002. 0-7808-0439-2. $78.

"Organizes into one concise volume the answers to the most common questions concerning vegetarian diets and lifestyles. This title is recommended for public and secondary school libraries." — *E-Streams, Apr '03*

"Invaluable reference for public and school library collections alike." — *Library Bookwatch, Apr '03*

"The articles in this volume are easy to read and come from authoritative sources. The book does not necessarily support the vegetarian diet but instead provides the pros and cons of this important decision. The *Vegetarian Sourcebook* is recommended for public libraries and consumer health libraries."
— *American Reference Books Annual, 2003*

◼

Women's Health Concerns Sourcebook, 2nd Edition

Basic Consumer Health Information about the Medical and Mental Concerns of Women, Including Maintaining Health and Wellness, Gynecological Concerns, Breast Health, Sexuality and Reproductive Issues, Menopause, Cancer in Women, the Leading Causes of Death and Disability among Women, Physical Concerns of Special Significance to Women, and Women's Mental and Emotional Health

Along with a Glossary of Related Terms and Directories of Resources for Additional Help and Information

Edited by Amy L. Sutton. 748 pages. 2004. 0-7808-0673-5. $78.

ALSO AVAILABLE: Women's Health Concerns Sourcebook, 1st Edition. Edited by Heather E. Aldred. 567 pages. 1997. 0-7808-0219-5. $78.

"Handy compilation. There is an impressive range of diseases, devices, disorders, procedures, and other physical and emotional issues covered . . . well organized, illustrated, and indexed." — *Choice, Association of College and Research Libraries, Jan '98*

SEE ALSO Breast Cancer Sourcebook, Cancer Sourcebook for Women, Healthy Heart Sourcebook for Women, Osteoporosis Sourcebook

Workplace Health & Safety Sourcebook

Basic Consumer Health Information about Workplace Health and Safety, Including the Effect of Workplace Hazards on the Lungs, Skin, Heart, Ears, Eyes, Brain, Reproductive Organs, Musculoskeletal System, and Other Organs and Body Parts

Along with Information about Occupational Cancer, Personal Protective Equipment, Toxic and Hazardous Chemicals, Child Labor, Stress, and Workplace Violence

Edited by Chad T. Kimball. 626 pages. 2000. 0-7808-0231-4. $78.

"As a reference for the general public, this would be useful in any library." *—E-Streams, Jun '01*

"Provides helpful information for primary care physicians and other caregivers interested in occupational medicine. . . . General readers; professionals."
— Choice, Association of College & Research Libraries, May '01

"Recommended reference source."
—Booklist, American Library Association, Feb '01

"Highly recommended." *— The Bookwatch, Jan '01*

Worldwide Health Sourcebook

Basic Information about Global Health Issues, Including Malnutrition, Reproductive Health, Disease Dispersion and Prevention, Emerging Diseases, Risky Health Behaviors, and the Leading Causes of Death

Along with Global Health Concerns for Children, Women, and the Elderly, Mental Health Issues, Research and Technology Advancements, and Economic, Environmental, and Political Health Implications, a Glossary, and a Resource Listing for Additional Help and Information

Edited by Joyce Brennfleck Shannon. 614 pages. 2001. 0-7808-0330-2. $78.

"Named an Outstanding Academic Title."
—Choice, Association of College & Research Libraries, Jan '02

"Yet another handy but also unique compilation in the extensive Health Reference Series, this is a useful work because many of the international publications reprinted or excerpted are not readily available. Highly recommended." *—Choice, Association of College & Research Libraries, Nov '01*

"Recommended reference source."
—Booklist, American Library Association, Oct '01

Teen Health Series

Helping Young Adults Understand, Manage, and Avoid Serious Illness

Cancer Information for Teens

Health Tips about Cancer Awareness, Prevention, Diagnosis, and Treatment

Including Facts about Frequently Occurring Cancers, Cancer Risk Factors, and Coping Strategies for Teens Fighting Cancer or Dealing with Cancer in Friends or Family Members

Edited by Wilma R. Caldwell. 428 pages. 2004. 0-7808-0678-6. $58.

■

Diet Information for Teens

Health Tips about Diet and Nutrition

Including Facts about Nutrients, Dietary Guidelines, Breakfasts, School Lunches, Snacks, Party Food, Weight Control, Eating Disorders, and More

Edited by Karen Bellenir. 399 pages. 2001. 0-7808-0441-4. $58.

"Full of helpful insights and facts throughout the book. ...An excellent resource to be placed in public libraries or even in personal collections."
—*American Reference Books Annual 2002*

"Recommended for middle and high school libraries and media centers as well as academic libraries that educate future teachers of teenagers. It is also a suitable addition to health science libraries that serve patrons who are interested in teen health promotion and education."
—*E-Streams, Oct '01*

"This comprehensive book would be beneficial to collections that need information about nutrition, dietary guidelines, meal planning, and weight control. ... This reference is so easy to use that its purchase is recommended."
—*The Book Report, Sep-Oct '01*

"This book is written in an easy to understand format describing issues that many teens face every day, and then provides thoughtful explanations so that teens can make informed decisions. This is an interesting book that provides important facts and information for today's teens."
—*Doody's Health Sciences Book Review Journal, Jul-Aug '01*

"A comprehensive compendium of diet and nutrition. The information is presented in a straightforward, plain-spoken manner. This title will be useful to those working on reports on a variety of topics, as well as to general readers concerned about their dietary health."
—*School Library Journal, Jun '01*

Drug Information for Teens

Health Tips about the Physical and Mental Effects of Substance Abuse

Including Facts about Alcohol, Anabolic Steroids, Club Drugs, Cocaine, Depressants, Hallucinogens, Herbal Products, Inhalants, Marijuana, Narcotics, Stimulants, Tobacco, and More

Edited by Karen Bellenir. 452 pages. 2002. 0-7808-0444-9. $58.

"A clearly written resource for general readers and researchers alike." —*School Library Journal*

"The chapters are quick to make a connection to their teenage reading audience. The prose is straightforward and the book lends itself to spot reading. It should be useful both for practical information and for research, and it is suitable for public and school libraries."
—*American Reference Books Annual, 2003*

"Recommended reference source."
—*Booklist, American Library Association, Feb '03*

"This is an excellent resource for teens and their parents. Education about drugs and substances is key to discouraging teen drug abuse and this book provides this much needed information in a way that is interesting and factual." —*Doody's Review Service, Dec '02*

■

Fitness Information for Teens

Health Tips about Exercise, Physical Well-Being, and Health Maintenance

Including Facts about Aerobic and Anaerobic Conditioning, Stretching, Body Shape and Body Image, Sports Training, Nutrition, and Activities for Non-Athletes

Edited by Karen Bellenir. 425 pages. 2004. 0-7808-0679-4. $58.

■

Mental Health Information for Teens

Health Tips about Mental Health and Mental Illness

Including Facts about Anxiety, Depression, Suicide, Eating Disorders, Obsessive-Compulsive Disorders, Panic Attacks, Phobias, Schizophrenia, and More

Edited by Karen Bellenir. 406 pages. 2001. 0-7808-0442-2. $58.

"In both language and approach, this user-friendly entry in the *Teen Health Series* is on target for teens needing information on mental health concerns." —*Booklist, American Library Association, Jan '02*